PROFESSIONAL SKILLS FOR LEADERSHIP

Foundations of a Successful Career

PROFESSIONAL SKILLS FOR LEADERSHIP

Foundations of a Successful Career

Michelle Morrison, RN, BSN, MHS, FNP

Nurse Educator/Consultant
Health and Educational Consultants
Williams, Oregon

Mosby

St. Louis Baltimore Boston Chicago London Madrid Philadelphia Sydney Toronto

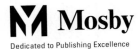

Mosby

Dedicated to Publishing Excellence

Executive Editor: Linda L. Duncan
Developmental Editor: Kathy Sartori
Project Manager: Barbara Bowes Merritt
Editing and Production: The Bookmakers, Incorporated
Designer: John Beck
Illustrator: Erva Zabel

Printed in the United States of America

Composition by The Bookmakers, Incorporated
Printing/binding by RR Donnelley/Crawfordsville

Mosby–Year Book, Inc.
11830 Westline Industrial Drive
St. Louis, Missouri 63146

Library of Congress Cataloging in Publication Data

Morrison, Michelle.
    Professional skills for leadership : foundations of a successful career / Michelle Morrison.
        p.   cm.
    Includes index.
    ISBN 0-8016-7235-X
    1. Nursing services—Administration.   2. Leadership.   I. Title
RT89.M63   1993
362.1'73'0683—dc20
                                                    93-27862
                                                    CIP

93 94 95 96 97   /   9 8 7 6 5 4 3 2 1

REVIEWERS

Susan A. Ruzicka, MSN(R)
Adjunct Professor
St. Louis University
St. Louis, Missouri

Cordelia J. Schaffer, RN, MSN
Clinical Nurse Specialist
Gerontology
Nursing Faculty
Butler County Community College
El Dorado, Kansas

Carol Smith, RN, BSN
Director of Education
Swope Ridge Geriatric Center
Kansas City, Missouri

Mary Ann Shea, RN, Attorney at Law
Medical/Legal Consultant
St. Louis, Missouri

PREFACE

For years, I have observed nurses and other health care providers assume the responsibilities of supervision without the benefit of the basic skills and knowledge necessary to do the job well. The educational preparation of health care workers ranges from a few weeks to many years, and few of these programs include supervision or leadership training. This book was written to fill the health care provider's need for a practical, easy-to-use manual of supervisory and leadership skills. The examples and case scenarios relate to nurses in long-term care settings; but the principles and concepts are universal and may easily be applied to acute care, home health, and numerous other health care settings. This book is appropriate for students in basic nursing, social services, and other allied health courses as well as currently practicing health care providers who are in need of practical, easily applied management principles.

This text contains 15 chapters divided into two units. For the purpose of this book, a supervisor, manager, or leader is defined as a nurse, CNA, or other health care employee who is responsible for the work (output) of one or more persons. Therefore, the success of a supervisor depends on the efforts of other people. Following this line of thought, Unit One focuses on the basic people skills needed for effective supervision. Chapter 1 discusses the personal outlooks and attitudinal traits of successful supervisors. Verbal and nonverbal communication techniques that are of special importance to the supervisor are covered in Chapter 2. Work groups, their characteristics, and dynamics are the focus of Chapter 3, while Chapter 4 explores the concepts of leadership, power, and empowerment. Chapter 5 introduces five common motivational theories and suggests several techniques for motivating one's self as well as others. The objectives of Chapter 6 are to provide the reader with effective conflict resolution skills, while Chapter 7 concludes Unit One with an overview of the five basic functions of management.

Unit Two addresses the daily application of supervisory and leadership skills. Chapter 8 discusses the characteristics and theories of the formal work organization, its culture, lines of authority, and the application of standards of care to client care (nursing) delivery systems. Techniques for making sound individual and group decisions are covered in Chapter 9. Chapter 10 focuses on developing effective planning skills and includes a discussion of the change process as well as techniques for acting as a successful change agent. Then, management by objectives is offered as an example of a system for defining, implementing, and evaluating change.

The focus of Chapter 11 is the creation of a productive, efficient working environment through the application of positive leadership, time management, negotiation, and supervisory techniques. Chapter 12 follows with an exploration of organizational morale — its principles, characteristics, and importance to the work environment. The four developmental stages of a new supervisor and techniques for building morale (while, at the same time, avoiding the 'Superperson syndrome') are offered. The all-important skill of delegation is the topic for Chapter 13. Delegation is a component of the broader management function of 'directing' and helps provide the connecting link between planning and actually getting the job done. The importance of using job descriptions, policies, skill levels, and standards of care when delegating is emphasized. Chapter 14 presents the principles and processes necessary for effectively evaluating programs, procedures, and people. The use of established criteria, data-collection tools, and performance standards as integral components of the evaluation process is encouraged. The last chapter focuses on the legal implications of nursing and health care supervision. Basic legal definitions are applied to nursing practice. Legal implications of the nursing process are discussed and specific legal duties explained within the framework of the 'reasonable and prudent nurse' theory. The incorporation of quality assurance and risk management programs in monitoring client care and, thereby, reducing or avoiding potential liability is discussed.

Features

Because this book is meant to be used as a resource for practicing health care providers as well as a teaching text for students of nursing, it contains several convenient features:

- Clearly stated and measurable learning objectives that allow the reader to easily understand the chapter's important concepts.
- A list of key concepts following each chapter, which provide a quick reference to material covered in greater depth.
- Learning activities, which encourage the reader to apply selected chapter concepts to real-life situations. Both individual and group activities are included.
- Annotated additional readings, which provide a short summary of each resource. It is hoped that the reader's interest will be stimulated, thus encouraging further exploration of topics.
- Key points (including sentences, phrases, and headings) have been highlighted with boldface print to allow the reader quick and easy access to important information contained within the chapter.

- Two appendixes, which provide an example of a Certified Nurse Assistant's job description accompanied by specific performance standards.
- A conceptual framework that weaves the use of the nursing process as well as concepts of worth, respect, and integrity throughout the text.
- Explanations of and frequent referral to the importance of quality assurance, risk management, and standards of care as applied to health care supervision and leadership.

Acknowledgments

The encouragement and support of several people were integral to the composition of this book. A special thanks goes to my husband, Russell, for his continuing patience and unexcelled manuscript preparation; Linda Duncan and Kathy Sartori, Mosby's knowledgeable and upbeat editors; Erva Zabel for her lively illustrations; Marian Masters and Fran Cardoza of Rogue Community College's library for ferreting out resources and maintaining my knowledge connection with the world; and Linda Morris for challenging me to write this book.

CONTENTS

UNIT ONE: THE PEOPLE SKILLS

PSYCHOSOCIAL
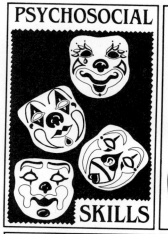
SKILLS

COMMUNICATION
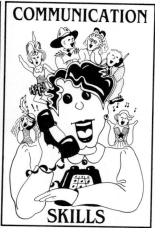
SKILLS

GROUP
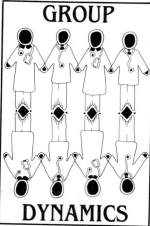
DYNAMICS

LEADERSHIP
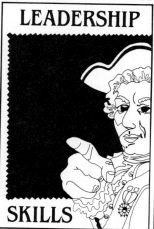
SKILLS

MOTIVATIONAL
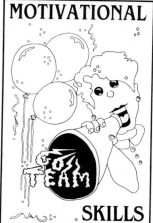
SKILLS

CONFLICT RESOLUTION
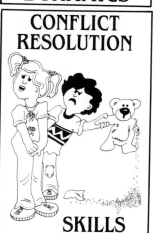
SKILLS

MANAGEMENT
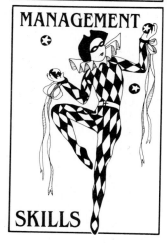
SKILLS

PSYCHOSOCIAL

1

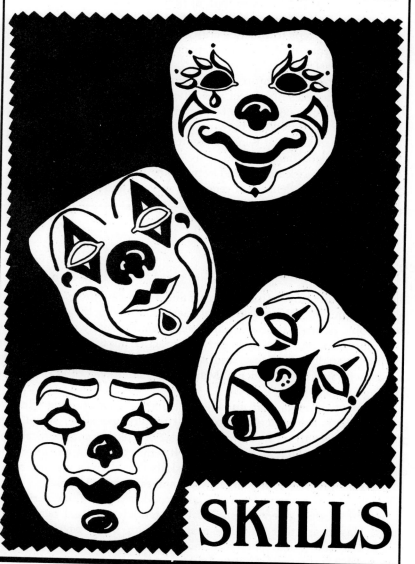

SKILLS

✒ Learning Objectives

Upon completion of this chapter, the reader will be able to:

1. Identify six basic personal skills important for effective management.
2. List three steps for directing your own change process.
3. Discuss three techniques for developing a positive mental attitude.
4. Explore four new ways to look at failure.
5. List four techniques to improve risk-taking behaviors.
6. Follow five steps to practice critical thinking or problem solving.
7. Compare four traits of 'caring' people with five traits of 'sensitive' people.
8. Identify three motivators for workers.
9. Explain the roles of respect and integrity in management.
10. Recognize four suggestions for developing a high level of integrity.
11. Compare the difference between achievers and sustainers.
12. List eight qualities of winners (achievers).
13. Describe eight 'image killers.'
14. Discuss how risk taking and networking assist the nurse manager.
15. Identify five guidelines for renewing energies and coping with stress.

The People Skills

Nursing is commonly defined as an art and a science. Nurses spend years in school studying natural and social sciences, applying the nursing process to solve patients' problems, and perfecting the many new skills and techniques they must master in order to practice nursing. Technology in nursing is rapidly expanding, and it is important that one work to stay abreast with new developments. Many universities even offer degrees in Nursing Science.

Remember, though, that nursing is also an art. Developing effective people skills is a long-term process that requires personal, social, and professional growth, as well as a knowledge of effective communications, group dynamics, and human behaviors. It is the constant application and development of psychosocial (people) skills that defines nursing as an art, and the practice of this art is what makes nursing unique.

Today, the definition of nursing has broadened to include caring for all aspects of the patient's *response* to potential or actual health care needs. This means that the nurse practices using many psychosocial as well as scientific skills. Therefore, **nurses already possess many of the skills needed to become effective leaders and managers.**

A manager coordinates resources and organizes them in order to meet goals. A leader influences other people to work toward those goals. Hence, an effective manager is also able to use people skills to inspire and lead others. Because of many changes in the health care delivery system, nurses are now commonly being thrust into management roles with little or no preparation. Do not fear, for many important management abilities dwell within. With practice and a willingness to apply knowledge you already possess to new situations, you will grow and develop into an effective manager of health (nursing) care delivery.

Commitment

The first step in developing managerial psychosocial skills is to begin working with the psyche, or personal skills. As human beings, we reveal our emotions and attitudes every time we interact with others. By consciously taking charge of personal growth, we are able to direct our energies and 'grow into,' or become, capable nurse managers.

Perhaps the most important trait of the competent nurse leader/manager is commitment. The definition of commitment is "an intellectual or emotional bond to some course of action" (Morris, 1976). The first commitment must be to yourself. If you refuse to grow, then you cannot empower or encourage growth in others. Self-commitment involves a promise to yourself to do the best you can in every situation—**to be the best you can be.** Everyone has different personalities, talents, and areas that need improvement. We also have the ability and even the need to challenge ourselves.

Change is certain, and as a result, growth will occur. By setting goals and directing energy toward meeting those goals, we are able to *choose* the directions in which we grow. This is an important point because it allows us to look at life, careers, skill development, and the like as a *process* that requires a little growth every day rather than mastery in a moment. Begin by looking at your behaviors objectively (without emotion), then list those behaviors you would like to enhance as well as those you want to change or replace.

Change process

To direct your own change process (growth), you need to do the following:

Set goals. The best managers were not born into their positions, complete with all the qualities of dynamic leaders. They set their goals and then slowly moved toward them. They stayed focused and persisted. Goals can include personal commitments (e.g., I will read for 30 minutes a day) or professional objectives (e.g., I will develop effective management skills).

Develop a plan of action. It is useful to list the steps needed to meet the goal, especially if the goal is broad. For example, to improve your public speaking skills, you may read information on the subject, attend lectures or discussions given by dynamic speakers, practice in front of the mirror, deliver a speech to your pet, and so on. Listing the steps also allows you to watch your progress in working toward the goal. *Work toward self-awareness.* Mary Poppins describes herself as a 'practically perfect person.' That is an example of a positive self-awareness. Learn to look at your own strengths and weaknesses without guilt or emotion. Become comfortable with both the positive and negative aspects of yourself. Look at your values. Are they reasonable, realistic, and right for you? Reject the values, traits, or behaviors that are unhealthy. Make the best of your strengths and commit yourself to work on the areas that need improvement (but remember to be patient with yourself). Following these steps will help you to become a practically perfect person.

Humor

Another important trait of great leaders is a sense of humor. A nurse's work is serious, but **gentle humor is essential** in relieving stress and discomfort. Gentle humor is not hostile. Laughter should not be generated at the expense of others (laughing at someone's inferiority or hurting someone). The ability to laugh at yourself also helps to put the situation in perspective. Humor is an appreciation of the human condition. A dog, for example, has absolutely no sense of humor, no matter what one may find funny. Through humor, humans are able to share thoughts and experiences. Humor can lighten the load when shared with others. It is also a reminder to remember the child that still dwells within each of us.

Positive mental attitude

A positive mental attitude is one of the most powerful tools for leaders. A person with a positive outlook radiates energy and cheers up everyone in the vicinity. People are attracted to those with positive outlooks and hope that some of that energy will be passed on to them. Positive mental attitudes (PMAs) can be developed by replacing the negative feelings that stand in the way of self-growth. This requires persistent, patient effort because our habits and attitudes are deeply ingrained, but we can begin by following this process (Husted, Miller, Wilczynski, 1990):

1. *Listen to yourself talk.* Pay attention to the words you use. Statements such as "it will never work" or "that's impossible" only become self-defeating. The human brain is programmed by thoughts. Thoughts become feelings, which become words and actions. Many nurses complain of becoming "burned out" or "stressed to the max." No one denies that the profession of nursing has its stressors; however, it is *how* each

stressor is perceived or viewed that determines the outcome. Practice listening to yourself. You may be surprised at what you discover.

2. *Change recurrent negative themes.* Changing any self-defeating thought, word, or action to a positive, empowering one requires practice (see box on p. 8). For example, do you awaken every morning with the thought "Good God, Morning!" or "Good Morning, God!"? Is today just another day at the same old grind, or is today an opportunity to be explored and discovered? Releasing and replacing negative attitudes leads to greater self-esteem, confidence, and happiness. Practice this skill first and frequently, for it lays the foundation for everything else you will do.

   Now that you are practicing your positive mental attitude, let us look at some tips for building your confidence:

3. *Be your own cheerleader.* Give yourself pep talks every morning and when dealing with daily stresses. Give yourself positive, inspiring thoughts. "I *can* handle this situation" is much healthier than "I can't wait to get out of here." The brain does not question any thought. It only stores it in case it may be needed in the future. Positive thoughts become the basis for effective actions.

4. *Visualize future successes.* Take a moment each day to picture yourself achieving a goal. See yourself as a dynamic leader and capable nurse manager. Besides, it is fun to do.

5. *Act the part.* Picture yourself as a person with confidence and ability, then act the part. Your confidence will grow each time you project that imagined confidence. Developing confidence and a positive outlook are skills that will serve you well. They are worth the effort.

Positive mental attitudes build self-esteem; and self-esteem builds self-respect, self-knowledge, and self-care (an emotional acceptance of yourself). The Greeks call this wholeness of self *oikos*. I like to think of this word as the basis for "OK".

Why is all of this important to nursing management or leadership? Because the person who is out of touch with self cannot touch others, and management is the art of focusing others toward a goal. Managers need to nurture (emotionally nourish) both their staff and themselves. This ability to nurture expands and eventually becomes the cornerstone for the facility's human relations.

Organization

Effective managers are organized. They realize that time is like money in the bank. It is usually very limited, and how you spend it is important. Your time in any given day is limited to 24 hours. How you choose to spend it can make the difference between a highly effective nurse manager, parent, etc., or someone who is always trying to catch up during the day.

✒ STEPS TO POSITIVE OUTLOOK

- Recognize the negative attitude and turn it away. Reject it and throw it out.
- Replace the negative attitude by frequently repeating positive statements.
- Use warm, enthusiastic, upbeat words that help build a feeling of success.

Fortunately, organizational skills can be learned. Organization will be discussed in greater depth in Chapter 7. For now, practice setting a few goals each day and work toward meeting them. A "Things To Do Today" list is a great help. If you do not finish everything on your list, figure out why you did not. Perhaps there were too many items on the list. Maybe one task required more time than you planned for it. Do not feel guilty. Be realistic. This tool will assist you in looking at *how* you spend time and prepare you for the more complex time-management skills required of the nurse manager.

Risk taking

Now let us look at risk taking and failure. Without a willingness to take risks and possibly fail, we will not encourage growth.

For most of us, the word failure has a negative meaning. It implies defeat, a 'you lose' attitude, nonfulfillment, and a lack of success; but failure can be a positive, growth-promoting experience. It can provide opportunities for change, encourage creativity, stimulate learning, and sharpen judgment. Failure is the price of improvement, and, when used as a learning tool, the experience can provide feedback for the next step. A manager that makes no mistakes or never fails is not taking any risks or working for improvement.

How do we grow from our failures? First, "realize that failure is a necessary part of change" (Vestal, 1991). Biologist Lewis Thomas (1979) maintains "that humankind is set apart from the rest of creation by our unique ability to make mistakes. If we were not provided with the knack of being wrong, we could never get anything useful done." **Failure is part of the growth process.** Learning to view it from this perspective is important.

Second, give yourself *permission* to fail. Guilt and feelings of inadequacy can paralyze you into denying yourself valuable opportunities. Believe that you have the right to make a mistake—to fail. The chances of living life with no mistakes are about zero. Failing, learning, and growing go hand-in-hand.

Next, consider failure as a learning experience. Examine the what, where, why, how, when, and who of the failure. Recognize what could have been done differently and what improvements could be made. Remember that this is an important aspect of self-education. There are valuable lessons to be learned from failure.

Last, discover the new options that are created by failure. By examining and learning from failure, we can find (or even create) options and new opportunities.

Now that failure has been recreated as opportunity, taking risks becomes easier. The willingness to risk the security and comfort of routine in exchange for improvement is a much needed attribute for nurse managers and leaders. Today's health care profession is crowded with uncertainty. The only things we can truly rely on are limited staff, limited resources, and an abundance of patients. Nurses will be called upon to use creativity and try new ways of solving problems. This involves taking risks and possibly failing, but taking risks benefits both you and the organization. Risk taking enhances your personal power, builds self-esteem, and contributes to self-confidence. Your staff and supervisors will also benefit by gaining solutions for problems and improving work performance.

Risk-taking behaviors. In her book, *Paths to Power*, Natosha Josefowitz (1980) encourages us to practice four techniques that assist in building effective risk-taking behaviors (see upper box on p. 10).

Finally, armed with a commitment, a sense of humor, a positive outlook, organizational skills, and a willingness to take risks, you are nearly ready to tackle the role of nurse manager. One more skill is necessary, however — the development of critical thinking.

Critical-thinking skills

Nurses who practice critical thinking know how to solve problems and seek new information. They maintain an open-minded and questioning attitude, and they realize that knowing the *process* for solving problems is more important than having all the answers.

As a manager, you will work with many large and small problems each day. With each problem, you have three choices:

1. Delay action, stall, ignore it
2. Make a quick decision with no thinking
3. Use the problem-solving process, logical steps, thinking

The first two choices both relate to the problem, but they usually create more difficulties in the long run because no real solution is found. The third choice may involve more effort, but the results are usually more effective.

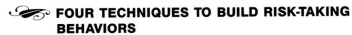 **FOUR TECHNIQUES TO BUILD RISK-TAKING BEHAVIORS**

1. **Express yourself.** Let others know how you think and feel, even if you do not agree. The skills here are having a well-thought-out message and presenting that message in a positive manner. Your opinions are valuable. Sharing them affirms your personal integrity and builds confidence.
2. **Make requests.** A higher risk level than expressing, asking for what you need and want involves sending clear messages, in addition to a willingness to explore alternatives and negotiate compromises.
3. **Learn to refuse.** Women in general and nurses in particular have been raised and trained to serve others, to be giving, and to put the needs of others first. Because of this, setting limits, stating objections, or saying no feels risky. However, exercising these behaviors when they are needed builds your credibility. The best managers are credible. Do not sell out your personal power in order to be well liked or buy approval.
4. **Expect to succeed.** Remember those positive mental attitudes? Use them to find the successes in whatever you do. Turn any negative emotions into motivators. Visualize that those risks you took paid off. Remember the saying: "When presented with a lemon, make lemonade." Anticipate success.

STEPS FOR CRITICAL THINKING

1. **Define the problem** — avoid the temptation to just make a quick decision. Gather all possible data (facts, opinions).
2. **List all possible solutions** — start with the ideal solution and then decide on the least acceptable solution as well. Then list all possible solutions.
3. **Compare each solution** — weigh the advantages and disadvantages of each possible course of action. Weed out those that seem less workable.
4. **Choose a solution and try it** — communicate the solution or plan to others.
5. **Evaluate the results** — how close to the ideal solution did it come? Has the problem been solved? Has the situation improved?

Problem-solving process. The problem-solving process, on the other hand, focuses on logical thinking to find the best solution (see lower box on p. 10). Practice these five steps. Keep an open mind and question what you do. These are the foundations upon which critical-thinking skills are built.

The Social Skills

The second area of focus for developing managerial psychosocial skills relates to the social aspect. Nurses by their nature and education have strong social skills. Our profession is directed toward caring for others, but what is caring really all about?

Caring

The dictionary description of the word *care* is: "to have a strong feeling or opinion, concern or interest" (Morris, 1976). Words such as caution (handle with care), protection, supervision (in the care of a nurse), and attention to detail (the resident was bathed with care) are also used. As one can see, caring is a concept that becomes an attitude.

Caring traits. Nurses who demonstrate a high degree of caring seem to practice four traits (see box on p. 12). Nurses demonstrate these traits in daily practice. We work diligently to monitor our clients' health and intervene rapidly to preserve life and promote wellness. We strive to meet the long-term care residents' needs for love, belonging, and respect as well as the physical needs. We show respect to families, physicians, and other health care professionals. We perform our duties with attention to details and follow high standards for nursing care. The next step for the nurse leader/manager is to apply the concept of caring to the work environment.

We in the health care profession, like other employees, work to satisfy our needs. Our paychecks help to secure basic needs such as food, shelter, and clothing. Needs to belong to a group and to give and receive attention are met to some degree by work. Work also provides stimulation and the opportunity to think. Fredrick Herzberg (1966) and other theorists believe that "to survive man must satisfy a need for cortical stimulation [thinking]." However, work in the health care field provides the additional opportunity to practice the art of caring. Naturally we care for, protect, and nurture our patients/residents. As managers, we now need to focus on applying the concepts of caring to our workers, assistants, peers, and supervisors. The director, administrator, and chief executive officer (CEO) all have the same needs we do. Caring for them is important, too, for when you know someone cares, it is much easier to cope with the daily difficulties.

✎ CARING TRAITS

1. **A concern for and an active interest in others.** They are interested in people in general and concerned about their well-being, not just patients but co-workers as well.
2. **A belief in the individual worth, uniqueness, and dignity of each person.** The caring nurse respects each person, not for what was accomplished or not done, but simply because each is a unique human being
3. **An accepting attitude.** Each person is accepted unconditionally, complete with strengths and weaknesses. The caring nurse is non-judgmental. He/she may not approve of the *behaviors*, but the whole person is accepted. Judgment or blame is not passed.
4. **Empathy.** Empathy is a willingness to try to understand how the other person feels. Although we may never be in the same situation, we care enough to show compassion for that individual. Empathy involves 'picking up,' or receiving, the messages being sent and placing them in the context (viewpoint) of the sender. It is an attempt to see the world from another person's point of view. Although you may never fully comprehend another person, the use of empathy allows you to accept, and perhaps understand, the other person's unique perspective.

From Travelbee J: What do we mean by rapport?, *American Journal of Nursing* 63(2):70, 1963.

Peers and co-workers need to be cared for also. They work hard and appreciate it when their efforts are acknowledged and encouraged. Learn to give praise generously and accept it graciously.

Perhaps the group that provides most of the patient/resident care is the one that needs the greatest amount of caring. Nursing assistants who provide daily hands-on nursing spend a great deal of energy caring for their patient/resident needs. They receive the least amount of pay for the hardest physical work. The nurse manager must demonstrate genuine concern, respect, and interest if an effective working relationship is to be developed, if needs are to be satisfied, and if growth is to be promoted in co-workers.

Sensitivity to people

Along with caring, a sensitivity to people is an important skill for the nurse leader/manager. H. C. Smith (1966), in his book, *Sensitivity to People*, defines sensitivity as "the ability to accurately sense what others think and feel."

Sensitivity traits. Many studies have been done to identify the traits or characteristics of sensitive people. Because this is a difficult area to study, some results are conflicting. However, when compared, a clear pattern of traits emerges: sensitive people are more tolerant, highly motivated, independent, responsible, and considerate.

Sensitive people are motivated: one learns what one *wants* to learn. Sensitive people approach learning with eagerness and are open to new experiences. They actively participate in the learning process.

'Sensitives' are involved with others. As H. C. Smith (1966) suggests, "The sensitive are people who find their greatest satisfactions in human relations, who are considerate and responsible in dealing with others, who want to give to others rather than to get something from them, but who are not dependent upon them." They enjoy the rich uniqueness of each individual without the anxieties related to others' opinions of them. To learn about people, you must be open to new experiences and willing to look at old knowledge about people in new ways. The more curious and nondefensive you are, the more you will learn.

An active attitude is important for developing sensitivity. Be eager to learn. Seek out new information and look at new ways of applying it. Test ideas in practice. Approach learning about people with "boldness—a willingness to approach people, ask questions, and express feelings" (Ludeman, 1989). As nurses, we do this when interacting with our patients, but we seldom apply this eagerness to learn about people to our fellow workers. The nurse who is a bystander does not learn.

Last, people with high levels of sensitivity have **empathy**—"an understanding so intimate that the feelings, thoughts, and motives of one [person] are readily comprehended by another" (Travelbee, 1963). To develop this level of understanding, one needs to listen more than talk. People will communicate what is foremost in their minds. The trick is to hear the message. Learn to listen with the heart as well as the ears and mind. Imagine yourself in the other person's situation. Although you may never be faced with the same situation, a deeper understanding of and empathy for others is developed by 'walking a mile in their shoes.'

How does sensitivity work in actual practice? Let us take an example:

Heather Harris is a staff nurse and day-shift wing supervisor for a long-term care facility. She is responsible for 24 residents and four certified nursing assistants (CNAs). Lately she has noticed that Angie Martin, CNA, has been arriving late for work, especially on Wednesdays, and seems preoccupied or worried. Also, she has been using the telephone several times a day, especially on Wednesdays. By observing these new behaviors in Angie, Heather senses a problem and becomes motivated to learn about it. Because Heather cares about her staff, she is involved and concerned. She arranges for some private time and space so that she and Angie may talk. During the discussion, Heather discovers that Angie and her husband have recently separated. She is now the sole support and parent for three small children. Arranging for child care was difficult, but she managed to find a sitter for every work day except Wednesdays. The only option each Wednesday was to arrange for the children to stay with her parents, an elderly couple with mobility problems due to arthritis. Although she would telephone them every few hours, she would worry about her parents' ability to provide safe child care and the energy these elderly people were expending to care for three small children.

Although Heather had never experienced Angie's dilemma, she could certainly understand and feel the discomforts arising from the situation. Together Heather and Angie developed some possible solutions, and after several attempts, Heather discovered a way to schedule Angie to have every Wednesday off. As a result, Angie's quality of work improved and she began to smile again. By using sensitivity, Heather was able to effectively manage a problem and improve the morale of at least one employee.

Thus, sensitivity to others can be increased by practicing the traits of sensitive people: motivation to learn about people; considerate and responsible involvement with others; an openness to new ideas, thoughts, or feelings; an active learning attitude; and empathy for others. These are some of the caring skills for working effectively with and leading others.

Caring for and sensitivity to other people, however, is not quite enough. Workers (including us) also need to have a sense of integrity and feel they are respected and valued.

The new work force

The work force is changing. We are no longer satisfied with just meeting the needs the paycheck provides. In earlier days, employees would work hard at any job because they feared starvation. Today, we work for different reasons: to prove our self-worth and to make a difference. The astute nurse manager recognizes these human desires (as well as tremendous untapped potential of each employee) and supports these inner motivations.

Many research studies of the work environment have been done to find what motivates workers. Results of these studies have proven that people are

- more cooperative and harder working when they receive attention, praise, and recognition from others;
- more committed when given a measure of control over their work;
- more loyal and excited about new opportunities when encouraged to grow and develop their potential.

In short, they are respected. Words that are used to define respect include esteem, honor, consideration, regard, and appreciation. Respected people are treated with consideration and regard for who they are and what they have done.

Respect. To create a climate of respect, the nurse manager needs to treat employees as people — talk with them, listen to their ideas, stay positive, involve them in projects early, and get in touch with their emotional needs (empathy). As Kate Ludeman (1989) states in her book, *The Worth Ethic,* "When we include our employees in the process of devising workable solutions to problems, we meet their needs to take part, make a contribution and feel valuable. Because we listen to their concerns, consider the validity of their objections, and integrate their ideas as much as is practical, our employees come to trust [and respect] our good judgment." This climate, in turn, creates a bond of mutual trust. Because we are working empathetically with our staff, we respect each other. That **respect helps to release the motivation, commitment, cooperation, loyalty, and energy** of our employees.

Integrity. Respect also involves integrity — rigid adherence to a code of behavior. Integrity is usually taken for granted. We are shocked when we discover scandals and products that do not live up to their claims, but we seldom consider our own small lapses in integrity such as the roll of tape we 'accidentally' took home or the promise we 'forgot' to keep. As nurse managers, we demonstrate the ethical fiber of the facility by our behaviors. The top management creates policy and sets the tone, but the individual nurse manager interprets policies and decides how actions are to be taken. Doing things the honorable way may take more time and energy. It is easier to come up with a simple solution just to keep everyone happy. However, in the long run, the price for expedient, unethical actions is loss of integrity. Employees will then view management with distrust and suspicion.

We earn the respect of others by holding ourselves accountable for what we do. Fortunately, we can practice acting with integrity. Suggestions for developing a high degree of integrity include:

Recognize areas that need improving and choose a more ethical way of working. Perhaps you may need to follow through on those items you told your staff you would explore, or maybe you may want to be more straightforward in working with people. Positively identify the change you want to make and pat yourself on the back every time you engage in the new behavior.

Be a model of integrity. Hold yourself accountable for your decisions. Do what you say you will do. Your staff is watching, and they notice the little everyday decisions. Tom Peters (Peters, Waterman, 1982), a well-known author and manager urges, "Do not make any commitment, starting right now, internal or external, that you cannot live up to."

Operate with honesty and openness. Ask yourself if you are willing to disclose your action or decision to your supervisor, your staff, or society as a whole. Trust others and encourage your staff to trust you by being open and honest. They will keep you informed about potential problems, which, in turn, will promote greater productivity.

Be consistent. Practice ethical behaviors every day. You may not be responsible for other people's ethics, but if you act with honor, you "will convey two very important messages to your staff: that you expect them to act honorably toward both the client and the facility, and that they can expect to be treated honorably by you and your organization" (Ludeman, 1989). Integrity and respect are two vital elements of effective management.

Achieving skills

Outstanding managers also possess a number of achieving skills — abilities to successfully accomplish something, to meet a goal. Dr. Julie White (1986), the first woman director of Virginia's Old Dominion University Institute of Management, believes there are three groups of people in the workplace: failures, sustainers, and achievers. Most of us move back and forth between the sustainer and the achiever groups.

Good student model. In this society, women have been taught to be sustainers. We follow the 'good student' model we were taught in school. The good student

- finds out exactly what is expected,
- works hard to do a good job, and then
- waits to be graded or rewarded.

As adults in the workplace, sustainers *unconsciously wait for recognition.* They spend over 70 percent of their work time doing the job well and 30 percent waiting for recognition. When (if) they are not graded or receive recognition, they become angry and envious. These emotions lead us to becoming victims. Victims sit and complain about the patients, other staff, the boss, the working conditions, the facility, and society in general. They become resigned to their fate and enter into the vicious circle of victim, complaints, and resignation that nothing will improve.

Achievers, on the other hand, spend about 60 percent of their work time doing the job and the remainder of their time practicing three crucial skills: projecting, positioning, and networking. Let us look at each of these in detail.

Self-projection skills. Self-projection skills follow the old saying of **"success breeds success."** Employers want proven winners—those people who present in the most positive manner and in a way that best meets the needs of the employer. This sounds easy, but many studies have demonstrated that women tend to present themselves as less than they are. For example, when asked to describe their bodies, women focused on the negative. "I'm fine except for my fat hips." Women tended to catalog their flaws, while men tended to focus on their attributes. "I'm a 40-year-old intelligent, good looking guy." Women have been taught from childhood, "You are not OK the way you are." Much of this results from advertising aimed specifically at women. Wear this outfit, drink this beverage, or drive this car and you will be better than you really are. Makeup covers flaws. Thin is beautiful, and if you are not thin, you are less beautiful. The sad part is that many of us believe this and limit ourselves time and time again.

Men, however, are expected to be aggressive, strong, and intelligent. They are expected to achieve and project success. An interesting study proves this point: A series of tasks was given to a group of both men and women. Several tasks were designed so that the only possible outcome was failure. When asked why they failed, men externalized or placed the blame outward, saying, "The directions were unclear" or "You did not allow enough time." Women, however, tended to internalize or place the blame on themselves, saying, "I'm sorry" or "I was never very good at this sort of thing." When the task was designed so that the only outcome was success, the researchers found that the reverse was true. Men internalized ("I've always been good at this." "I have a natural ability."), while women externalized ("I was lucky." "It's because the directions were so clear."). The women would not take credit for success, but were much too ready to accept the blame for failure. In other words, they projected themselves as losers and, as a result, were viewed as losers.

Winners project success. Winners focus on the positive and have special qualities that keep them positive and upbeat. We, as women, nurses, and managers, need to remember this and focus on developing these qualities (see box on p. 18).

A good professional image begins in the mirror. Like it or not, people judge others by the manner in which they dress and groom themselves. Nurses have moved from the starched white uniform to the do-your-own-thing style of dress. How a nurse manager dresses has an impact. It sets the tone for other staff members. If the nurse manager arrives at work with her hair flowing in the breeze, long red fingernails, and unpressed clothes, the staff will follow that lead. After all, "If she can do it, why

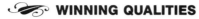 **WINNING QUALITIES**

1. **Positive self-expectancy.** As Henry Ford offered, "Whether you think you can or you think you can't, you're right." What you expect to happen usually happens.
2. **Positive self-esteem.** Believe in yourself. Take credit for and share your successes. Know you will do well because you *are* a successful person.
3. **Positive self-awareness.** Be aware of your strengths and weaknesses. Capitalize on the strengths and work on areas that need improving, but do not feel guilty about your weaknesses. Winners are aware that certain improvements are needed, and they expect to improve.
4. **Positive self-perspective.** Look at your whole self. Clarify the many roles you have and see how they fit into your life. See how others depend on you. Give freely of yourself but remember to renew your energies.
5. **Positive self-direction.** Define your goals and start taking steps to meet them. Be realistic and patiently persist toward each goal. Motivate yourself with the rewards that come with reaching each small goal.
6. **Positive self-control and discipline.** Limit or refuse negative thoughts. Accept positive encouragement from yourself and be honest. Take the credit or the blame for the results of your actions — just *your* actions — and not those of others. Learn to discern who owns the problem.
7. **Positive communications.** Listen more than you talk. Be clear and direct when you do speak. Clarify any area of potential misunderstanding. Communicate with 'can do' messages.
8. **Positive self-image.** Remember the 30-second, first impression rule: people form their impression of another in the first 30 seconds of the interaction (White, 1985). This impression can be stronger than physical evidence or data. It tends to last, and it colors other interactions. The impression we project depends on our clothing, our bearing (use of the space around us), our handshake, and our use of verbal and nonverbal messages.

Adapted from Barrett G: Are you a winner?, *Nursing 90* 20(9):120, 1990.

can't I?" Good grooming, neatness, and proper fitting conservative cloth-ing deliver a professional impression, a high level of confidence, and helps to build the image of all nurses.

Image killers. 'Image killers' are those mistakes that, when repeated, give messages that you do not want to send (White, 1986). By becoming aware of image killers (see box on p. 20), you can avoid sending the wrong messages. Be alert for them. They have no place in positive self-projection skills.

Positioning skills. Positioning skills are also important to achievers. Being in the right place at the right time is no mistake. **Achievers position them-selves to make things happen.** They become involved in many things, and when something works out, they are there to grasp the opportunity. The staff nurse who volunteers for different committees or activities is in a better position for advancement when a new position is created or a position opens.

Taking risks. Our society teaches women to engage in low-risk behav-iors. Finish school, marry well, and support your husband's endeavors. Be patient. Hang in there and, above all, do not fail. Achievers (both men and women) take risks but do not blame themselves for failures. They learn to minimize their losses and move on to the next opportunity. Fail-ure is viewed as an opportunity for growth.

Networking. Achieving skills also involves networking — the sharing of expertise, current challenges for the profession, and new learning. Net-working offers us the chance to gain input and support for our ideas or opinions. We learn from other nurses in the same position that we are not alone and can support and be supported by others. Often, we stop or prevent ourselves from making vital connections with other professionals due to anxiety or insecurity. Meeting and sharing with others assists in developing confidence in ourselves, our abilities, and our ideas.

Energy

Finally, achievers (and competent nurse managers/leaders) have energy. They are bright, energetic people who handle crisis and stress without blaming themselves. They focus on the positive side of things instead of finding fault or placing blame. Their experience and creativity are used to make things happen, nurture others, and maintain the balance between caring for others and self-care.

Nurses, by their very nature, are givers. Self-sacrifice is a large part of our daily work. Everyone else (i.e., patients, staff, family, church, etc.) comes first. As nurses, we give without asking for anything in return.

IMAGE KILLERS

Dressing inconsistently. Maintain a standard of dress. Showing up in a tailored suit one day and a baggy T-shirt with leggings the next day sends mixed messages to everyone around you.

Dressing beneath you. Remember the old saying, ''If it looks like a duck, walks like a duck, and quacks like a duck, then it is a duck.'' It may sound silly, but if you present like a manager and dress like a manager, people will relate to you as a manager. Dress simply in tailored styles. Ruffles, bows, lace, and 3-inch heels project femininity, not competence or leadership. (See Chapter 2.)

Having a negative attitude. 'Can't do' attitudes go nowhere. Even if you feel an idea is bad, do not work against it. Use the positive side and offer another approach. Working *toward* something focuses energies in a positive direction. Working *against* something requires much more energy and seldom pays off. Remember: work toward, not against.

Projecting anxieties or nervousness. Work to appear confident, collected, and composed. Even if you do not feel self-assured, act as if you do. If you cannot make it, fake it. Pretend to have all the self-confidence you need. Remember that people do not know what you are thinking. They will judge you by what they see.

Not making decisions quickly. Noted feminist, Helen Gurley Brown, put it well when she said, ''The worst bosses I've had and the ones other people complain about the most, are those that can't seem to get back to you with anything, even answers you don't want to hear. Don't leave anybody dangling. Decide'' (White, 1986).

Allowing others to interrupt you. It has been said that the hierarchy of an organization is established by the number of successful interruptions one can make. Allowing others to interrupt gives the impression that what you have to say is not important or that others have more important ideas or thoughts. When interrupted, be polite, yet firm, and finish your statement.

Not joining your professional association. To become known and respected takes networking. Being active in your professional association is an investment in your future.

Being cheap. Most nurse managers are not in the position to give financial rewards, but they are able to give praise and recognition. In her book, *Having It All,* Helen Gurley Brown states that ''some bosses are so greedy they forget underlings are not thirteenth century peasants who can be satisfied with a glass of mead and three festivals a year. 'Cheap' is almost worse than nothing'' (White, 1986). Remember, workers thrive on respect and recognition. Avoid being cheap.

Adapted from White J: *Image and self-projection*, Boulder, Colo, 1986, Career Track (audiotape).

Sometimes the intensity of the trauma, illness, despair, and death we face daily can wear us down and sap our energy. Nurses need to learn to re-charge their energies by nurturing and caring for themselves.

Renewing energies. Practice working with the following guidelines and you will find higher levels of energy and lower levels of stress (Yovanovich, 1991):

1. *Accept your needs no matter how small or insignificant.* By fulfilling these needs and caring for yourself, you will be better able to meet the needs of others. Take the time to identify and accept your own needs.
2. *Share your feelings* (with an appropriate person). Especially difficult or traumatic situations can have a strong negative impact. By sharing the feelings associated with the episode, you are allowing yourself to experience and work through them, to let them go, and to move on. Sharing helps to resolve emotions and focus energies in more positive directions.
3. *Be kind to yourself.* Enjoying life's simple pleasures is a superb way to energize yourself. The old cliché, "Take time to smell the roses," holds much truth. Be gentle with yourself.
4. *Accept imperfections in yourself and others.* Throw away that emotional roller coaster called the 'perfect syndrome.' Besides, think of how dull you would be if you (or anyone else) were perfect.
5. *Practice good health.* Meet your physical and emotional needs. Neglecting your needs leads to self-denial, anger, resentment, and finally, physical illnesses. A nurse who neglects the self cannot help others. Self-care renews, recharges, and revitalizes our energies. It provides the basis for our outlooks and attitudes and supplies the energy reservoir for the development of all those psychosocial skills discussed in this chapter.

A final reminder: do not become overwhelmed. Each topic discussed here is a skill, and because they are skills, each can be developed. Changing behaviors or developing new ones is a long process. It takes at least 40 days to change an old habit. Do your best each day. Challenge yourself with one skill at a time; and with practice, you, too, will become a highly competent leader, manager, and a practically perfect person.

Summary

Nurses, especially those in management, draw upon many skills and talents when working with others. Developing effective people, or psychosocial, abilities as a manager is a growth process that begins with developing the personal skills of commitment, humor, a positive outlook, risk taking, and critical thinking. Social skills that are important for effective management include caring, sensitivity, respect, integrity, and energy. Persons who have high levels of achievement possess effective self-projection, positioning, and networking skills. Practicing the techniques discussed in this chapter is the first step in the process of developing effective managerial and leadership abilities.

∞ **Key Concepts**

- Nurses possess many of the skills necessary for effective management and leadership.
- Personal commitment involves doing your best in every situation.
- Directing your growth involves setting goals, focusing energies, and becoming self-aware.
- An important trait for effective management is a gentle sense of humor.
- A positive mental attitude is one of the most powerful tools for leaders.
- Effective nurse supervisors are organized and willing to take risks.
- There are no failures; there are only opportunities for learning.
- The problem-solving process is an important critical-thinking skill for managers.
- Important social skills for nurse leaders include caring, sensitivity to others, respect, and integrity.
- Workers function better in an environment that fosters self-worth, respect, and creativity.
- In this society, women have traditionally been taught to sustain or support success rather than achieve it.
- Dynamic leaders and managers project success.
- Image killers are traits and behaviors that send unfavorable messages.
- By becoming involved, nurse managers are practicing positioning skills and developing opportunities.
- Achievers have well-developed self-projection, positioning, risk-taking, and networking skills as well as a high level of energy.
- Nurses and their managers need to replenish their energies by nurturing and caring for themselves.
- Psychosocial skills are abilities that, with persistent practice, can be developed and enhanced.

∞ **Learning Activities**

1. Wake up each morning and decide that you are going to have a good day.
2. Pick one suggestion, hint, help, or guideline presented in this chapter and practice using it until it becomes comfortable and natural.
3. Write a list of all your personal and professional commitments. Compare the similarities and differences with your work group or class.
4. Discuss the following statements:
   a. Be the best you can be.
   b. Whether you think you can or you think you can't, you're right.
   c. Failure is a necessary part of change.
   d. Walk a mile in my shoes.
   e. Women have been taught to be sustainers, not achievers.

References

Barrett G: Are you a winner?, *Nursing 90* 20(9):120, 1990.

Herzberg F: *Work and the nature of man*, Cleveland, 1966, World Books.

Husted G, Miller M, Wilczynski M: Five ways to build your self-esteem, *Nursing 90* 20(5):152, 1990.

Josefowitz N: *Paths to power*, Reading, Mass, 1980, Addison-Wesley.

Ludeman K: *The worth ethic: how to profit from the changing values of the new work force*, New York, 1989, EP Dutton.

Morris W, editor: *The American heritage dictionary*, Boston, 1976, Houghton Mifflin.

Peter LJ, Hull R: *The Peter principle*, New York, 1969, William Morrow.

Peters TJ, Waterman RH: *In search of excellence: lessons from America's best run companies*, New York, 1982, Harper & Row.

Smith HC: *Sensitivity to people*, New York, 1966, McGraw-Hill.

Thomas L: *The medusa and the snail: more notes of a biology watcher*, New York, 1979, Viking Press.

Travelbee J: What do we mean by rapport?, *American Journal of Nursing* 63(2):70, 1963.

Vestal K: Making a failure a positive experience, *Nursing 91* 21(9):111, 1991.

White J: *Image and self-projection*, Boulder, Colo, 1986, Career Track (audiotape).

Yovanovich L: A caregiver's guide to self-care, *Nursing 91* 21(10):149, 1991.

Additional Readings

Anderson K: Making a good first impression, *Nursing 91* 20(10):145, 1991. *A short article which outlines five tips for making a favorable impression when first meeting others.*

Durald MM: Toward positive attitudes and feelings, *Nursing Management* 20(10):64A, 1989. *The author, a NeuroLinguistic Programming counselor, explains a process for replacing negative attitudes.*

Goetz C, Von Froliol L: Five steps to help you feel good about yourself, *Nursing 91* 20(5):112, 1991. *This is another short article which presents several suggestions for boosting self-esteem.*

Hamilton J: Personal power: your key to success, *Nursing 91* 20(10):146, 1991.

Hangert T: Presenting yourself successfully, *Nursing 91* 21(6):146, 1991. *Advice to help prepare for an interview is offered.*

Kotite E: Personal best, *Entrepreneur* 19(4):154, 1991. *An inspiring article which tells four success stories of people most unlikely to succeed.*

LaBella A, Leach D: *Personal power: the guide to power for today's working woman*, Boulder, Colo, 1985, Career Track. *This is an excellent book for learning to recognize and develop the power unique to women.*

Layden M: Responsibility to self: first step to leadership, *Nursing Leadership* 2:26, Sept 1979. *To foster growth in others, nurses must learn to be critically aware of themselves as individuals.*

Milliken ME: *Understanding human behavior*, ed 3, Albany, NY, 1981, Delmar. *This text was written for beginning-level health care providers. It is a study of the basic principles of human behavior as applied to health care workers and their clients.*

Pinkleton N: Commitment to nursing and self, *Nursing Management* 13(2):39, 1982. *The author contends that nurses need to analyze and review their commitment to nursing in order to provide the framework of our practice.*

Rutkowski B: Six steps to building your confidence, *Nursing Life* 6(1):26, 1986. *Six simple techniques for generating a cycle of self-confidence are described.*

Silber M: Nursing management starts and succeeds with self-esteem, *Supervisor Nurse* 12(3):42, 1981. *Nurse managers who make defensive decisions and live by reacting with self-protecting behaviors pay a heavy price in self-esteem.*

COMMUNICATION 2

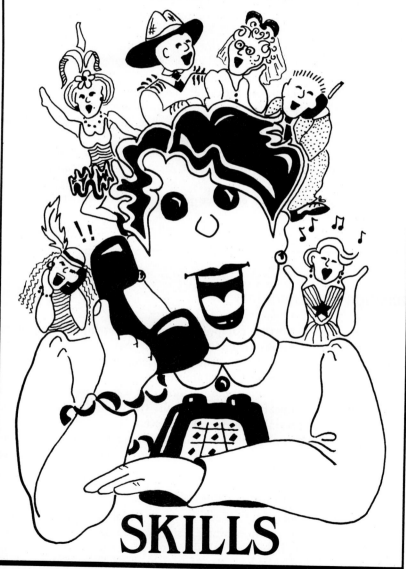

SKILLS

Upon completion of this chapter, the reader will be able to:

1. Identify at least seven factors affecting communication.
2. List six characteristics of a clear and effective message.
3. Compare four techniques for sending verbal messages with five tech-techniques for receiving verbal messages.
4. Identify five guidelines for developing effective nonverbal communication skills.
5. Describe nine keys for career dressing.
6. Define the concept of rapport and its four basic ingredients or elements.
7. Discuss four strategies for creating rapport.
8. Identify seven techniques for developing expert listening abilities.
9. Describe six purposes for the client's health care record or chart.
10. List 10 guidelines for the manager to use when assessing or reviewing nursing documentation.
11. State six key points for effective written communications.
12. Describe nine hints for giving and receiving a clear and concise change-of-shift report.
13. Compare eight rules of effective phone manners with nine phone taboos.
14. Discuss 10 telephone techniques for communicating with physicians.

Communication Fundamentals

Perhaps the most important component of the leadership/management process is communication, an exchange of information that takes place on several levels and that is constantly occurring. Richard Bandler, co-developer of NeuroLinguistic Programming states, "You cannot NOT communicate. We are always communicating, at least nonverbally. Even thoughts are communications with the self" (Bandler, Grinder, 1979). Good communication skills are essential to effective management. Without them, leadership is not possible. Thus, an understanding of the components and process of communication is of great value in developing management and leadership skills.

Factors affecting communication

Communication is dynamic. It affects everyone involved in the exchange. The actual process of communicating is simple: a message is sent and received. A closer look, however, reveals many influences on this dynamic process.

The message. Every message contains content (the actual message) and relationship (information on how to interpret the message). Consider the following situation: Ivy Jones, a wing supervisor for a long-term care facility, is checking the progress of the CNAs in assisting residents with their showers. She asks Marge Brown how they are coming along. "Just fine," says Marge with a frown while rushing past her. If Ivy were to receive only the message's verbal content, she would assume that the CNAs were doing well and had no problems. However, if she also considered the message's relationship (Marge's frowning facial expression and rapid body movements), she would realize that everything was not fine and that a problem may exist. By considering both aspects of a message, she was able to develop a greater understanding of the entire communication, which may either reinforce the verbal message or convey an entirely different message. Most of the nurse manager's time is spent communicating. This makes it especially important to learn to receive the whole message.

Each person is unique and, thus, responds to thoughts, emotions, and communications from a unique point of view. Because of this, **communication is not what is sent, but what is** *received*. Remember this important premise when sending as well as receiving messages. Other factors that have an impact on the communication process are listed in the box below.

Level of development. Children develop increasingly complex language skills as they grow. By adulthood, one is usually quite fluent in a language. As one grows older or deals with health problems, language abilities may be affected. When communicating, the nurse should take into account each person's level of development. The nurse manager who applies this element when communicating within the work setting may give the same

---

🖎 FACTORS THAT IMPACT COMMUNICATIONS

- The message
- Level of development
- Individual background: culture, attitudes
- Emotions
- Past experiences
- Relationships and roles
- The grapevine
- Space and territory
- Environmental factors

Adapted from Potter P, Perry A: *Fundamentals of nursing: concepts, process and practice*, ed 3, St Louis, 1990, Mosby.

message to the supervisors as to the aide staff, but it may be presented in a different style for each group.

Individual background. The background of the individual includes one's culture, language, attitudes, and values. **Culture influences the subject of the communication,** its style, the gestures used, and the values placed on the messages. To be truly effective, the nurse manager needs to be aware of his/her personal values and not allow them to interfere when communicating. **Attitudes strongly influence communications.** Staff members with negative attitudes are less likely to receive complete messages, especially if those messages involve changes. By paying attention to the backgrounds of the people with whom you communicate, you are better able to send messages that will be more completely received.

Emotions. Emotions are feelings, and how one feels about the subject strongly influences the sending and receiving of messages. Emotions can be easily misunderstood; thus, it is important to be aware of both your emotions and what you perceive of others' emotions. Keep an open mind. Observe how your staff interacts with others and how you interact with them. Develop an awareness of your own emotions. These hints encourage clear communications and save many wasted emotions that result from misunderstood messages.

Past experiences. Past experiences can have an impact on communication. If, for example, your staff was promised a day off for working a double shift and that never materialized, the next communication about working overtime will be less likely to be received positively. They will 'turn off' the message. The outcomes of similar situations one has experienced in the past colors many present communications.

Relationships and roles. At work, **communications are affected by the roles people assume.** As a first-line supervisor, you will communicate with people in different roles. According to Douglas (1991):

1. Downward communications occur when you direct and coordinate activities with your staff. It also includes listening and gathering information from them.
2. Upward communications occur when you are interacting with your supervisor. Messages are then sent up to various authorities. This line of communication motivates employees and encourages effective problem solving, for employees frequently have a better grasp on a problem than managers.
3. Lateral communications are most frequently used when coordinating activities with persons on the same level. For example, every client

or resident in the facility requires a TB skin test. Wing/unit supervisors meet to plan the details that will accomplish the goal.

4. Communications are diagonal when they occur between employees or departments who are not on the same level in the organization. A housekeeper interacting with the nursing supervisor is an example of diagonal communication.

The grapevine. The grapevine is by far the most important informal communication system in any organization. Communications within the grapevine are usually based on relationships rather than roles. The grapevine fills the need for people to communicate. It occurs at all levels in the organization and can have a strong influence on attitudes and behaviors. The grapevine carries information that is of interest. Unfortunately, that information can become distorted or incomplete. People will naturally want to fill in the missing pieces, thus distorting the communication even further. Grapevines can have a negative impact on workers, especially when the information carried is ignored by supervisors. Here are a few guidelines for nurse managers to work with the grapevine (Douglas, 1991):

1. **Keep your staff well informed,** especially when the information affects them. Your data are usually more accurate and complete, and well-informed workers spread fewer rumors.
2. **Keep communications open with your staff.** Listen and learn from the grapevine. Encourage feedback from workers.
3. **Encourage the use of the formal communication channels** for important work-related messages. If a CNA or food service worker, for example, has an idea that saves time and you hear about it via the grapevine, the use of formal channels for communicating that idea may result in a change of procedure as well as recognition for the idea's owner.

The grapevine is alive and well in all organizations. Many managers wish it would go away. Your effectiveness as a leader and manager is improved when you learn to use the grapevine to prevent problems and promote organizational goals.

Space and territory. When people interact they keep a certain amount of space or distance between themselves (see box on p. 32). Territoriality is the need to claim an area of space as one's own. It can be defined by barriers such as walls, fences, or curtains, or it can contain no physical features — just an agreed-upon area belonging to a specific person like a desk, a certain wing in the facility, or even a particular group of clients. People tend to defend their territory. The CNA who works with a particular group of clients for five days a week needs to be assured that, during the two days off, his/her clients will receive care that is of the same standard

✒ INTERACTIVE DISTANCES

Intimate distance (18 inches or less). It is usually reserved for mates, lovers, close relatives, and friends. Hugging is an example of communication at the intimate distance. Nurses involved with direct client care frequently work at the intimate distance levels, but team leaders and other managers are usually more removed from client care and, thus, work at less intimate distances.

Personal distance (18 inches to 4 feet). This is the space at which most managerial communications take place. They are usually one-on-one interactions (e.g., performance evaluation meetings, giving directions) but they can involve small groups (e.g., several people huddled together). Messages delivered at 18 inches are usually more forceful than those delivered at a distance of 4 feet. The alert nurse manager is aware of this when considering the impact the message may have on staff members.

Social distance (4 feet to 12 feet). It is commonly used when working in groups. Staff meetings and giving work assignments are examples. Communication at this distance is usually less threatening than on other levels because it is less personal. However, some people can be intimidated by groups and may limit their communications.

Public distance (more than 12 feet). This is employed when addressing large groups. The speaker usually requires a microphone, and little group interaction occurs. To be an effective speaker, the nurse manager 'tailors' his/her communications by using space and distance.

Adapted from Hein EC: *Communication in nursing practice*, Boston, 1973, Little, Brown.

as the regular CNA provides. Territoriality is an important consideration when communicating, assigning work, staffing, or scheduling.

Environmental factors. The sending and receiving of messages is much more effective when people are free of physical and emotional discomfort. The best physical environment for communicating is one that is private, warm, and free of noise or distractions. When several people are talking at once or there are other distractions, the effectiveness of the message is greatly reduced. In such situations, be sure to get the attention of the other person *before* attempting to communicate. This will help to reduce the confusion that results from an unclear message.

The effectiveness of communications is also decreased when one's internal environment is uncomfortable. A staff member who is hot, cold, tired, hungry, or worried is much less likely to send or receive messages effectively.

Several factors affect the effectiveness of communications. Developing an awareness of these factors assists nurse managers to improve their communication skills and leadership abilities.

Verbal communications

We continually send and receive two types of messages: verbal and nonverbal. Both types of messages involve the idea to be communicated, the sender, the message, the channel or method of sending the message, the receiver, and, most importantly, the *understanding* of the message. Although we will consider each component of communication separately, one must remember that they are all intricately entwined. When receiving verbal or spoken messages, we are also processing nonverbal cues (messages) to confirm or deny the verbal message that is being sent. The result is a unique impression, a mixture of messages.

The need for the manager/leader to accurately and reliably send and receive verbal messages is critical for effectiveness. Verbal messages that are vague or unclear promote confusion and poor job performance.

Effective verbal messages. According to Potter and Perry (1990), clear, effective verbal communications contain messages that are:

- **Brief.** Use the fewest words that send the message. Keep it short, simple, and to the point. Using too many words can muddy the message and confuse the receiver.
- **Clear.** Speak slowly and clearly. Repeat important points. Use words or vocabulary that are simple enough to be understood. Watch the use of slang, medical jargon, and 'nurse-esse' (our particular brand of slang words, abbreviations, and symbols). Unless the meaning of the terms is agreed upon, the message will be unclear.
- **Paced appropriately.** The speed with which a message is delivered has an impact on the communication. A message that is sent too rapidly increases anxieties in the receiver. Awkward pauses or the use of too much or too little silence can convey messages other than what was intended. For example, Mrs. Smith asks the wing supervisor if her father's condition is improving. The nurse gazes at the floor and responds with silence for about 45 seconds before speaking. No matter what the nurse now says, Mrs. Smith has interpreted the nurse's pauses as an indication that her father's condition is deteriorating. Learn to think about what to say before speaking. This will allow for proper pacing.

- **Effectively toned.** The tone of a person's voice can have a strong influence on the message being sent. Vocal tones can also indicate one's emotional state. To send an effective message, the tone of voice must match the words that are sent.
- **Relevant.** Communications that are important have more impact. If the message has little relevance or importance, it will be casually received and soon forgotten.
- **Well timed.** In order to be received fully, verbal messages need to be sent at advantageous times. During a break in the staff lounge is not the time to speak with a CNA about job performance. Messages that are personal or relate to performance need to be timed so that they can be sent in private, with time for discussion. Communications that praise a staff member should be sent in public, thus encouraging recognition and worth. A good rule of thumb for timing messages: "Praise in public; criticize in private."

Nurse managers are in the unique position of already possessing and using many therapeutic communication skills through their work with clients. As a manager, techniques for transmitting or sending messages now need to be polished. Remember, your staff members are people who will also benefit from the use of therapeutic communication techniques.

Sending verbal messages. Most of the nurse manager's time is spent communicating. This makes the art of sending and receiving clear verbal messages vitally important. Gilmore and Fraleigh (1980) offer these suggestions to assist in sending verbal communications:

- **Make a clear purpose statement.** As a manager, you must communicate reliability. You must be predictable to others. Staff members who are honestly informed of your intentions will cooperate. However, if your purposes or motives are unclear, you could potentially be 'the enemy,' and workers will actively or passively become defensive. If your purpose is clear, others are aware of what you want to do, and this fosters communication and cooperation. Purpose statements are goals. Most managers assume that others somehow know what their purposes are. That is usually incorrect. Be clear about what you want to accomplish (your goal) and share that with the staff (see box on p. 35). Once the purpose or goal has been stated, make every effort to accomplish whatever is necessary to meet the goal. Workers watch to see if their managers actually do what they say they will do. Reliability and credibility can rapidly be gained or lost in this area.
- **Describe the behaviors.** A behavioral description is used to specify what actually happened or what specific actions need to be taken to meet the goal. When used to explain what occurred, behavioral descriptions

---

✍ WORDS INDICATING PURPOSE STATEMENTS

- My goal for . . . is . . .
- My purpose is . . .
- Objectives for today are . . .
- The purpose of this meeting is . . .
- My intention is . . .
- I am trying to . . .

---

chronicle the actual actions of those people involved. Listing the behaviors is an excellent tool for removing the emotionally laden parts from the actual behaviors. This can be of great assistance when resolving disputes or making highly emotional decisions.

When working with others, behavior descriptions will list each step or action to be taken in order to meet the goal. Many times, directions or explanations can be crystal clear to one person and foggy or vague to another. By comparing their expectations with the behavioral description, staff members will have a clear idea of what is expected and the steps that need to be taken to meet the goal.

- **Describe the feelings.** Feeling descriptions focus on the inner, emotional state. Although others may guess at what one is feeling, the only person who can send a feeling description is the one who owns the emotions. Because our profession involves caring for clients, feeling descriptions can be important tools for working with the emotions we frequently encounter. By monitoring your own feeling descriptions, you are better able to work with others. Assisting others to use feeling descriptions promotes the release of stress and anxiety. The following situation illustrates this point:

> Sara Lang, the team leader for Wing A, has lately noticed that Brenda Bradshaw, a CNA who has worked at the facility for 5 years, has been slipping in her job performance. Brenda repeatedly denies that anything is wrong. Sara decides to meet with Brenda in order to discuss her job performance. When she asks Brenda for a feeling description, she discovers that Brenda lost her favorite patient, a lady for whom she had been caring for 3 years. By using a feeling description, Brenda was able to share her feelings of grief and loss, while Sara discovered the cause of Brenda's poor job performance. Together they were able to focus on actions that would resolve Brenda's grief and promote growth by coping with the loss.

- **State the preference.** By letting others know what you would like to see happen or what you prefer, a clear message is sent, and possibilities for ways to meet the goal are suggested. Most people, however, are reluctant to share their preferences. Some do not have strong inclinations. Others are either unaware of their preferences or unwilling to share them. Knowing what you and others prize and prefer adds to constructive communications and promotes realistic problem solving. Be careful not to state your preferences so forcefully that others feel coerced by your message. As a manager, wing supervisor, coordinator, or the like, you are also a leader, and your statements have strong impact. Be careful to elicit or draw out the preferences of each of your staff members first. In this way, information is shared, creative ideas may be offered, and communication is constructive. Most importantly though, the people you supervise feel respected and valued as members of the team.

By using the four major sending, or transmitting, skills (stating the purpose and preferences, describing behaviors and feelings), your verbal messages will be clear and hopefully encourage others to communicate more accurately.

Receiving verbal messages. Receiving verbal messages also requires attention and practice. There are five receiving skills that will assist in improving your reception of verbal messages. They are as follows (Gilmore, Fraleigh, 1980):

1. **Observing** — the proverbial art of 'people watching.' As a manager and leader, your people watching becomes purposeful. Learn to employ the tools of scanning and focusing. Scanning is looking over a wide area quickly but thoroughly. It is a technique that allows you to survey the scene to catch the action (interactions) or assess the situation. Focusing improves understanding. It is the practice of closing out distractions that may interfere with receiving the message. Practice these two techniques at your next meeting and you will find how valuable they are.
2. **Empathizing** — putting yourself in your worker's place. How does he/ she feel about . . .? What is it like to do this job? The answers will assist in choosing different strategies for interacting and working with each person. By observing and empathizing, your receiving of verbal messages becomes more effective.
3. **Paraphrasing** — a technique learned during the study of therapeutic communications, paraphrasing is a very useful tool for increasing the nurse manager's understanding of verbal messages. Paraphrasing is a technique of restating the verbal message you received, using your own words. It is a brief description of what was communicated to you. This tool accomplishes several communication tasks:

- It helps develop active listening skills. In order to accurately reflect the message being sent, one must be attentive and listen carefully.
- It states that you respect the speaker enough to listen carefully. People are much more inclined to share information when they feel someone is really listening.
- It allows the speaker to correct or clarify the message. This avoids many unnecessary problems of miscommunication because it allows the speaker to hear the message you received and revise or modify it to improve your understanding.
- It allows the speaker the opportunity to share a personal experience or emotion. Intensive listening and paraphrasing assists in sharing the emotional aspect of the experience.

In summary, statements that contain the elements of good paraphrasing are brief; focus on the speaker's experience; and contain both facts and feelings, but not judgments. Good paraphrasing skills improve the quality of your communications and interactions many times over.

4. **Summarizing** — 'capturing' the message by arranging it in some order and reducing it to one or more main points. Summarizing has several purposes:

- It weaves together separate and different pieces of information and allows patterns to emerge.
- It helps to define and agree on expectations.
- It encourages communication and movement in a conversation.
- It presents the main points at the close of a communication.

Summarizing avoids communication errors because it allows both the receiver and the sender an opportunity to agree upon the message.

5. **Checking perceptions** — perceptions arise from all the verbal, nonverbal, and other data we receive from the message. They include the feelings or energies of another's attitude or emotional state. When you check or validate these impressions by communicating them, you are using the tool of perception checking. To develop this skill takes practice, but it is worth the effort. Guidelines for the use of effective perception checking encourage you to

- signal that you want to check your perception (e.g., "Before we go on . . .").
- share your purpose (e.g., "I'm confused." "My perception is . . .").
- speak slowly and avoid being judgmental. Mary may be behaving like a jerk, but that perception is not shared. Instead, focus on

your impression of her *behaviors*, not her attitudes or emotions. (e.g., "When I see Mary staring at the wall, I get the message that she is not interested. Is that accurate?").

- accept whatever the other person has to say, even though it does not agree with your perceptions.
- use perception checking when the communication process appears blocked or when paraphrasing fails to move the interaction constructively.

Developing and practicing the verbal receiving skills (observe, paraphrase, summarize, and check perceptions) will greatly improve your competency as a nursing manager and leader. Clearly sent and received communications provide the foundation for effective job performance.

Nonverbal communications

Just as important as verbal messages is the constantly occurring nonverbal communication. These messages are considered to be a *more* accurate description of emotions than verbal messages. It is easier for us to control our words and speech than the nonverbal messages we send. Researchers (Mehrabian, 1971) found that nonverbal signals had a greater impact on communications than verbal messages. Fifty-five percent of one study's subjects felt that facial expression had the greatest impact, followed by tone of voice (38 percent). The words used had only a weak effect (7 percent). Data like these demonstrate why nonverbal communication techniques are such powerful tools.

Techniques for developing effective nonverbal communications focus on the use of personal appearance, professional appearance, body language, distance and territory, attending behaviors, and touch.

Personal appearance. First impressions, most of them nonverbal, are formed within the first 30 seconds of an interaction. Like it or not, how one appears to others has a strong impact on the whole relationship. One's personal appearance is the combination of one's physical characteristics, style of dress, hygiene, hairstyle, and use of cosmetics or accessories (jewelry, scarves, etc.). It is this mixture that creates an impression. As a leader and manager, your **personal appearance will stimulate responses in staff members.** To communicate professionalism and leadership as a nurse manager, try these tips:

1. Use your physical characteristics to your advantage. Stand up straight whether you are short or tall. If you are tall, remember that high heels can make you look overpowering or unapproachable, especially to short people. If you are short, be sure to get eye contact before speaking. Project confidence but do not become cocky. Choose eyeglasses (if they are needed) that project intelligence.

✐ FIVE TYPES OF NURSES' ATTIRE

Traditional dress — the starched white uniform, stockings, shoes, and cap. Hair is worn off the collar; and jewelry, makeup, and nail polish are avoided. These nurses give the message that they are clean, controlled, and competent but not very imaginative, powerful, or important.

Cute little girl — those who wear puffed sleeves, frilly blouses, ruffles, lace, and shoes with colorful laces and trim. They are neat, clean, and tend to wear cute, little girl hairstyles and moderate amounts of makeup. Their nonverbal messages say they are nice, conscientious little helpers with little authority or competence.

I-don't-care style — includes a variety of clothing. The hit-or-miss combination of jeans and sneakers to odds and ends of uniforms plus the long and stringy or short and uncombed hairstyle sends the message that these nurses are not attentive, concerned, or caring.

Sexy dress — nurses who wear tight-fitting uniforms or street clothing, heavy makeup, and large items of jewelry convey the message that they are more interested in themselves and attracting the attention of others than working with patients.

Career dress — focus is on neatness and quality. Hairstyles are neat and usually simple. Makeup and jewelry are used conservatively. The person, rather than the outfit, is presented. The message is one of competence, commitment, and authority.

Adapted from Kalish B, Kalish P: Dressing for success, *American Journal of Nursing* 85(8):887, 1985.

---

2. Learn to 'career dress.' Kalish and Kalish (1985), in their article "Dressing for Success," have identified five types of nurses' attire (see box above).

Professional appearance. Clothing communicates. To convey the message of an effective nurse leader/manager, consider these guidelines:

1. Tailored lines are more business-like than frilly or flowing lines. Choose simple, classic styles.
2. Skirt length should be at the knees or lower. Skirts that display a high percentage of leg send a sexual message.
3. Shoes should be of quality materials with a heel no higher than 1 inch. No tennis or jogging shoes, sandals, or spiked high heels should be worn. They all send a casual, unprofessional message. Clean and polish shoes often enough to cover scuff marks.

4. Lace, ruffles, and highly colorful clothing is not recommended. The message is casual or helplessly feminine.
5. Denims and jeans are out. No matter how casual the facility's dress code, you are not 'down home.' These pants destroy the message that you are a competent leader or manager.
6. Jewelry, if worn, should be one (or, at the most, two) small items. Large pieces, those with several stones, dangling, and noisy jewelry is not appropriate for the business message you want to send.
7. Keep fingernails well manicured. Use polish of muted or conservative colors. Keep the length fairly short. Hands, especially the fingernails, send many messages. In the Orient, long fingernails were once considered a sign of status. In fact, those people of very high status were afraid to do anything with their hands for fear of breaking a fingernail. Today, we are not so extreme, but long fingernails (natural or artificial) still convey the message of leisure and not having to do much work.
8. Makeup should be used sparingly. Its purpose is to enhance natural features, not to remodel the face. The 'painted lady' looks superficial and will seldom inspire others to do their best.
9. Hygiene is paramount. Bad breath and body odors send a strong I-don't-care message. Nursing is a profession that values cleanliness highly. The nurse manager must lead by example in this area.

By understanding the nonverbal messages that personal appearance conveys, you are able to present the image of a competent, caring manager.

Body language. The sending and receiving of nonverbal messages through the use of bodily movements and facial expressions is referred to as body language. Remember that these messages sometimes have a greater impact on communication than the verbal messages. The nurse sends many distinct messages using body language. Learn to make use of the following guidelines:

1. **Body position.** People who take up as little space as possible send signals of being small and insignificant. Women especially send this message. Notice how men and women sit in a group. Men rest one ankle on the knee and spread the arms out to the sides. Women cross their legs and sit with their hands in their laps. The use of space influences how powerfully each person is viewed.
2. **Posture.** Posture communicates attitude. People who walk with slumped shoulders, look at the ground, and avoid eye contact send a closed message. "I'll interact with you if I must, but I won't like it." Nurses, especially their leaders, need to stand and walk with heads up and shoulders straight — the open position. This communicates a readiness and willingness to interact as well as an I-am-approachable attitude.

3. **Gait.** Walking communicates by its pace and gait. If someone is stag-
gering, we assume he is ill or intoxicated. The worker who stomps
rapidly into the staff lounge is assumed to be angry. Rapid walking
signals one is too busy to stop or be interrupted. A very slow pace
may indicate wanting to put something off or delay involvement. A
stomping gait usually means the walker is not happy. The 'rolling hips'
gait expresses sexuality. Awareness of what you are communicating
while walking will assist you in sending appropriate messages.

4. **Gestures.** The use of our bodies, especially the hands, to communicate
or emphasize verbal messages serves several purposes (Potter, Perry,
1990):

   - To illustrate an idea — the client points to an area of pain, or the
     CNA draws a circle in the air to describe the size of a client's skin
     lesion.
   - To express an emotional state — covering the eyes or heart; point-
     ing a finger to accuse. Each gesture sends information.
   - To signal — by using an agreed-upon sign, gestures can convey
     such messages as "Come here!" (moving the hand rapidly toward
     one's self), "You've had it" (tracing the first finger in a line across
     the throat), or "Good job" (making a circle with the thumb and
     first finger). Gestures emphasize speech or send their own specific
     meanings. Astute managers will work to cultivate gestures that
     match with the other messages they send.

5. **Facial expressions.** The face is a powerful communicator. Social scientists have been studying facial expressions and their impacts on children and adults for years. Their research shows that in all cultures, six
primary emotions are revealed by facial expressions: anger, disgust,
fear, happiness, sadness, and surprise. Facial expressions are frequently
the basis for judgments, although their meanings may be difficult to
judge or they may contradict verbal messages. In this culture, eye
contact is important. The eyes reveal subtle cues that add to the overall message. The amount of eye contact during an interaction influences
the outcome of the communication. Managers who maintain eye contact (but do not stare) during a communication are perceived as concerned and believable.

Distance and territory. Learn to match each type of communication
with the most effective distance: intimate (18 inches or less), personal (18
inches to 4 feet), social (4 feet to 12 feet), or public (12 feet and greater).
In general, the more private or personal the communication, the closer
the distance between people.

✐✐ PURPOSES OF POSITIVE TOUCH

- Serves as a coping behavior to handle stress
- Assists in compensating for a loss
- Communicates value and worth
- Stimulates and encourages involvement with others

Attending behaviors. These are a combination of behaviors that indicate if (and how) you are listening to the speaker. They include eye contact, focusing on the speaker's message, and attentive listening techniques.

Touch. Touch is a powerful tool that conveys both positive and negative expressions. Sometimes it becomes the most effective form of communication. People need touch. We provide for this with our clients but rarely for our staff members. Positive touching serves several purposes (see box above). The need for touch does not diminish with age, and its meaning is highly individual. Its interpretation depends on the cultural background and emotional state or mood of the people and the nature of the relationship or interaction. Awareness of space and territory is essential when communicating with touch. Touch is a learned behavior based on sound theories and concepts. Staff members who receive frequent, appropriate touch from their managers respond with greater performance and express more satisfaction with their work.

Nonverbal communications encompass many aspects. By practicing and applying the discussed techniques, you will develop many of the nonverbal communication skills necessary for competent management and leadership.

Rapport

An often overlooked aspect of communication is rapport—a particular manner in which we perceive, relate to, and interact with another. It is a group of genuine thoughts and feelings. When in rapport with another person, communications 'match,' and there is a flow of verbal and nonverbal messages being sent and, most importantly, received.

In 1963, Joyce Travelbee wrote an article titled "What Do We Mean by Rapport?" In it she described rapport as "the catalyst which transforms a series of contacts into a meaningful relationship." This description is still relevant 30 years later. As managers, we need to be in rapport with those people we supervise.

Basic elements. Look at your interactions with staff members with the basic ingredients (elements) of rapport in mind (see box on p. 43). These

---

🐦 ELEMENTS OF RAPPORT

- A concern for and active interest in others
- An accepting, nonjudgmental approach
- Empathy and sympathy
- A belief in the dignity, worth, and uniqueness of each individual

Adapted from Travelbee J: What do we mean by rapport?, *American Journal of Nursing* 63(2):70, 1963.

---

attitudes allow you to promote the growth of each staff member while meeting organizational goals.

Emotional involvement. Being in rapport with others also includes a certain degree of emotional involvement, but it is important that it be a controlled type of involvement to maintain a therapeutic level of emotional objectivity. Keep these points in mind:

- **Be clear regarding your goals.** As manager, your basic goals are to supervise the delivery of nursing care, maintain standards, and promote unity and harmony among staff members.
- **Develop a sense of proportion.** Do not become so emotionally involved that you become ineffective. Remember who owns the problem.
- **Keep in mind the difference between the professional role of manager and the social role.** The goals of the manager's role are to meet the needs of the organization and its workers. In contrast, social role goals are focused on sharing, having fun, and enjoyment. If you choose to socialize with staff members, remember these two roles are very different and may sometimes produce conflicts.
- **See persons as they are.** All people are not alike. Do not perceive them as someone in your past or associate them with Uncle Louie, for example. Each of your workers must be treated as individual and unique human beings.

Staff members (workers) who believe they are in rapport with their supervisors state the following:

1. They feel a sense of trust and confidence in the manager.
2. They can predict how the manager will behave.
3. They can obtain emotional support from the manager when needed.
4. The manager is accessible and will listen.
5. The manager projects a together-we-can-see-it-through attitude.

 TECHNIQUES FOR ESTABLISHING RAPPORT

1. **Define your goals for the relationship.**

   Are my goals positive and attainable? (Can Mary, the grumpiest CNA on the staff, participate constructively in staff meetings?)

   What will I see/hear/feel when I reach the goal? (Mary offering several suggestions in a pleasant manner during staff meetings.)

   What do I want now and long term? (I want Mary to be a cooperative, productive worker.)

2. **Listen for the 'rapport alarm.'**

   What do I see/hear/feel when I know I have lost rapport? This involves being in touch with the messages being sent by the other person. Work on receiving skills.

   What are the nonverbal messages I am receiving? Do they agree with the verbal messages?

3. **Use rapport builders.**

   To share another's experience, try to 'match' or identify with their:

   - body alignment and postures. Match the direction of attention (e.g., sit next to the person rather than 'facing off'). Match part or all of the person's stance, gestures, etc.
   - emotional state. Assess the person's emotional state. Then verbally identify the emotions (e.g., "You seem happy today.").
   - rhythm. Parallel the rhythm of movements and the tone, pitch, and tempo of speech.
   - feelings. First ask, "How do I want those who work with me to feel when I am around?" Then sincerely feel or experience these emotions. Third, remember these feelings when interacting with others. A manager who has a positive rapport with his/her staff can lead them to accomplish many goals.

Creating rapport. Obviously, some people, nurses, and managers form rapport more easily than others. To apply the principles of rapport, see the box above for techniques.

Effective listening

An important component of effective communication and rapport building is the skill (art) of effective listening. Poor listening (receiving) habits can cause misunderstandings, conflicts, and decreased managerial effectiveness. Unfortunately, most of us were not taught to listen effectively. We have developed poor listening habits such as letting the mind wander or planning how to respond before the speaker finishes talking. In fact, statistics reveal that only 10 percent of people listen properly (Raudsepp, 1990). Also, how much of the message was garbled by the listener's interpretation?

Expert listening abilities. Eugene Raudsepp (1990), president of Princeton Creative Research, offers these basic listening skills for developing expert listening abilities:

Take time to listen. Stop what you are doing and look the speaker in the eye. Nod your understanding. Ask questions to clarify messages. These behaviors reassure the speaker that you are listening and will help you to stay focused on the interaction.

Teach yourself to concentrate. We think three to four times faster than people speak. That leaves much time to become impatient with the slow pace of the speaker and then allow the mind to wander. A helpful technique that overcomes this habit is to adapt your thinking speed. Keep analyzing the speaker's point. What is he trying to tell me? Has he looked at all sides of the question?

Do not interrupt. Breakdowns in communication occur when you interrupt the speaker or finish his/her sentences. One technique to prevent these habits is to apologize every time you interrupt. After a few apologies, you will be reminded to allow the speaker to complete the message before you interrupt.

Listen to *what* the speaker is saying, not *how* it is being said. Do not get involved with the speaker's style, especially if it is disagreeable. Keep focused on the *message.*

Do not judge. When reacting emotionally to a word or phrase, you may miss the message. Learn to listen to ideas you may not want to hear. Try not to unconsciously tune out ideas that you perceive as anxiety-provoking or threatening. Selective hearing helps protect us from ideas which are disagreeable, but it becomes a negative mechanism when it interferes with communications.

Listen 'between the lines.' Nurses are trained to focus on the facts in the message, but this is not always an effective technique. Sometimes the true message lies *behind* the facts. People often repeat themselves because they are unsure of how to send the real message. When communications appear garbled, vague, or repetitious, ask yourself, "What do the facts mean? How do they relate to the other messages I am receiving? What key idea binds them together?" Matching facts with ideas and other incoming messages gives a clearer picture of what the speaker is saying.

Listen with your eyes. Pay attention to the other modes of nonverbal communication—the gestures, facial expressions, and the like. Be alert for behaviors that may indicate conflicts between feelings and words. Developing effective listening skills and replacing poor listening habits takes time; every time you practice these techniques, though, you move a step closer.

Professional Communications

As nurses and managers, we are also responsible for a special type of communications — those with other health care professionals. Professional communications are messages that focus on being accurate, concise, and descriptive. Both written and verbal communications should meet these criteria. Nurse managers are responsible for the quality of communications among nursing staff members as well as between staff members and other professionals. Let us look at two of these specialized areas in detail.

The health care record

The patient/client/resident health care record is commonly known as 'the chart.' It is an account of the client's health history, treatment, progress, and current status.

Purposes. The health care record serves important purposes (Christensen, Kockrow, 1991):

It is a communication tool. The chart documents any service or care received. All health care professionals involved with the client will leave a written record on the chart. As a nurse manager, it is prudent to assure that each service the client receives is documented. The chart commonly will include notations from staff members from these departments: Medical (MD or NP), Dietary, Laboratory, Radiology, Special Studies, and possibly Surgery, Post-Anesthetic Care Unit, other specialized units, or different facilities. The chart is also an important tool for communication within the nursing department by allowing the nursing staff to convey data among shifts. An accurate, up-to-date chart prevents errors by documenting all medication doses and treatments received.

It serves as a legal document. The chart is admissible as evidence in court. It is highly confidential, for it contains very personal information about the client. The agency in which services are provided usually retains the chart after the client is discharged. Policies regarding the client's right to the chart's information vary. Know and follow your agency's policy.

It provides statistical information and data for research. Statistical data helps the facility's manager anticipate and plan for future needs. Also, the law requires the reporting of certain statistics (e.g., certain communicable diseases). These data then become part of local, state, national, and international data bases. Research data may also assist the nursing team in focusing on a current problem or yield information that would assist job satisfaction or performance.

It is a tool that educates. The health care record provides a comprehensive view of the client, his/her condition, treatments, and responses. By comparing data in the chart with expected normals, the nursing staff is able to plan appropriate individualized care for each client.

It is used to monitor client care and the competence of those people giving the care. The method used to accomplish this is called a nursing audit, where the care given the client is measured with established standards. It serves as an in-house tool for monitoring quality and solving problems early. As the manager (supervisor) of your wing/unit, etc., you will probably be involved with audits. Cooperate fully and honestly. The results will assist you in coping with small problems before they become large dilemmas.

It is a vehicle for planning client care. The chart is used by the entire health team to plan care. Each specialty views the client's problems from a particular point of view. As nurses usually have the most comprehensive perspective, it is their responsibility to coordinate each specialty with the delivery of safe, competent care. As the nurses' supervisor, it becomes your responsibility to assure this happens for every client.

Today, client documentation has many forms. Whether you use the traditional narrative style of record keeping or one of the newer methods, the standards remain the same. Most managers or supervisors have some degree of responsibility for assuring appropriate documentation.

Guidelines for assessing nursing documentation. Use the checklist in Figure 2-1 when reviewing charts to assure that each chart has:

1. **Restricted access.** Because the client record is a legal document and contains highly personal information, only those health care workers who actually care for the client are allowed access to it.
2. **Accuracy.** Notations must consist of objective data. Information gathered by the five senses is objective. If one can see, hear, feel, smell, or taste to gather the data, then it is considered objective. Objective data can be shared; opinions and interpretations cannot. Look for facts and observations of the client's behaviors (Table 2-1). Re-

Client's Name: _____

Room: _____

Date Reviewed: _____

Does this health care record (chart) contain:

	YES	NO	DATE TIME	CONTACT PERSON
Access restricted to caregivers				
Accurate entries				
Appropriate notations				
Blanks filled				
Brief, concise entries				
Complete notations				
Dates and times documented				
Errors noted and corrected				
Ink used for all entries				
Standard abbreviations, symbols				

Total _____

Comments: _____

_____

_____

Date of Review _____

Reviewer _____

FIGURE 2-1   Health care record (chart) review.

Table 2-1 Examples of Objective Data

Inappropriate	Accurate
Appears confused	Wandering in room. Oriented to person only. Thinks he is on the farm. Calls nurse Mom. G. Jones—LPN.
Wound healing well	Wound pink, clean, and dry. Edges aligned. No redness or drainage. S. Smart—LPN.
Fell and fainted when walking	While walking in hall unassisted, fell onto L. side. Eyes gazing upward. Became unresponsive to voice × 15 sec. VS 120/90-90-24. I. Good—LPN.

member that client records are used in court cases as evidence. Accurate, objective notations provide legal protection for you, your staff, the facility, and the client.

3. **Appropriateness.** Only information that directly relates to the client's health problems and care is recorded. Other information is usually personal and may be considered an invasion of privacy if written in the chart. For example, a client just shared with your staff member that he was in prison as a young man. Unless this information directly relates to his current health care problems, it should not be charted.

4. **Blanks.** The chart should contain no blank spaces. Make sure that all blank spaces have lines drawn through them. If large areas of a page are blank, draw an "X" to cover the space.

5. **Brevity.** "Say it in as few words as possible" is a good rule of thumb. Names and the words *client* and *patient* are not used because the whole chart is specific to each client. Check for a period at the end of each thought or sentence.

6. **Completeness.** Client records are used to indicate the quality of care provided according to accepted standards. Data recorded should contain a complete description of the event, observation, etc. Emphasis should be on facts or observations that may indicate a change in the client's condition. Essential information that needs to be recorded includes:

- Visits by health team members (e.g., MD, therapists, dietician).
- Any changes in physical functioning or abilities to perform the activities of daily living.
- Any changes in behavior (e.g., mood, relationships, level of consciousness).
- Any sign or symptom that persists, worsens, becomes severe, is not normal, or indicates a possible complication.
- Any nursing intervention or care provided.

7. **Dates and times.** Always check for dated entries. If time is recorded in the conventional manner, ensure that A.M. or P.M. follows each entry. If using 24-hour, or military, time, A.M. or P.M. is not needed.
8. **Errors.** Never erase or blot out an error. When an error is made, draw a line through it and write the word "correction" above it. Then initial it. Each facility has a policy relating to charting errors. It is your responsibility to know and follow this policy.
9. **All entries in ink.** Most facilities require the use of black or blue ink for charting. It is permanent and copies well. In some facilities, each shift records with a different color of ink (e.g., black for day shift, green for evenings, and red for night shift). Check your agency's policy.
10. **Standardized abbreviations, terms, and symbols.** Only commonly accepted symbols and abbreviations specified by the facility should be used. If the nurse is unsure of the symbol or abbreviation, the term should be written in full to prevent confusion. Some medical terminology can be confusing. For example, P.N.D. can mean paroxysmal nocturnal dyspnea or postnasal drip. Be sure you and your staff are clear on the use of abbreviations and symbols.

By keeping these 10 guidelines (Kozier, Erb, 1987) in mind and using the checklist, you will be able to quickly and accurately review clients' health care records.

Other written communications

Nurse managers have numerous duties that involve written communications. Memos, client summaries, and notes to health care providers or staff all require effective writing skills, but even the most talented writer must remember that words are only symbols. There is no meaning attached to them until someone reads them. **It is the *value* given to words that influences the communication.** To prove this to yourself, look at each of these words and identify the feeling you associate with each word:

important	imperative	at your convenience
urgent	depressed	uncooperative
incompetent	excitable	boring

Words have emotional impact. Be careful with their use.

Guidelines for written communication. Wlody (1981) lists six criteria for every communication (see box on p. 51). These are especially helpful when sending written messages. Practice with these guidelines will yield clear, accurate written messages for both you and your staff.

> ### ✎ GUIDELINES FOR WRITTEN COMMUNICATION
> 1. Have a clear idea of what is to be communicated.
> 2. Know the essential facts. The receiver needs them to help form a conclusion or take action.
> 3. Consider the receiver. Think about the reader's attitude, feelings, and educational level.
> 4. Decide on the medium. Telephone, personal interaction, and written message all have a different impact on the receiver. Be guided by the type of message you want to send. For example, you certainly would not review an employee's job performance over the telephone.
> 5. Write clearly (legibly). If your writing cannot be easily read, print.
> 6. Use clear language. Choose words carefully. Be clear and organized. If unsure of a meaning, do not use the word.

Professional verbal communications

Health care givers constantly interact with clients, families, and other professionals. Verbal messages are the basis for most of these communications. You as the first-line supervisor (manager) can do much to encourage clear, accurate communications by keeping the guidelines in mind. Two often overlooked areas of professional communications are the change-of-shift report and the use of the telephone.

Change-of-shift report. The change-of-shift report (shift report for short) is defined as an exchange of client information between nurses completing the shift and the staff coming on duty. The shift report may be given orally in a meeting of staff from both shifts, by audiotape, or during 'walking rounds' where the caregivers from both shifts visit each assigned client. Whatever method is employed, a well-prepared and well-presented report provides vital client data in a short time.

Guides for client reports. Kozier and Erb (1987) list several guidelines for client reports (see box on p. 52). Practice using these techniques when exchanging client information. You will find them valuable in providing much data in a short time.

Telephone communications. A very important, but often neglected, area of professional communications is use of the telephone. First impressions

GUIDELINES FOR CLIENT REPORTS

1. **Follow a specific order.** If the report includes clients in rooms 1A to 8A, begin with room 1A.
2. **Provide identifying client data.** Include the client's name, room, and bed number. Knowing the client's age and sex is also helpful.
3. **Note medical diagnosis (diagnoses).** This is a must for acute care settings. In long-term care settings, medical diagnoses remain important, for they provide information on which body systems are impaired and allow the nurse to focus on providing safe, individualized care.
4. **Report any diagnostic tests and their results,** any therapies, the administration of any nonroutine drugs, or any out-of-the-ordinary events.
5. **Identify any changes in the client's condition.**
6. **Present assessment data** (s/s, v/s, complaints, etc.), nursing diagnosis or problem, plans to help, how the nurse intervened (or what was done), and how the client responded (evaluation). Work on applying the nursing process when giving the report. It is an excellent organizational tool that allows nurses to share in the process of planning client cares.
7. **Provide objective information.** Give times, dose amounts, test results, vital signs, and the like. For example, "Mrs. Bea Brown was medicated for pain" is incomplete. A more complete statement would be, "Mrs. Bea Brown was medicated for left leg pain at 0910. She received 50 mg of Demerol in the right hip. At 1000, she stated her pain was much better." This report includes specific data and saves other staff members time.
8. **Do not include data that are unremarkable** (within normal range) unless they indicate a change in condition. Always compare new information with previous data to determine any changes.
9. **Report any emotional responses or behaviors that may need attention.** This assists other staff in providing support for the client.

From Kozier B, Erb G: *Fundamentals of nursing: concepts and procedures,* ed 3, Menlo Park, NJ, 1987, Addison-Wesley.

count. A person calling your unit forms an opinion about the facility in the first 4 to 6 seconds. Telephone manners communicate much about the concern and professionalism of the entire organization. As Stephanie Barlow (1990), a writer for *Entrepreneur,* states, "Whether your business is large or small, good phone etiquette is essential." Many businesses are currently making telephone training a part of employees' orientation. As

GUIDELINES FOR TELEPHONE ETIQUETTE

1. **Answer the phone with your unit (or facility's) name.** Then identify yourself and state your title. For example, "ABC Nursing Center. This is Mary Nurse, RN. How may I assist you?" gives a much stronger impression than "Hello."

2. **Project a positive attitude.** Do not share any negative emotions over the phone (even if you are in a bad mood). Take a deep breath. Become calm and composed before you answer the phone.

3. **Allow the caller to tell his/her story.** Try to understand his/her point of view. Use remarks such as "I see" or "uh-huh" to draw out the details of the story. Ask yourself, "What does the caller want?" If unsure, ask about and clarify the purpose of the call.

4. **Listen.** Use the techniques for effective listening. Look for ways to solve problems (if one exists). Ask questions to clarify any misunderstandings.

5. **Speak with respect.** Use your phone manners to show the caller respect and courtesy. Make the caller feel important.

6. **Speak the caller's language.** Translate any medical or nursing words or expressions into language the caller is able to understand.

7. **Be prepared.** Be sure the information that is given via telephone is accurate. Know the latest facts. If you do not have the needed information, be honest with yourself (do not fake it). Refer the caller to someone who can supply the information.

8. **Return all phone calls,** even the ones you would rather not return.

9. **End each call with courtesy and tact.** "Thank you for calling" reinforces the caller's importance.

10. **Teach your staff to take complete messages.** Each message should include time of call, the name, organization, department, phone number, and any other information the caller may care to leave. Initialing the message helps identify who recorded it.

Barlow S: Dial "M" for manners: good calls, *Entrepreneur* 18(4):175, 1990.

a nurse manager, your knowledge and use of proper telephone techniques will encourage others to practice positive telephone communications.

Telephone etiquette. Most of us were not taught to use the telephone correctly. Fortunately, we are capable of learning new, more effective techniques (see box above).

Complaints and angry callers. Handling angry callers and complaints requires extra sensitivity. Encourage the caller to talk about the problem. Do not interrupt. Try to define the problem or complaint. Take notes, writing the important details, and make sure that you both clearly agree on them. Apologize for any difficulties he/she may have experienced. Tell the caller what you will do with the complaint, to whom you will refer it, and when a response can be expected. End the conversation with a "Thank you," then be sure to follow through by communicating with the appropriate person. People remember how their complaints/problems are handled. **Turning anger and frustration into cooperation is a highly valuable management technique.**

Killer phrases. Certain phone behaviors and phrases cause callers to immediately cool their opinions of your organization. Ensure that your staff members do not answer the phone with 'mouth noises' (i.e., smacking, chewing, swallowing), put the caller on hold abruptly, keep the caller on hold for longer than 20 seconds, or speak impolitely.

According to Nancy Friedman, owner of The Telephone Doctor (a management firm specializing in telephone skills), there are five forbidden phrases that no caller should ever hear when telephoning your company (Barlow, 1990):

1. **"I don't know"** destroys confidence. It is usually your business to know. If the information is not readily available, refer the caller to the appropriate person or let him/her know you will find the data and return the call.
2. **"You will have to. . . ."** The caller does not *have* to do anything. Soften the message with "The best thing to do . . ." or "I recommend. . . ."
3. **"We can't do that."** Try to focus on what *can* be done instead. Explore other options.
4. **"Hang on; I'll be right back."** No one is ever put on hold for a second. If asking the caller to hold, tell the truth about how long they may have to wait. "I may be 5 minutes finding that information. Can you hold for that long or would you prefer that I call you back?" allows the caller to make the choice.
5. **"No" at the start of a sentence.** It is difficult to work your way out of a negative position once it has been established. Before saying no, think how you can phrase the statement positively.

Good telephone skills are an art. Patience and practice reward the staff members as well as administrators by projecting a high level of competency and caring to all callers.

Communication with physicians. Good communications with physicians is vital to the clients' welfare. We have (or will have) all suffered through a vague, uncomfortable phone conversation with a doctor. Several nurse telephone techniques are offered by Terry Murphy, RN (1990), in her article, "Improving Nurse/Doctor Communications." To promote more effective telephone communications with physicians:

- Identify yourself immediately. The MD has a right to know who you are and which facility you are representing. If you are calling with patient information, identify the patient by name and room number.
- Do not apologize for calling. You have a good reason.
- Give your message briefly but completely. Have all the needed data available *before* you place the call.
- Ask for specific orders if needed. Tell the physician what you need and why you think it is necessary. If you feel the client needs to be seen, say so. Write all orders verbatim and *repeat each order* for clarity.
- If the doctor is coming to the facility, ask when he/she can be expected. This may help reassure the client/family and allow you to prepare for the visit.
- If you get cut off, call back immediately. Remember to stay polite and calm.
- Document all attempts to contact a doctor. Note the date, time, and method (i.e., phone, visit, message via another person).
- If, after several attempts, you are unable to reach a doctor, contact your supervisor.

The goal of all professional communications is to send and receive accurate information. It is essential, and even vital, to communicate professionally when planning and implementing quality health care for each client.

Summary

Good communication skills are one of the most important assets for the effective manager. Many factors affect the communication process. To send and receive accurate verbal messages, the nurse manager ensures that each message is clear and brief, using appropriate vocabulary, tone, pacing, and timing. Nonverbal communications are a combination of personal appearance, body language, distance, attending behaviors, and touch. Communications also involve rapport or being 'in tune' with another. By practicing the discussed strategies, the manager is able to create rapport with staff members. Seven guidelines for improving poor listening habits are offered. Accurate, concise, descriptive, written professional communications are vitally important for the nurse manager. The client's health care record documents all data relating to the client's diagnosis (diagnoses), care, and responses. By using the discussed suggestions, the nurse manager is able to assess health care records for accuracy and completeness. All written professional communications should state the idea clearly, include facts and understandable language, be written legibly, and consider the receiver.

Effective, professional verbal communications for nurses include clear reports about client conditions, good telephone etiquette, and techniques for improving communications between nurses and physicians.

Key Concepts

- Communication is a constantly occurring process in which an exchange of information takes place on several levels.
- Ten factors that affect communication within the work setting relate to the message: the developmental levels, individual backgrounds, past experiences, roles and relationships, and emotions of the communicators; the grapevine; space and territory; and environmental factors.
- The grapevine is an informal communication system that exists in every organization. To become effective managers, nurses need to be aware of and work with the grapevine.
- The distance between persons has an impact on communication.
- The most effective verbal messages are brief, clear, paced appropriately, effectively toned, relevant, and well timed.
- Sending and receiving verbal messages require attention to and practice with specific communication skills.
- Nonverbal communications include appearance, body language, distance, territory, touch, and attending behaviors.
- Clothing communicates professionalism.
- Body language encompasses position, posture, gait, gestures, and facial expressions.
- Touch is a powerful communication tool.
- Rapport is a catalyst that transforms a series of interactions into a meaningful relationship.
- Effective listening, an important component of the communication process, is a developed skill.
- The client's health care record (the chart) serves several purposes. Nurse managers are usually responsible for assessing the staff's documentation in the chart.
- Words have an emotional impact. Nurse managers should be careful to understand the value given to certain words or phrases.
- Change-of-shift reports exchange important information among health care providers in a short period of time.
- Good telephone skills are imperative for effective management and a professional impression.
- Effective communication with physicians is vital to the client's welfare. Managers should encourage the nursing staff to practice good communication skills, especially when phoning physicians.

Learning Activities

1. Write each of the following words on a separate piece of paper: happiness, sadness, surprise, anger, disgust, fear. Fold each piece of paper. Have six people each choose a folded paper and then act out or portray

the emotion using facial expressions only. The objective is to accurately 'read' the nonverbal expression.
2. Role play two people discussing Mrs. Wright's latest treatment, first with poor listening habits, then using the seven active listening techniques.
3. Pick a partner. Converse with him/her at the intimate, personal, social, and public distance. Discuss your reactions.
4. Write a memo to your staff that would encourage them to attend the monthly staff meeting, Tuesday, June 15, 2 P.M. in the classroom.
5. Role play calling a physician at 2 A.M. to report a significant change in a client's condition.

References

Bandler R, Grinder J: *Frogs into princes: neurolinguistic programming*, Moab, Utah, 1979, Real People Press.

Barlow S: Dial "M" for manners: good calls, *Entrepreneur* 18(4):175, 1990.

Christensen B, Kockrow E: *Foundations of nursing*, St Louis, 1991, Mosby.

Douglas LM: *The effective nurse leader and manager*, St Louis, 1991, Mosby.

Gilmore SK, Fraleigh PW: *Communication at work*, Eugene, Ore, 1980, Friendly Press.

Hein EC: *Communication in nursing practice*, Boston, 1973, Little, Brown.

Kalish B, Kalish P: Dressing for success, *American Journal of Nursing* 85(8):887, 1985.

Kozier B, Erb G: *Fundamentals of nursing: concepts and procedures*, ed 3, Menlo Park, NJ, 1987, Addison-Wesley.

Mehrabian A: *Silent messages*, New York, 1971, Wadsworth.

Murphy TG: Improving nurse/doctor communications, *Nursing 90* 20(8):114, 1990.

Potter P, Perry A: *Fundamentals of nursing: concepts, process and practice*, ed 3, St Louis, 1989, Mosby.

Raudsepp E: Seven ways to cure communication breakdowns, *Nursing 90* 20(4): 132, 1990.

Travelbee J: What do we mean by rapport?, *American Journal of Nursing* 63(2): 70, 1963.

Wlody G: Effective communications techniques, *Nursing Management* 12(10):19, 1981.

Additional Readings

Burnside IM: Touching is talking, *American Journal of Nursing* 73(12):2060, 1973. *In this classic early article on therapeutic touch, Ms. Burnside describes her results with touch for elderly, regressed clients.*

Castillo HM: *The nurse assistant in long-term care: a rehabilitative approach*, St Louis, 1992, Mosby. *Chapter 3, "Communications, Care Plans, and Charting," provides a review of the basic communication techniques taught to nursing assistants.*

Grau L: What older adults expect from the nurse, *Geriatric Nursing* Jan/Feb:14, 1984. *This article is the result of the data analyzed from 496 essays written by authors over age 70. Expectations, grouped into four categories, provide some eye-opening insights into the reality of being cared for by nurses.*

Greenlaw J: Documentation of patient care: an often underestimated responsibility, *Law, Medicine and Health Care* (9):172, 1982. *A nurse/lawyer reminds us of the importance of following accepted principles of documentation.*

Iyer PW, Camp NH: *Nursing documentation: a nursing process approach*, St Louis, 1991, Mosby. *The authors provide an excellent text focused on current information about the documentation of client care in the 1990s.*

Kelly LS: Looking good: the pendulum swings, *Nursing Outlook* 33(3):114, 1985. *If nurses want to improve their image, they need to look at how they dress and appear to patients.*

Krieger D: Therapeutic touch: the imprimatur of nursing, *American Journal of Nursing* 75(5):784, 1975. *"Research by the author showed that the laying-on of hands with the intent to heal raised hemoglobin levels in ill persons."*

Marrelli TM: *Nursing documentation handbook*, St Louis, 1992, Mosby. *The goal of this book is to "facilitate succinct documentation that assists the nurse in thoroughly documenting the care given to patients while minimizing the time required for that documentation."*

Phippen ML: Winning through communication, *AORN Journal* 34(6):1043, 1981. *Mr. Phippen discusses the importance of intraorganizational communications and the need for nurses to speak and be heard within the organization.*

Reeves DM, Underly NK, Goddard NL: How to improve your image, *Nursing Life* 31 (May/June):57, 1983. *The authors list three tips for working with unfair stereotypes of nursing.*

Schacht R, Anastasi J: How to break down communication barriers between you and your co-workers, *Nursing Life* 30 (Sept/Oct):17, 1982. *This article, written by managers, offers numerous suggestions for coping with six different barriers to communication.*

Smith S: *Communications in nursing (caring)*, ed 2, St Louis, 1992, Mosby. *The author explores the communication process from a humanistic point of view. Several excellent suggestions for developing both personal and professional skills are offered.*

Tobiason SJ: Touching is for everyone, *American Journal of Nursing* 81(4):728, 1981. *Results of an investigation into the attitudes and feelings of nursing students regarding touching newborn and aged clients yields strong data supporting the use of touch as a planned therapeutic nursing intervention.*

Worthington J: The art of effective communication, *Nursing Management* 13(11): 47, 1982. *Using the Peter Principle to describe motivational differences in managers, the author presents the view that effective managers use communication techniques which encourage self-discovery in others.*

GROUP

3

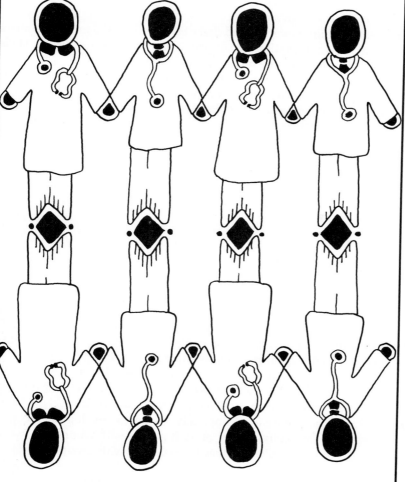

DYNAMICS

Upon completion of this chapter, the reader will be able to:

1. Define the word *group* and list three of its characteristics.
2. Compare the functions of primary and secondary groups.
3. List three levels of group formality.
4. Identify five purposes of groups.
5. Discuss the three stages of group development and describe the characteristics of each stage.
6. Define *group dynamics* and describe three roles of group members.
7. Identify five suggestions for developing strong group leadership skills.
8. Discuss three roles members assume in groups.
9. State six criteria for productive conflict and describe three tasks of the group leader for resolving conflict.
10. List six common group problems.
11. Discuss the influences of hidden agendas on group dynamics.
12. Explain at least three techniques a leader may use to influence nonproductive behaviors of group members.
13. Identify seven criteria for assessing group effectiveness.
14. List 12 suggestions for proficient group communications.

Groups and Management

Managers function by getting work done through the efforts of others. This involves not only excellent communication skills but also an intimate knowledge of group behavior. **To be a nurse is to work with groups.** To be a nurse manager is to direct and guide the work group toward meeting its goal of providing caring, quality nursing.

One of the joys of long-term care nursing is the relative stability of the groups. Clients remain at the facility for longer periods, and staff turnover is usually less than in acute care facilities. Staff members and supervisors get to know each other and, hopefully, begin to develop appreciation and respect for the individuality of each person with whom they work. Knowledge of effective techniques for working with groups allows the nurse manager to meet organizational goals as well as promote harmony, respect, and feelings of worth among the staff members. How well the group works together often determines the 'personality' of the unit (or groups), and it is the manager who 'sets the tone,' or creates the environment, for the group.

Types of Groups

A group, as defined by Kozier and Erb (1987), is "two or more persons who have shared needs or goals, take each other into account in their actions, and are thus held together and set apart from others by virtue of their interactions." Health care workers, for example, have the shared needs of all workers: the need to contribute, feel respected, and receive adequate compensation (e.g., salary, good relationships, recognition, etc.). Our main goal is to provide high-quality, individualized care to meet our clients' needs. Health care workers who provide direct client care are set apart from others in their interactions (we even use a different language at times). Who has not thought, "If I do not get this done now, someone on the next shift will have to do it"? Because nurses work so closely with clients and staff, we usually consider the impact of our actions on others and interact frequently with various groups of people.

Primary groups

Most people belong to two types of groups. The first group with whom one associates is the family, the first primary group. Primary groups are small, intimate, and supportive. They not only set and enforce standards of behavior but also nurture and support each member. They assist in working with stresses that would be too much for one person, and they have a strong sense of unity, or 'oneness.' Successes and failures of one member are shared by all members of the group. The group has value unto itself; it needs no goals. It exists to provide limits on behaviors and support for its members. In addition to the family, examples of primary groups are friendship groups, children's play groups, and some informal work groups.

Secondary groups

Secondary groups are larger, less personal, and more task-oriented than primary groups. The goal of these groups is to get something done, to accomplish a task, or to meet a goal. Members may or may not know each other. Thus, these groups usually provide little support for individual members. Once the goals or tasks have been achieved, the group usually dissolves. Examples of secondary groups are committees, task groups, professional associations, and business groups. Supervisors frequently work within secondary groups.

Groups can also be classified by their levels of formality. The three levels of formality are formal groups, semiformal groups, and informal groups (Kozier, Erb, 1987).

Formal groups. Formal groups, such as the work organization, exist primarily to meet goals or carry out tasks. Traditionally, the leadership is formal with a well-defined chain-of-command. Decisions are made at the top, and managers remain aloof from the workers. Many rules and regulations enforce the standards of behavior expected from the employees.

Semiformal groups. Semiformal groups help to satisfy the social needs of many people. They are similar to formal groups in that their structure is formal and the chain-of-command is established. The goals are usually less rigid, however. They differ because membership in the group is usually voluntary, but it may be difficult to achieve (e.g., country club, social club). Group members often enjoy status and prestige. Examples of semiformal groups include lodges, societies, churches, social clubs, and sports clubs.

Informal groups. Informal groups help provide educational, social, and cultural values. We are all members of several informal groups. These groups have no set of written rules and regulations, but a strong code of ethics and unwritten laws do exist. Basic group objectives can be recognized, the leadership role may rotate, and duties are assigned to the best qualified member. Interactions are comfortable and spontaneous. Conformity is important to help protect and preserve the group. Rules are enforced by sanctions — punishment by the group (e.g., removal of group privileges). There are many kinds of informal groups (see box on p. 65).

To work effectively with groups, **the nurse manager must be aware of each group's**

- **Goals.** What is the purpose for the group?
- **Communication patterns.** How do members interact?
- **Ability to get things done.** Are the goals being met?

This knowledge, combined with your communication skills, will assist in making every group of which you are a member a productive one.

Purposes of Groups

Man is a social being. We *want* to be around each other. As a consequence, groups are formed. Groups may be joined on a voluntary basis (e.g., your choice to become a health care worker) or on an involuntary basis (e.g., attendance at this meeting is mandatory). Whatever the group, it serves one of several purposes: achieves goals, provides power, acts as

---

✐ TYPES OF INFORMAL GROUPS

1. *Hobby groups.* The goal is to share and enjoy a hobby. Individual personalities and backgrounds are less important than the enjoyment from the hobby (e.g., model airplane club, needlework club, bowling or tennis league).
2. *Convenience groups.* These groups meet to fill a need. Groups that carpool to work or travel to workshops together are examples.
3. *Friendship groups.* Common interests provide the motivation for this type of group. They are first formed early and continue throughout life. Many friendship groups are derived from the work organization, semiformal, or formal groups.
4. *Self-protective groups.* This type of group is formed to cope with a threat. It is commonly found in the workplace, especially if workers feel the need to present a united front. When the threat subsides, the group dissolves. Examples of self-protective groups include staff members walking to their cars in a group after leaving the facility, self-defense programs, and managers encountering united resistance from their staff.

Adapted from Kozier B, Erb G: *Fundamentals of nursing: concepts and procedures,* ed 3, Menlo Park, NJ, 1987, Addison-Wesley.

---

an information center, provides support, or solves problems (Kozier, Erb, 1987).

Achieve goals

Groups meet to achieve one or more common goals. This can be as simple as deciding to walk every day after work with a friend or as complex as redesigning a health care delivery system.

Provide power

Groups supply the power to achieve goals that are not attainable by a single person's efforts. Strength and power are increased as the number of group members grows. Also, groups will often take more risks than individuals.

Act as an information center

Groups act as information senders and receivers. Data can be disseminated to groups much more quickly than to individuals. Information gathered by the efforts of individual members is shared with the group, thus preventing wasted time and effort.

Provide support

Groups provide support and a sense of belonging for members. Some groups, such as Al-Anon and other support groups, exist primarily to provide encouragement and emotional support for their members.

Solve problems

By pooling their ideas and knowledge, group members can often solve problems more effectively (and creatively) than a single person. Also, groups are more willing to tackle more complex problems because the success or failure reflects on the group, not the individual.

Each group can have more than one purpose, and each person in the group may play one or more roles — member, leader, learner, teacher, etc. Understanding the purpose of each group is important. If you do not know where you are going, how will you know when you get there?

Group Development

One characteristic of groups is that **they are dynamic.** They are changing. Groups routinely form, work together, and terminate. Nurse managers need to know where the group is in its development in order to promote effectiveness.

Phases of growth

Beginning phase. During the beginning stage, members meet and become familiar with each other. Roles are established, and a method of operation is chosen. Tasks are the central focus at this stage. Behaviors are tested as people seek a place within the group in relation to others. Members gradually begin to exchange viewpoints, values, and attitudes. The group may appear harmonious, but it is superficial.

✐ GROUP PROPERTIES

- Tone — a pleasant or unpleasant atmosphere
- Degree of likeness (or differences) among members
- Degree of unity (cohesiveness) among members
- Norms and sanctions — expected standards of behavior (norms) and measures used to enforce the standards (sanctions) are established
- Conformity — actions of individual members are revised to fit the group's behaviors.

Working phase. The working stage begins when members feel comfortable with each other. Group properties (characteristics) will be determined during this stage (see box on p. 66). During the working stage, members move toward a common goal, and individual behaviors become less obvious. Attitudes and beliefs blend. The group is unified and works to achieve its tasks and meet its goals.

Ending phase. When group members no longer sense a need for the group, the ending phase has begun. The group's goals may or may not have been met. Members may feel a sense of relief that it is over or may feel frustration because of the loss of group support.

Effective groups

Groups that are highly functional have certain characteristics (traits) in common. To promote a group's effectiveness, the nurse manager periodically assesses the group for these traits (see box below).

Group Dynamics

The term *group dynamics* was coined because of a need to look at the social forces operating within a group. As you read earlier, communica-

---

 GROUP CHARACTERISTICS

1. Goals and tasks are clear, understood, and accepted by the group.
2. Group members share ideas, accept and discuss disagreements, and provide feedback that is constructive.
3. Solutions are based on group input.
4. Decisions are made with group consensus.
5. Assignments are specific, understood, and accepted by each member.
6. Leadership focuses on moving the group toward the goals.
7. It has the ability to evaluate its own effectiveness.
8. There is a degree of support for and loyalty to the group.

From Kozier B, Erb G: *Fundamentals of nursing: concepts and procedures,* ed 3, Menlo Park, NJ, 1987, Addison-Wesley.

tions involve a complex interaction of many factors. Each individual brings to the group a unique psyche or personality, an array of verbal and nonverbal habits along with varying abilities and motivations for communicating, interacting, problem solving, achieving tasks, working harmoniously, and the like. The communication and behavioral patterns established by the group members is referred to as the group's dynamics. Each group has its own dynamics because each group is composed of unique individuals.

Meetings

In the work setting, two basic types of group interactions are used: *meetings* for solving problems, discussing ideas, or planning; and *teams* for working on tasks together. Meetings are of two types: committee meetings and staff meetings.

Committee meetings. Committee meetings are those in which each member's role and function is structured. The authority of the group is delegated to solve one or more problems. Standing committees, such as a nursing quality assurance committee, meet routinely to monitor and solve problems such as those associated with the delivery of nursing cares. Ad hoc committees meet for a specific purpose, and once the goals have been accomplished, they are discontinued.

Staff meetings. Work teams frequently have staff meetings for informational, educational, and problem-solving purposes. Usually, workers from all shifts attend. They are less formal than committee meetings and serve to fill some social needs. Both types of meetings, however, provide the same function: to solve problems, discuss ideas, or plan to meet goals. **Nurse managers who function effectively in meetings are powerful change agents.**

Good meeting management

As the chairperson of a committee or meeting leader, you are responsible for moving the group forward, toward meeting its goals. Follow these hints to help yourself develop the vitally important skills of effective meeting management:

Atmosphere. Provide the best environment possible. The meeting room should be large enough for the group to sit or work comfortably but not so large that it overwhelms a small-sized group. Lighting should be bright. Room temperature is most comfortable between 68° and 74° F. Make the atmosphere psychologically comfortable by making a comment to each member of the meeting and providing introductions when necessary. Encourage an atmosphere that encourages group work.

Introductions. Identify the purpose(s) for the meeting. Remember to begin and end the meeting on time. People who must sit and wait for a meeting to begin are less likely to be cooperative during the meeting. Also, keeping within established time limits behaviorally (nonverbally) demonstrates respect for others by recognizing that their time is also important.

Agenda. This aspect focuses on the actual process of the meeting. Be prepared in advance to define each agenda item, its importance, time allocated for discussion of each item, the method of presenting the information, resource materials, and the person responsible for each item.

When introducing each agenda item, clarify the objectives. Be as specific and concrete as possible. For example, compare each of these statements:

1. "We seem to have a problem with staff clocking in for work late."
2. "For the past 6 months, 90 percent of the staff on the day shift has arrived for work on an average of 10 minutes late."

Which statement is more specific and concrete? The more specific the agenda item, the easier it becomes to focus group attention and energy.

As the meeting moves through each item, keep the discussion focused on the goal. Clarify any areas that are unclear. After discussion, summarize the main points and clarify what outcome is expected. If the agenda item is for information purposes only, communicate this. If a decision is required, specify the type of decision-making method used (i.e., majority rule, unanimous consent, etc.), state the final decision, and obtain specific commitments to action (if needed) before moving to the next agenda item. Follow this process for each item. Also, remember that the first and last 10 minutes of any meeting are the most important. By spelling out the meeting's objectives clearly and eliciting commitments from the members before adjournment, every meeting can be more productive.

Monitor progress. Follow up. Do not neglect it. It is a pivotal area of focus during and after the meeting. Without follow-up, all objectives and commitments are useless because there is no thread to weave them into action.

During the meeting, note the follow-up action required for each agenda item. Each item should include:

1. *WHAT* the plan of action is,
2. *WHO* is responsible for the plan, and
3. *WHEN* the action is to be completed.

This allows each person at the meeting knowledge of the important points and focus of each item. It also facilitates communications by providing clear, specific information to everyone involved.

After the meeting, *coordinate* the efforts of the people responsible for each agenda item. Assist them to meet the goals, if necessary, and be sure to recognize their extra efforts. Then begin the cycle once again and prepare for the next meeting. By developing good meeting management skills, the nurse manager can make meetings enjoyable and highly productive.

As a member of a committee or meeting, you are still responsible for arriving prepared, participating in the discussion, and contributing to the goal. As a manager, even though you may not be taking an active leadership role, you are being watched. Your staff subconsciously observes your behavior in various situations and then adapts according to the tone or atmosphere you create. By taking an active member role in meetings, you are quietly encouraging others to follow your example.

Group roles

In meetings, work teams, and other group interactions, members take certain roles. The interactions of the members assuming these roles make up the *dynamics* of each group. According to Sullivan (1990), members of a group usually assume one or more of the following roles:

Task roles. These involve the job to be done and the means to accomplish it. The task role provides the structure and focus for meeting the goal. Group members who assume task roles keep the interactions focused on the business at hand.

Maintenance roles. Members assuming these roles are concerned with how the group is functioning. They tend to focus on individual attitudes and behaviors of group members. They want group members to get along.

Self-serving roles. Members who take on these roles are usually motivated by personal needs that have nothing to do with the group or its goals. An example of this is the group member who would rather discuss his/her personal problems than focus on the task at hand. An awareness of the roles group members assume will assist the nurse manager to promote effective group interaction and function.

Group leadership skills

Because nurse managers participate in a wide variety of groups, it is important to develop effective skills as both a leader and a follower. Although we will explore leadership skills more thoroughly in a later chapter, here are a few suggestions for developing strong *group* leadership skills:

Set workable goals. Both individual and group behaviors are goal directed. If each group member feels the goal is worthwhile, participation will be high.

Provide adequate resources. Nothing is worse for a group than to establish a goal and then discover that few or no resources are available. Effective group leaders consider the tools, money, time, and other resources necessary *before* setting goals. Members need support in terms of materials or supplies and in terms of psychological support as well. Leaders that provide support for members improve group effectiveness.

Clarify. Clarify goals, roles, and tasks with each group member. This is a simple but important step. By taking the time to communicate and clear any misconceptions in the beginning, you are saving much (possibly wasted) time and effort in the future. Also, when each group member is aware of the others' tasks and roles, a higher degree of cooperation is encouraged.

Monitor progress. Follow up, follow up, follow up. Monitor the group's progress toward the goal. Be generous with praise and stingy with criticism. Troubleshoot any possible problems. Assist each member, if needed, to meet the goal.

Offer recognition. Offer praise, respect, and recognition for a job well done as well as encouragement when needed.

Group followership skills

A good follower is just as important as a good leader. Nurse managers are leaders of the staff and followers of the administration and, therefore, have ample opportunities to practice skills in both areas.

Brakely (1991) asserts that good followers have many traits in common with effective leaders. She lists the traits of an effective follower as:

Respect. You do not have to always agree with your leader. In fact, to do so would be boring, but disagree with your leader in a respectful manner. Point out the facts as you see them. Avoid the personal arena. Avoid being defensive.

Loyalty. Be loyal to the facility, organization, and profession. 'Bad mouthing' or complaining, both on and off duty, fosters nothing but negative feelings. No one works for the perfect organization. Focus your energies toward improvement, and loyalty will be fostered.

Self-management. Capable followers can work with little supervision. They understand the goal and can direct their time and energies productively in order to attain it.

Honesty. Admitting a mistake is taking a risk, but effective followers are willing to admit when they are wrong and take steps to correct the situation or prevent a recurrence.

Enthusiasm. People who like what they do are positive and upbeat. Problems become challenges and opportunities for improvement. They approach difficulties with a 'can do' attitude. This rubs off on other members, and the group becomes more productive and successful. An enthusiastic follower is a priceless addition to any group.

Appreciation. Remember the saying, "It's lonely at the top." Leaders, managers, and administrators seldom hear from their staff when things are going well, but they are the first to know when something is not as it should be. Remember to thank your leader when the goal has been met or when everything is going smoothly. We all need and appreciate recognition.

Common Problems

Each group is comprised of unique individuals, all interacting with others from a unique point of view. Each member brings to the group a distinct set of abilities, attitudes, and behaviors. As a result of all these individuals, each interacting from a different perspective, problems are bound to arise. Kozier and Erb (1987) list conflict, ineffective decision making, apathy, and nonproductive interactional behaviors as the most common group problems. Let us look at some techniques for coping capably with these events.

Conflict

Disagreement and controversy are normal and valued components of group interactions. Whenever two or more people repeatedly interact, conflict will arise. During the working phase of group development, disagreement and arguments are inevitable. These are valuable components of group interactions when the leader keeps the focus on positive, productive results. Conflict can be productive by assisting group problem solving or nonproductive by altering the group's focus.

Productive conflict. According to Sampson and Marthas (1977) a group's conflict is considered productive when:

- Members are working toward a common goal. Each member clearly understands the goal and willingly devotes energy to meeting it.
- Comments made by group members relate to the task.
- All group members are encouraged to participate even though they may disagree or hold different opinions.
- All group members listen to each other and consider everyone's point of view.
- The reasons or bases for the conflict are openly and critically evaluated.
- Problems are solved. Decisions, action plans, or solutions are reached through rational decision making, compromise, and agreement (p. 160).

Techniques to manage conflict are discussed in Chapter 6.

Ineffective decision making

This is a common group problem that usually stems from a perceived threat relating to the decision or a decision that is too difficult for the group to make. If the objectives are unclear or the group fears the consequences of the decision, they will attempt to leave the decision making to others, refuse responsibilities, and wander away from the topic during discussions. The **conflict must be uncovered and addressed** if the group is to be productive. Apply the skills for keeping conflict productive. Support group members to share their anxieties and perspectives, then clarify the problem, objectives, tasks, and available resources. With all data available to the group, discuss possible options and negotiate each issue. If the group is still unable or unwilling to reach an adequate decision, outside assistance may be necessary, or the group may discontinue or alter its dynamics by changing members.

Apathy

Nonparticipation in group activities can vary from boredom and lack of interest to complete indifference and the inability to accomplish even simple tasks. Apathy can be traced to several sources.

Causes of group apathy. Bradford, Stock, and Horowitz (1974) identify four common causes for group apathy. They are as follows:

1. **The task (goal) is not important to the group.** Someone attaches importance to the task, but it is not the group members. To cope with this, acknowledge the general atmosphere of boredom or indifference and then ask each group member to explain why the task seems unimportant or irrelevant. Then ask what things the group would prefer to do.
2. **Conflict.** If individuals within the group are mainly concerned with

achieving status or fulfilling their own interests first, others will become 'turned off' and withdraw. If conflict is continual and members refuse to compromise, it becomes unproductive and leads to frustration and apathy.

3. **The group is unable to problem-solve in order to reach a decision.** Resources may be sparse or unavailable. No one is able or willing to apply the process for solving problems or consider the consequences of possible decisions. This group needs help if it is to function. The nurse leader can review or teach the problem-solving process, acknowledge any feelings of inadequacy or anxiety, and gently begin to focus the group on the work to be done. Divide the goal, task, or project into smaller parts. For each part, decide which issues are important and devise possible methods or solutions. This will assist the group with solving problems by presenting the data in manageable units.

4. **Powerlessness.** When group members feel their time is wasted because a higher authority will not listen or consider their decision as worthwhile, they become powerless. If the group's decision is considered reasonable and justifiable, the leader has the duty to follow the decision through the appropriate administrative channels and report back to the group regarding its progress, disposition, or action taken. The group needs to know that their decisions are worthwhile and deserve consideration. Once a group has experienced success, it invests itself with power to tackle the next objective.

Hidden agendas

Because individual needs, ideas, and behaviors play a part in group interactions, two kinds of goals influence a meeting's process. The stated or official goal, objective, or reason for the meeting is referred to as the official, or public, agenda (Tappen, 1989). Goals arising from individual or group needs, preconceived ideas, special interests, or conflicting loyalties influence the group process and are referred to as the hidden agenda. "Although their existence is not recognized, they can be strongly felt by group members and greatly influence the outcome of the group process" (Tappen, 1989). Hidden agendas can slow or prevent the group's progress if they go unrecognized by the leader.

Coping with hidden agendas. To assist the group in discovering and working with conflicts that may exist between the public and hidden agendas, try the following:

1. **Recognize that a hidden agenda exists.** This involves the assessment of the leader's motivations and then the group's behaviors. Some hidden agendas are easy to define, while others are more subtle and

become evident only after many frustrations and failures. Identify the goals of the hidden agenda.

2. **Determine if the official agenda is genuinely accepted** by the group members. Does the group feel that the goals are important and relevant?

3. **Compare the goals of both agendas.** Are they agreeable and compatible? How do they conflict?

4. **Decide on a course of action.** If the hidden agenda is an attempt by the group to meet needs that were not included in the official agenda, or if the group is using the hidden agenda to defend itself from actual or perceived threats, find a direct way to meet those needs. Consider the following example:

A meeting of staff representing each work shift was called in order to develop a plan to put into effect the new peer review process. Members of the group have misconceptions and negative attitudes about peer review. Some members believe (and have stated), "One poor peer review and you are out." As a result, the group feels anxious and threatened. The hidden agenda here is to protect group members from losing their jobs. This is in direct opposition to the official goal of implementing the peer review program. This group will make very little progress, if any, until these needs and feelings are addressed. The nurse leader acts to meet these needs directly by providing members with clear, understandable data about the peer review process and following up with a group discussion focused on relieving anxieties and correcting misconceptions.

In deciding how to deal with a hidden agenda, several options exist. First, the leader can find a direct way to meet the group's covert needs. Next, open discussion provides the group with the opportunity to discuss both the official and hidden agendas. Last, the leader can use the tactic of confrontation, which must be used with great care. "The leader needs to judge how much confrontation the group is ready to handle" (Tappen, 1989). By directly attacking hidden agenda issues, the leader may bring about a defensive, hostile response. The maturity of the group and its ability to handle confrontation must be first assessed by the leader. One of the most tactful ways to use confrontation is to present information only. Do not interpret or color the data. If the group is willing to address the issues relating to the hidden agenda, then problem solving can begin. Hopefully, open discussion will help to align the goals of both the hidden and public agendas.

Groupthink

When a group works so closely together that the members overconform to the group's values, excessive cohesiveness develops. Individuals within the group begin to talk, think, and behave alike. The group becomes nonreceptive to new ideas or opinions. No one wants to 'rock the boat.' Consequently, ideas and behaviors remain within prescribed limits. The group leader should remember that the best cure for excessive group cohesiveness is prevention. From the beginning, keep the group open to new ideas, opinions, and points of view. This promotes both self and group growth, problem solving, and creativity.

Nonproductive interactions

Because individual needs sometimes become more important than group progress, members will play a role within the group that is nonfunctional. Tappen (1989) identifies seven of these roles (see box on p. 77).

Tactics for leader. The group leader can use one of several tactics to interrupt the nonproductive behavior and redirect the group's focus back to the task:

1. **Interrupt directly but positively.** Let the member know the idea may be valuable and interesting but that in order to hear from everyone, the discussion must include other points of view.
2. **Reflect the member's or the group's behavior.** Focusing on an individual is an attempt to help the member become aware of the behavior. With the 'zipper mouth' type, for example, the leader may say, "Mary, I have noticed that for the past three meetings, you have said nothing. I would like to hear your opinion on. . . ." Focusing on the group's behavior encourages the individual to become aware of how his/her behavior affects the group. To work with a 'dominator,' the leader may say, "Sandy, I have noticed that the group becomes uncomfortable when you tell us what to do. I wonder if you are aware of this?"
3. **Confront the member or the group.** A word of caution here: never confront or attack the person, only the behavior. A nonproductive interaction is only a role or set of behaviors. The individual is not the problem; the behavior is. To use individual or group confrontation, describe the negative behaviors and focus on possible solutions. Take the following situation, for example:

Angie is a bright, quick-thinking nurse. During group interactions, Angie becomes the aggressor with overly critical remarks and attacks on others' suggestions. During a meeting called to discuss new staffing schedules, the group leader, Chris, decides to confront Angie's behavior. She says, "Angie, you seem to be responding critically to most suggestions. Perhaps a more effective use for your ability to analyze things critically would be to develop a plan for your unit's staffing schedule."

NONFUNCTIONAL GROUP ROLES

1. **Aggressor.** Makes hostile, attacking remarks, criticizes others, is overly assertive.
2. **Recognition Seeker.** Does things to call attention to himself/herself; uses group as a personal audience.
3. **Monopolizer.** Talks so often or so long that others do not get a chance to speak.
4. **Dominator/Usurper.** Tries to take over leadership of the group; wants to have his/her own way and tells the group what to do.
5. **Blocker.** Obstructs progress of the group by making non-constructive contributions, being negative, and resisting beyond a reasonable point.
6. **Playboy.** Makes irrelevant and silly comments; whispers, plays around, and does not take the group task seriously.
7. **Zipper Mouth.** Does not participate even in nonverbal behavior; demonstrates no acceptance of the group (as follower does); may sulk.

From Tappan R: *Nursing leadership and management: concepts and practice,* ed 2, Philadelphia, 1989, Davis.

Although nonproductive group interactions are to be expected when working with groups, the astute nurse leader learns to quickly recognize ineffective behavioral patterns and to intervene early.

Assessment of Group Dynamics

As with other areas in nursing practice, the group leader needs to **evaluate the effectiveness of both the group and leader.** Evaluation is begun early in the group's development and continued until the group terminates. Evaluations have more impact if the group is also involved. To evaluate a group's dynamics and effectiveness, consider the following areas.

Goals

Is the group's purpose clearly stated? What are the group's goals? Are they clearly understood and accepted by each member? Are group goals integrated and compatible with individual needs and goals (hidden agendas)? Are they realistic and achievable?

Commitment

Do the group members willingly give time and energy to the group? Are contributions of members valued? Is there a sense of belonging and support for members? Are members loyal to the group? Does the group believe that its goals are important, worthwhile, and achievable?

Decision-making abilities

Kozier and Erb (1987) list eight criteria for evaluating the effectiveness of group decisions:

1. The atmosphere and energies of the group are positive.
2. Time is used to focus on the problems and solutions of the task.
3. All ideas from members are heard, discussed, and considered.
4. The group uses its talents and expertise to full advantage.
5. Problem solving is encouraged and facilitated.
6. Group members participate and feel satisfied with their contributions to the decision-making process.
7. The *group* makes the decision.
8. Members are committed to the decision, and they are willing to share responsibility for implementing or providing follow-up.

Communications

Are the members focused on the subject? Do they show respect for others' ideas? Does everyone in the group participate? Are ideas shared and discussed? Do disagreements or conflicts result in positive outcomes? Do members interact freely and comfortably?

Cohesiveness

Are members friendly, willing to interact, and supportive of each other? Are problems and activities handled by group action? Are members' actions cooperative, complementary, and focused on the goal? Are difficult problems or achievements met with persistent effort? Are communications, participation, and productivity high?

Leadership style

Who makes the majority of decisions? Is the leader's style autocratic (only the leader decides), democratic (leader facilitates and encourages decision making by the group), laisse-faire (little leadership, group makes decision), or diffused (leader varies with function and expertise)? Does the leader direct the group process toward the goals?

Power

Does the group have the power to work with the problem or formulate the goals? Does the group have the ability and willingness to decide on a change (solution, goals)? What actions is the group willing to employ in order to meet the goal or solve the problem? Power is often viewed negatively, but the effective group is aware of its power and is capable of using it wisely.

A quick, simple method for evaluating a group's effectiveness is illustrated in Figure 3-1. The checklist focuses on group goals, communications, problem solving, power, leadership, and evaluation by the members. Use it early to assess how well the group is beginning to function and to uncover any areas of potential problems. If the group is experiencing difficulties or not making progress, have each member use the checklist to evaluate the group. This process assists everyone in identifying problems and assuming responsibility for the group's growth. Last, use the checklist when the group terminates. It will provide you with future opportunities to develop and improve your skills and abilities for working with groups.

Techniques to Improve Group Productivity

Working effectively with groups takes practice and experience. Group productivity is directly related to the ability of its members to cooperatively focus their time, effort, and energies in order to meet a shared goal. Groups vary in effectiveness just as individuals do. As a member of some groups and a leader of others, a positive image as an effective and dynamic group participant encourages group resourcefulness.

Presenting positively

In order to present yourself positively in groups, practice the following techniques:

Project confidence. About 15 minutes prior to the actual group interaction, prepare yourself psychologically by visualizing yourself during the meeting. Dress professionally. Note your facial expression, eye contact, and body language (see Chapter 1). Picture yourself as another group member may see you. Then project warmth, respect, and confidence in your (and the group's) ability to get the job done. Try it; it works.

Be prepared. As a group member or leader, do your homework. Gather any data that may assist the group to meet the goal. Be ready to share your findings completely but concisely. Keep your promises and fulfill your commitments.

Appreciate others. Acknowledge the contributions of your co-members. Listen genuinely to what they say. Make eye contact and smile. Do not be hesitant to express appreciation. Two of the most powerful

Group: _____

Evaluator: _____

Date: _____

Function	Yes	No	Problem?	Comments

1. Clear Goals
   accepted by members
   written with time table				

2. Constructive Communications
   share ideas
   share disagreements
   provide feedback				

3. Solves Problems
   group consensus
   offers solutions				

4. Use of Power
   responsibilities shared
   follow up on decisions				

5. Assignments
   specific
   accepted by members				

6. Leadership
   shared
   directed to goals				

7. Evaluation
   decisions made
   own effectiveness				

# of No Responses _____

Problems: _____

Interventions: _____

Reevaluate by: _____ (date)

FIGURE 3-1 Checklist for evaluating group effectiveness.

words in the English language are "thank you." They communicate respect and value for what was done and appreciation for time, effort, and energy spent.

Respect differences. Groups are composed of individuals, each arriving with a unique set of abilities and behaviors. Differing opinions, values, and outlooks *will* occur. They are a vital part of the group's working process. It is only through the distinctive contributions of each member that solutions to problems are reached and goals are attained.

Admit mistakes. Errors are a part of the growth process. By admitting a mistake openly, you are gaining respect by accepting responsibility for your actions. Also, a climate of openness and support for risk taking within the group is encouraged.

Think positively. Think of the problem as a challenge to be met by employing the creative energies and abilities of each group member. If the goal or problem seems overwhelming, break it down into small, attainable steps. Use every available resource. If you have a criticism, make it constructively and offer suggestions for improvement. Griping, complaining, and focusing on negative aspects drag people down and waste time and energy. Directing both individual and group energies *toward* the goal is a much more productive process than working *against* the situation. Besides, it is a much more enjoyable process. Stay positive.

Make an extra effort. Pitch in and help, even if it is not your task. Observe what needs to be done and offer to do it. Do not wait to be asked. Remember that cooperation is contagious—the more you give it, the more you receive it.

Improving group communications

Now that your group 'image' is polished and positive, let us consider some approaches to proficient group communications. Potter and Perry (1989) offer several suggestions:

Listen attentively. Practice the techniques discussed in Chapter 2 to become an active, attentive listener.

Convey acceptance. Give the speaker eye contact and nonverbal cues that indicate understanding. Be sure verbal and nonverbal messages compliment and match each other. Respect the speaker's opinion, even if you disagree with the message.

Ask related questions. Questions serve to clarify or expand the information being discussed. They also "set the tone of the verbal interaction and control its direction" (Potter, Perry, 1989). Using open-ended questions will encourage the speaker to elaborate. Examples include such questions as "Would you explain . . .?", "Could you describe . . .?", or "What do you think?" Questions also assist the group in maintaining its focus and keeping the discussion on track.

Paraphrase. Restating the speaker's message in your own terms helps to clarify the communication and clear up any misunderstandings. Be careful not to change or distort the meaning of the message when returning the communication. In the group setting, paraphrasing is useful because it may help to simplify information for members who hesitate to ask questions or enter into discussions.

Seek clarification. During active group discussions, members may tend to drift away from the topic, or so much information is presented that confusion results. At these times, simplifying the message is a valuable tool for refocusing the group. Messages such as "I'm not sure I follow what you said" or "What would you say is the main point of this discussion?" assist members to understand vague, abstract, or complex communications.

Share observations. Feedback allows the speaker to learn if his/her communication was clearly sent. As communications take place on both verbal and nonverbal levels, so does feedback. If a group member says, "I'm willing to listen," and then sits with legs crossed, arms folded, and head bowed, the nonverbal feedback becomes the dominant message. When interacting with groups, making observations is an effective method for providing feedback. "You appear . . .", "I noticed that whenever we discuss . . . you seem to become tense" are examples of making observations.

Provide focus. Reminding the group of its purpose helps when the discussion begins to drag or has drifted into less related areas. Focusing helps to limit the discussions to areas directly related to the group's task or objective.

Encourage comparisons. When attempting to solve a problem or move toward a goal, the group has to weigh and evaluate the merits and disadvantages of each proposed solution. By comparing the possible outcomes of each alternative, the group is encouraged to devise realistic, workable decisions.

Use silence. A powerful communication tool, silence serves several purposes in group interactions. The use of silence allows one to organize thoughts, process information, and plan responses. More importantly, in group communication silence also conveys interest, acceptance, and a willingness to wait for a response. The effective use of silence requires skill and timing. A period of silence in order to emphasize a point is appropriate as long as group members do not become uncomfortable. A few seconds of silence followed by a deep, slow breath can diffuse a potentially emotional situation.

Be assertive. Group members who are assertive can stand up "for one's own rights without violating those of others" (Stanhope, Lancaster, 1988). By expressing emotions, observations, and opinions freely and clearly, members of the group are able to explore creative alternatives. Be careful, however, to keep the communications respectful of others.

Seek consensus. This is not to say that everyone must fully agree. Dynamic group members seldom speak as a single voice, but decisions or plans of action must be generally agreed upon and supported by all group members. The magical key to gaining consensus is to concentrate on the commonalities of each idea. Compare the similarities first. It motivates the group to move toward considering the differences.

Summarize. A review of the main points should follow each topic of discussion. Summarizing helps members to understand the key aspects of a discussion. Summaries given at the close of a meeting also list the tasks and responsibilities of group members between meetings. In addition, summarizing sets the tone for the next group interaction.

Communication techniques are important for working well with groups. Equally important, however, is a **knowledge of group dynamics and its applications to nursing.** Understanding group process and dynamics assists the nurse to

- become a more competent and capable leader and manager,
- become a more active and effective group member,
- coordinate groups to meet both individual and organizational goals,
- tactfully manage conflict and assist with problem solving,
- develop awareness of any hidden agendas, and
- focus the group in a positive direction.

Working effectively with groups takes practice, patience, and persistence. Keep trying. The rewards (for both you and others) are worth the efforts.

Summary

An understanding of group process and dynamics is critical for any supervisor. Groups may be *primary*, as in the family, or *secondary*, as in the work group. Another method of classifying groups is by their levels of formality. Groups serve several important purposes. The energies of members, directed toward a common goal, can achieve goals that are unattainable by one individual. In groups, members solve problems, provide support for each other, and give and receive messages. As they grow and develop, groups pass through three stages: beginning, working, and ending. Effective groups have several traits in common. A group's dynamics are influenced by the social forces operating within it. When people come together for a purpose, the leader has the responsibility for moving the group toward a goal. Good meeting management requires careful planning, preparation, and capable group leadership skills. Effective followers are important, and they have many traits in common with good leaders. Common group problems include conflict, poor decision making, apathy, hidden agendas, and nonproductive behavioral interactions among group members. Group leaders need to frequently assess and evaluate the groups dynamics. Techniques to increase group productivity focus on positive self-presentation and effective group communication techniques.

◒ Key Concepts

- Groups consist of two or more people coming together for a shared purpose.
- Primary groups are small, intimate, and supportive.
- Secondary groups are task-oriented. They include formal, semiformal, and informal groups.
- Groups serve several purposes. They provide support, power, and information; solve problems; and achieve goals.
- Because each member is unique, groups are dynamic and progress through beginning, working, and ending stages.
- Highly functional groups have several characteristics in common that can be used by the nurse manager to increase effectiveness.
- Group dynamics are the social forces operating within the group.
- To manage meetings efficiently, the nurse needs to consider the atmosphere, agenda, and follow-up tasks.
- Members of groups usually assume task, maintenance, or self-serving roles.
- It is important for the nurse manager to practice developing both good leadership and followership skills.
- Problems common to groups include conflict, ineffective decision making, apathy, hidden agendas, groupthink, and nonproductive interactions.
- To evaluate a groups dynamics and effectiveness, the nurse manager assesses the group's goals, level of commitment, decision-making skills, communications, cohesiveness, leadership style, and use of power.
- Presenting positively and improving group communications are two important techniques for improving group productivity and harmony.

◒ Learning Activities

1. Attend a self-help group meeting (A.A., Al-Anon, Weight Watchers). Assess the group's level of formality, purpose(s), and effectiveness. Present your finding to your group.
2. Develop an agenda for a meeting called to discuss the problem of short staffing.
3. Role play a staff meeting in progress. Elect a leader. The purpose of the meeting is to vote on a solution to the short staffing problem. Develop a hidden agenda (e.g., to end the meeting without the vote) for two members. Have observers monitor the group's progress.
4. Divide the class into two groups. One group will act as observers and evaluators. Divide the remaining group into teams of two. One person will play the nonproductive group role of aggressor, recognition seeker, monopolizer, dominator, blocker, playboy, or zipper mouth.

The other will use tactics to refocus the behaviors positively. The observing group will evaluate.

5. Listen to a conversation for 5 minutes, then summarize the major points. Evaluate your effectiveness by checking your accuracy with the speakers.

References

Bradford LP, Stock D, Horowitz M: *How to diagnose group problems.* In Bradford LP, editor: *Group Development,* La Jolla, Calif, 1974, University Associates.

Brakely MR: Are you a good follower?, *Nursing 91* 21(12):78, 1991.

Kozier B, Erb G: *Fundamentals of nursing: concepts and procedures,* ed 3, Menlo Park, NJ, 1987, Addison-Wesley.

Potter P, Perry A: *Fundamentals of nursing: concepts, process and practice,* ed 3, St Louis, 1989, Mosby.

Sampson EE, Marthas MS: *Group process for health professions,* New York, 1977, John Wiley & Sons.

Stanhope M, Lancaster J: *Community health nursing: process and practice for promoting health,* ed 2, St Louis, 1988, Mosby.

Sullivan M: *Nursing leadership and management: a study and learning tool,* Springhouse, Pa, 1990, Springhouse.

Tappen RM: *Nursing leadership and management: concepts and practice,* ed 2, Philadelphia, 1989, Davis.

Additional Readings

Anderson K: Making a good first impression, *Nursing 91* 20(10):145, 1991. *Outlines five tips for making a good impression when first meeting.*

Bernard L, Walsh M: *Leadership: the key to professionalism of nursing,* ed 2, St Louis, 1990, Mosby. *Discusses the theories, components, and processes of organizing, teaching, and decision making for the nurse/leader.*

Bond M: Dare you say no?, *Nursing Mirror* 10:40, Oct 1982. *The author describes several methods for assertively making and refusing requests.*

Bradford L: *Making meetings work,* La Jolla, Calif, 1976, University Associates. *Offers several suggestions for planning, developing, and presenting effective meetings.*

Calabrese R: Interactional skills for nurse managers, *Nursing Management* 13(5):29, 1982. *Dr. Calabrese focuses on the social concerns of managers and suggests five behavioral techniques for creating a supportive climate.*

Chapman EN: *Supervisor's survival kit: a mid-management primer,* ed 2, Chicago, 1975, Science Research Associates. *An excellent text for beginners, this book explores the management process and offers many techniques for the neophyte supervisor.*

Chartier M: Clarity of expression in interpersonal communication, *Journal of Nursing Administration* 10(6):42, 1981. *The author first defines clarity in com-*

munication. Sending and receiving skills, as well as seven principles for increasing the clarity of messages are then explored.

Chivaetta L: Group communication: when I speak no one listens, *Nursing Management* 13(5):36, 1982. *The unit conference can be a valuable tool for sharing information when not used as an exchange of defense mechanisms. Explores six defensive role behaviors and their more positive counterparts.*

Douglas LM: *The effective nurse: leader and manager*, ed 4, St Louis, 1992, Mosby. *This we''-written text provides information and tools for the beginning manager.*

Durald MM: Toward positive attitudes and feelings, *Nursing Management* 20(10):64A, 1989. *The author, a NeuroLinguistic Programming counselor, explains the process of replacing negative feelings through persistent effort.*

Fast J: *Body language*, New York, 1970, M Evans. *The author explores the topic of kinesics, the study of nonverbal communication.*

Gilmore SK, Fraleigh PW: *Communication at work*, Eugene, Ore, 1980, Friendly Press. *This book focuses on the basic premise that, to be successful in your work, you must be able to communicate effectively. An easy-to-read book designed to improve group communications in the work setting.*

Grensing L: A formula to avoid miscommunicating, *Nursing 90* 20(9):122, 1990. *A three-stage approach for minimizing misunderstandings is described. The importance of "I" messages is stressed.*

James J: Learning the art of verbal self-defense, *Nursing 92* 22(1):108, 1992. *The author discusses four criteria for recognizing a verbal attack and six strategies for responding to them.*

Korobow L: Think you're powerless? Think again, *Nursing 89* 19(11):103, 1989. *Overcoming the feeling of powerlessness by assuming responsibility for personal power is the basic premise of this article. Explores four myths related to powerful people and describes five guidelines for attaining personal power.*

Leebov W: Getting along with co-workers better. *Nursing 91* 21(1):113, 1991. *Ms. Leebov presents 10 principles for working harmoniously with groups.*

Liberatore R and others: A group approach to problem solving, *Nursing Management* 20(9):68, 1989. *The authors discuss the procedure, advantages, and pitfalls of the survey-based, problem-solving process.*

Nawrocki H: Whatever happened to common courtesy?, *Nursing 88* 18(9):43, 1988. *A review of four tactics to help a newcomer feel welcome in the work group is offered.*

Raudsepp E: Six steps to becoming more assertive, *Nursing 91* 21(3):112, 1991. *To project a more confident, professional image, practice these techniques.*

Scully R: Staff support groups: helping nurses to help themselves, *Journal of Nursing Administration* 11(3):48, 1981. *The author contends that a nursing staff support group can reduce stress, manage conflict, and prevent burnout.*

Smallegan M: How to communicate effectively with groups, *Nursing Life* 3:16, 1983. *Several suggestions for working with groups of varying size and maintaining control are described.*

Steven D: Profile of a good manager, *Nursing Management* 21(1):60, 1991. *The author examines eight important qualities needed for accomplished management.*

White J: *Image and self-projection*, Boulder, Colo, 1986, Career Track (audiotape). *Designed specifically for professional women, this workshop addresses image and self-projection problems faced by all working women.*

Widell J, Pitts C: Coping with problem personalities, *Nursing 90* 20(9):102, 1990. *This article presents nine types of problem behaviors and offers suggestions to preserve morale by working effectively with each type.*

LEADERSHIP

4

SKILLS

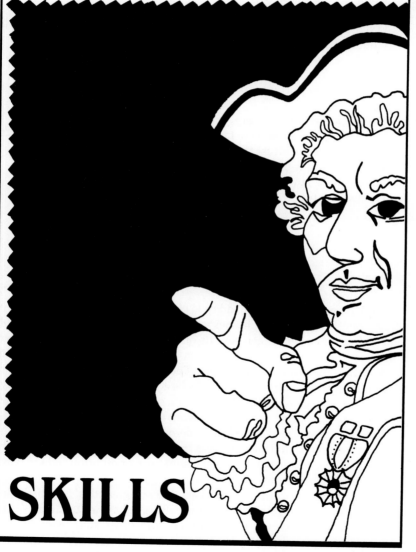

✒ Learning Objectives

Upon completion of this chapter, the reader will be able to:

1. Explain three ways in which the work force is changing.
2. Describe the three components of leadership.
3. Apply four theories of leadership to nursing situations.
4. Define *leadership style*.
5. Compare the characteristics, advantages, and disadvantages of three basic leadership styles.
6. Discuss three nursing situations in which a specific leadership style would be preferred.
7. Compare the characteristics and functions of formal and informal leaders.
8. Explain the importance of recognizing and empowering the informal leader.
9. Define *power* and identify your feelings in relation to its use.
10. Describe how women were taught to support, but not develop, power.
11. Compare and contrast personal power with position power.
12. List 12 qualities of a creative leader.
13. Identify five guidelines for developing the qualities of leadership.
14. Discuss the use of the 'nurturing role' as applied to leadership.

Today's Workers

The American work force of today is changing. Masses of people move away from their childhood homes in order to pursue work. More people tend to live alone for longer periods of time. As a result, many workers now supply most of their personal, as well as social and actualization, needs within the work environment. Today's workers are committed to their organizations. They want to do the best job possible. However, today's workers are also demanding. They want a sense of identity to the profession, organization, and group. They want to feel self-worth and personal fulfillment. To contend with these demands, American industry and business are slowly shifting emphasis from a 'task' orientation, where the focus was on goods produced, to an **'employee' orientation**, where trust, respect, and shared ideas are cultivated.

Nurses and other health care workers derive a great deal of satisfaction from providing care for clients. Historically, we have not paid attention to generalizing our caring to co-workers and other staff, though. The nurse, as leader/manager, is in an excellent position to encourage caregivers to thrive and grow by providing an atmosphere based on nurturing the self-esteem, integrity, trust, and respect of each employee. Develop your leadership skills with this in mind.

Components of Leadership

Bernard and Walsh (1990) state that "nursing leadership is a multidimensional process that depends on the relationship between a nurse leader and a group, the setting or organization of the interaction, and the theory of leadership chosen by the nurse leader." Campbell (1980) simplifies the definition by stating that "leadership is any action that focuses resources to create new opportunities." The *action* is the dynamic relationship with the group. The *resources* include the group and anything within the organization that will help to meet the goal. New *opportunities* are born when the leader and group both function capably and creatively.

Every leadership situation consists of three parts: the **group**, the **organization,** and the **leadership theory.** It is the *relationship* of the nurse leader to each component that determines the outcome (success or failure) of the situation.

The group

According to Bernard and Walsh (1990), nursing leadership is multidimensional because it combines the inherent (personality) and learned characteristics of the leader with characteristics of the situation. To simplify, each leader, each group, and each situation is unique. The nurse leader needs to assess two things when considering his/her relationship with a group: attributes of the nurse leader and composition of the group.

Attributes of the nurse leader. These include the characteristics of accountability, advocacy, assertiveness, and awareness (see Chapter 1). These, along with the leader's psychosocial skills, are acquired through an ongoing growth process. As the leader becomes more skilled, the leadership becomes more effective.

Composition of the group. The nurse leader who also provides direct patient care relates to two types of groups—those who seek out health care (clients) and those who give or provide that care (nurses and other providers). Because the composition of the groups differ, the purpose, goals, and dynamics will differ. When working with clients, the nurse is involved in a *therapeutic* relationship. The relationship between the nurse and other members of the health care team is, hopefully, a *collaborative* relationship. In long-term care settings, the collaborative, or team, approach is very important in providing quality patient care. The team strives to work together as a functional unit composed of caregivers with varied and specialized skills. Team leaders focus on coordinating members' energies and activities in order to work together on a defined task. The goal is to provide the best client care with the resources available; therefore, the nurse leader needs to analyze the composition and dynamics of the group as well as his/her relationship with each group.

The organization

All "health care organizations share a common goal: to provide, to maintain, and to restore the health of clients" (Bernard, Walsh, 1990). Each organization, however, establishes its own unique philosophy, policies, procedures, and structure. It is the combination of these variables that determines the nurse's leadership behaviors. For example, if the facility's policy was to keep each client as physically active as possible, the nurse team leader would encourage staff members to ambulate clients frequently. The type and amount of input or collaboration by team members is also determined by the organization. Some long-term care facilities allow the CNA to participate in client care conferences, while others do not. Team members (followers) have a wealth of information and like to be consulted. The nurse leader needs to be aware of the degree of staff involvement and make efforts to create an environment that encourages interest and promotes dialogue from *all* staff members.

The leadership theory

The third component of every leadership situation is the theory the nurse chooses. Although numerous leadership theories are available, the nurse leader should critically compare each theory with the philosophy and goals of the organization. Leadership theories are important, for they enhance the effectiveness of the leader by providing a framework for evaluating different situations. They deserve a closer look.

Theories of Leadership

A theory is a set of ideas that explain the nature or behavior of something. A theory is based on facts or observable and predictable behaviors. Because these facts and behaviors can be demonstrated and thus shared, they are assumed to be true. These evolve into general principles which, when applied, govern practice. To simplify, theories are ideas that help to explain reality, predict actions, and provide guidance for their users.

Theories of leadership (see box on p. 93) have probably been around in some form since one person led the group to the hunt. As long as there

---

✍︎ LEADERSHIP THEORIES

Great Man theory — belief that leaders possess innate characteristics that impel them to lead

Trait theory — defines essential characteristics that determine leadership

Situational theory — leadership is determined as a result of a particular situation

Interactional theory — leadership is the interaction between leader and group behaviors and a particular situation

---

are groups of people with common goals, there will be leaders. The major responsibility of the leader is to move the group toward the goal. In the health care setting, the basic goal is to provide the best nursing care possible. Leadership theories are important because they help to describe the *who, what,* and *how* of guiding others. They are also valuable in explaining which conditions or behaviors are needed by the leader in order to solve problems and attain goals.

During the past 50 years, theories about leadership have attempted to explain who leaders are, what they do, and how they do it. In an attempt to describe the relationship of a leader to a group, four levels of theories were developed.

Great man theory

The first and most simplistic theory is concerned with defining, identifying, and naming. It is one of the oldest theories in history and is based on Aristotle's philosophy that some people are born to lead and others are born to be led. The great leaders possessed innate, or inherited, characteristics that impelled them to lead—'born leaders.' Europe's history of monarchy rule is an excellent example. The families that produced kings and rulers were expected to have the abilities to be great leaders. Intermarriages among the monarchies was thought to encourage the creation of a superior class of leaders.

The advantage of this theory was an acceptance of a leader–follower system. People were comfortable knowing that when a ruler died, an heir to the throne was readily available, possessing all the traits and abilities necessary for a great leader. No questions existed as to who was the ruler.

Two disadvantages of this line of thinking were (1) the ruler may not have been capable of great leadership, and (2) people who were not leaders were assumed to be untrainable. Because leadership abilities were innate, no ordinary man could attain them. This first-level theory explained nothing. It only identified the requirements for leadership, namely, membership in a socially elite ruling class. The great man theory was accepted and followed for hundreds of years, up until the mid-1900s when the trait theory began to emerge.

Trait theory

Also based on naming or describing, the trait theory identified certain leadership qualities and stated a belief that they can be taught to others. Studies identified the essential traits of leaders as intelligence, energy, self-confidence, initiative, empathy, patience, and persistence. The trait theory expanded on the great man theory by attempting to define the essential characteristics of leadership — an explanation of who the leader 'is.'

The problem with the trait theory was that it did not lead to a comprehensive explanation of the leader's qualities because many of the same traits were found in both leaders and followers. Moreover, characteristics such as energy or intelligence were difficult to define and measure. Studies relating to traits considered essential for leadership revealed that most successful leaders possessed some, but not all, of the 'essential' leadership characteristics.

During the 1920s and 1930s, the trait theory generated many research studies. However, by 1940, theorists were looking for a theory that considered the interactions and relationships of the leader with the followers. They no longer believed that a single explanation of leadership traits was sufficient.

Situational theory

Because the great man and the trait theories could not offer a complete explanation of leadership, theorists expanded their ideas in an attempt to find relationships within a leadership situation. The two first-level theories considered the leader's personality. The situational theory states that it is the *situation* that determines the leadership behaviors. Leadership is "the process of influencing the group in a particular situation, at a given point in time, in a specific set of circumstances" (Cribben, 1972). This influence propels the group toward achieving objectives that meet the goal.

The major advantage of the situational theory was that it attempted to explore the context or the situation in which leadership occurred. The theory, however, states that a leader will emerge as a result of the situation; this is not always the case. A leader may not materialize in every situation, crisis, or problem. Even if a leader were to emerge, that does not guarantee effectiveness. Also, group leadership is fluid — the appropriate leader for one situation may be dismal under another set of circumstances. Because the situational theory was felt to be incomplete, further development by later theorists such as Fiedler, Hershey, and Blanchard has made the model a more useful basis for action. The situational theory represents a second theory level, factor-relating, which attempts to explain the relationships among the leader, the specific group, the organization, and the situation. By considering only one component, the situation, this theory remains inadequate and incomplete. More work was needed to provide logical and suitable explanations relating to leadership.

Interactional theory

The basis for this approach to leadership is the interaction between the personalities (the leader and the group) and the situation. An important aspect of this theory is a consideration of the followers as well as their needs and goals. The interactional theory focuses first on the group interaction. The behavior of one group member influences and causes a behavior change in another member. The leader's behavior affects the group, and, conversely, the group's behavior affects the leader. For example, a leader who is protective of the group is much more likely to be protected by the group when threatened. The group can impact leaders by supporting, threatening to rebel, protecting, or ousting them. "Thus, leadership involves a working relationship between the group members and the leader, who acquires leadership status through active participation and demonstration of his/her capabilities for completing, or helping the group to complete, cooperative activities" (Heimann, 1976).

Second, the interactional theory considers the leader. Building on the earlier trait theory, the interactional theory supports the idea that a group will choose a leader with characteristics that will help the group meet the goal. Leadership then becomes a process of mutual stimulation with a cycle of interactions that moves the group toward its goals.

A great advantage of this theory is that it takes into account the variable of change. Situations change rapidly. The group changes by gaining or losing members or by becoming involved in conflict. The task or goal for the group may change. Even the working conditions or economic situation will eventually change. "The only negative aspect of interactional theory is that is does not predict outcomes or prescribe actions that would direct leaders in their role" (Bernard, Walsh, 1990).

Level-three and level-four theories predict actions. Leaders' actions are judged by their effectiveness. Examples include McGregor's Theory X (the basis for managerial theory) and Theory Y (the basis for management by objectives), the path–goal theory (where the leader shows the group how their actions will lead to reward), the managerial grid (emphasis on the interdependence between people and production), and the tridimensional leadership effectiveness model (forces within the leader, group, and situation will determine the style of leadership).

Some of these theories can become complex due to the consideration of the many aspects of leadership. The most important factor for the nurse leader is to *choose* a theory and *work* with it. Heimann (1976) recommends the interactional theory as a good place to start. The theory is not difficult to understand or apply, and it is comprehensive enough to generalize to any leadership situation. In addition, the interactional theory directs the leader to assess his/her own personality, the group's dynamics, and the situation. These three assessments are repeated continually, then the results are combined with previous knowledge and used to improve effectiveness. No matter which theory the nurse leader chooses, the organization's goals, as well as individual group members, must be considered when applying a leadership theory to actual situations. Remember that leaders interact with people, not theories or productivity units.

Styles of Leadership

Style refers to the approach or manner a leader uses to influence workers' (group members') behaviors in various situations. Different styles are effective in different situations. Leadership style is the manner in which the leader influences the group to accomplish goals. A part of the growth process for nurse leaders is the development of an awareness of the most appropriate style for each particular situation.

Choosing a style

When deciding upon the most effective style for a given situation, the leader needs to consider the following:

The structure of the environment. What are the traditions and values (the unwritten guidelines) of the organization? Does the facility's philosophy support or discourage the leadership style?

The task or goal. Is the goal realistic and attainable? What are the resources and limitations relating to the task? How much time is needed or allotted?

The people to be led (the group). What is the group's level of maturity? How confident are members about the group's ability to get things done? Is the group interested, committed, and capable of making decisions?

The leader (you). What are your values and attitudes? Assess your amount of confidence in the group's abilities, your comfort with the leadership role, and, of course, any feelings of uncertainty about the situation. If the leadership style is inconsistent with your basic personality, it is unlikely to be effective. In the beginning, select a style that feels comfortable for you. It is better to be able to use a few styles effectively and consistently than to employ every style poorly. Try to adopt the leadership style that complements the situation, respects the group's abilities, and moves the group toward the goal.

Leadership styles directly relate to the amount of control or freedom allowed the group. The best style for any particular situation is one that "promotes a high level of work performance in a wide variety of circumstances, as efficiently as possible, and with the least amount of disruption" (Douglas, Bevis, 1983).

Common styles

Leadership styles range from total control to extreme permissiveness. A few of the most common styles of leadership are autocratic, democratic, and laisse-faire.

Autocratic. This style is also referred to as restrictive, authoritarian, or directive. In sum, the leader controls all the information and makes all the decisions. The emphasis is on the task or goal, while people are considered secondarily if at all. Input from the group is not encouraged nor considered in the decision-making process. The leader decides what is to be done, how it is to be accomplished, and who is to do it, then orders the workers to carry out specific tasks. Authoritarian leaders behave in a firm and dominating manner. They use power to ensure orderly, prompt, and predictable behaviors from group members. Their wishes and desires are most important when making decisions. The autocratic leader is at the center of attention and usually exercises power with little trust or confidence in the workers. McGregor (1960), in his book, *The Human Side of Enterprise,* describes the autocratic leader as "viewing the worker as a naturally lazy, unambitious person who dislikes responsibility and prefers to be led." Workers are not very bright or creative. They do not support organizational goals and are highly resistant to change—not a very pleasant viewpoint of the American worker.

As a result of this attitude, workers in this system fear and mistrust their leaders. They may feel pressured, forced, or exploited. Fear and threat of punishment motivate them to perform. Because their leader remains aloof from the group, members are unable to discuss their concerns or make any positive contributions.

Variations of the autocratic style range from the very rigid pure form to more benevolent practices. One common variation is known as *paternalism,* where the group members view the leader with a 'father knows best' attitude. The main difference between these two leadership styles is that the paternalistic leader has a greater consideration for the welfare of the group. These leaders have a personal relationship with the group, although they still make all the decisions. They feel responsible for the group's actions and want to prevent mistakes, thus protecting group members and providing them with a sense of security. Rewards are bestowed on members who follow directions and disciplinary actions for those who do not.

Another variation is the *mature autocrat,* or diplomatic style, of leadership. The mature autocrat is a highly competent, persuasive decision maker. Freedom is provided within strict limits, but group members are allowed input. This leader wants the group to feel satisfied and meet its needs but still retain all decision-making powers. Differences in status are still emphasized, and the leader, although interacting with the group, remains separate from the group in a higher position of status.

Some autocratic leaders are frequently referred to as *bureaucrats* because the organization always remains a higher priority than concern for individual workers. This type of leader employs a high-directive/low-supportive style by giving many orders and actively directing the group's activities. Support for the worker is minimal, and when given, the leader tends to use nonconstructive criticism and praise for *personal* traits rather than for *work performed.*

The bureaucrat is a system supporter who believes that the organization's system provides all the answers. This leader type wants all possible situations covered in the policies and procedures manual—a 'by the book' person. Individual judgment is minimized because every possibility is embodied in the manual. "This leader allows no violations of rules and procedures under any circumstances. If violation occurs, disciplinary action follows immediately" (O'Donovan, 1975).

The authoritarian, paternalistic, mature autocrat, and bureaucratic leader all practice high-directive/low-supportive behaviors. The leader's primary concern is for the task, and these types of leaders closely supervise their group members to monitor performance (high-directive behaviors). Some workers refer to this style of monitoring as 'snoopervision.' Low-supportive behaviors include an expectation that the job will be done because that is what group members are supposed to do—work. Feedback is provided in the form of praise for personal traits or criticism. Workers are not expected to question authority or offer suggestions for improvement.

Authoritarian leadership styles have been used in the nursing profession for many years. In fact, this basic style of leadership is the most traditional and common style utilized by nurses. Team leaders give orders and expect them to be followed. Adherence to the facility's policies and regulations is expected. Staff members are expected to conform with the directions and examples set by the leader.

Autocratic leadership styles are appropriate in some situations. During a crisis, in an emergency, or in a situation where a quick decision must be made, authoritarian leaders excel. For example, an air traffic controller cannot land airplanes by consensus or group decisions. The situation must be assessed rapidly; and instructions must be clear, specific, and organized. Chaos would result if the authoritarian style was replaced in this situation.

Staff members with limited technical skills and high needs for security and stability respond well to an authoritarian leader. Also, people who are unable or unwilling to accept responsibility require the watchful eye of the authoritarian. Last, autocratic leadership styles may be appropriate for some difficult, complex situations.

The disadvantages of this style are fairly obvious. Because the leader assumes that workers are unambitious and lazy by nature, much time and effort goes into supervision. By directing or controlling others, the leader is closed to communications from workers and, therefore, may miss important information. Most importantly, autocratic leadership styles do not consider the worth of the individual worker. All people need to feel respected and recognized for their contributions to the organization. As Carl Jung (1964), psychologist and analyst of human behavior, so aptly stated, "The supreme goal of man is to fulfill himself as a creative, unique individual according to his own innate potentialities and within the limits of reality." Authoritarian leadership styles are effective in their place. Use these styles cautiously and only when assessed as necessary.

Democratic. The autocratic leader's primary focus is the task, while the democratic leader's focal point is the people. This is a people-oriented leadership style designed to build effective work groups by emphasizing the value and dignity of the group member. The leader encourages the group to assume responsibility for establishing goals, setting policies, and solving problems. The role of the democratic leader is to stimulate and guide the group. These leaders empower workers. The underlying message is, "You are an important and valuable asset. I respect, encourage and promote your growth" (LaBella, Leach, 1985). Democratic leaders give the workers an overview of the task, explain all steps, and make suggestions but do not give orders. The group establishes policies, sets goals, defines the steps needed to meet the goals, and decides when the goals have been accomplished. Communications among group members and the leader are trusting, open, friendly, and considerate. Criticism focuses on behaviors, not personal traits, and is given in a matter-of-fact manner in an attempt to assist, not degrade, the individual. There are four principles of democratic leadership (Tappen, 1985):

1. Every group member should participate in decision making.
2. Freedom of belief and action is allowed within reasonable bounds that are set by society and by the group.
3. Each individual is responsible for himself or herself and for the welfare of the group.
4. There should be concern and consideration for each group member as a unique individual.

Obviously, the democratic leadership style does not work well with all groups. Mature groups whose members communicate and work together effectively are most suited for this type of leadership. Groups displaying the following characteristics are usually comfortable with the democratic leadership style (Bernard, Walsh, 1990):

- a need for independence
- a readiness to accept and work with responsibility
- a commitment to the group's common goal
- interest in the tasks of the group
- abilities or capabilities to get the job done
- a high level of tolerance for uncertainty and ambiguity
- an expectation of sharing in the decision-making process

Groups with these traits are usually quite successful with the democratic style of leadership. It is important for the nurse leader to look for these characteristics before deciding to employ a democratic leadership style.

Participatory leadership is much similar to the democratic style except that, while allowing the group to participate, the leader still retains control over the final decision. The leader may assume the role of member during the discussion or present the information, listen to alternatives or suggestions from the group, and then make the decision.

There are many advantages to the democratic leadership style. Group members are usually more committed to the task since they participated in its development. Motivation stems from the group, not from only the leader. When the task or problem is complex, the leader can employ high-directive/high-supportive behaviors in which the leader closely supervises the task while also praising and facilitating workers' performance. When the group is comfortable with the task, the leader can choose a low-directive/high-supportive style, which supports the goal and encourages the group to progress toward meeting the goal. Other advantages include a higher level of job satisfaction and a decrease in complaints, feelings of frustration, and submission. The group's morale, productivity, and participation are improved. Creativity is fostered, and unique solutions may be offered.

Although democratic leadership styles appear to be the perfect answer for the nurse leader, there are a few disadvantages. The group's maturity and capabilities must be taken into account. Dependence on the leader is minimized, and this may be perceived as threatening to the leader. If full decision-making responsibilities lie with the group, a new leader may be appointed. Nurses who need a firm control will feel uncomfortable. The democratic process is more cumbersome and time-consuming. This can frustrate people who only want to get the job done. Additionally, a greater number of disagreements will arise, which may require additional time and effort for resolution. Work performed by the group may be more original and creative, but many "studies indicate that democratic leadership is not as efficient quantitatively as authoritarian leadership" (Tappen, 1989). This indicates that, although workers may be happy and satisfied with this style, they are not as productive. Decisions made by the group may result from social pressures or a need to maintain the status quo. Group members may become more interested in winning an argument than meeting the goal. Excessive cohesiveness may lead to groupthink. Last, the nature of the task or problem may make close supervision difficult, if not impossible. The democratic style of leadership may be the most demanding, but it is usually worth the effort, for it fosters respect, dignity, and value for each group member.

Laisse-faire. This is the permissive, or free-run, style of leadership. We have all seen the laisse-faire parent who allows Junior to 'explore his environment' by screaming through the building, jumping on or at people, and otherwise behaving in a generally obnoxious manner. "Where is this child's control?" we wonder. This may be an extreme example, but not by much.

The **laisse-faire, or permissive, leader** is usually fairly laid back, that is, passive, inactive, and nondirective. The focus is on the individual, not the group (democratic) or task (authoritarian). The climate is permissive, with the leader wanting everyone to feel good. Virtually all control and decision making is left to the group. This leader may provide materials and information for the group but offers little else. No direction, suggestions, or ideas are provided. No attempt to evaluate the group or its progress is made. Power is relegated to the group, and few, if any, limits are imposed on workers' behaviors.

Permissive leadership is based on the premise that all workers are ambitious, creative, responsible, and willing to accept the organization's goals. Communications with the leader and the group are open and friendly but lack focus and direction. Group members commonly act independently and may be at cross purposes or repeating each other's work due to a lack of coordination, cooperation, or communication. Goals may be unclear and tasks confusing. The leader may answer questions when asked directly or refer the question back to the group.

Disadvantages of the laisse-faire leadership style are numerous. This is a low-directive/low-supportive style in which neither the task nor the worker is fostered. Members can become frustrated by the lack of direction, which, in turn, creates tension and anxiety throughout the group. Apathy and disinterest may become evident. This may lead to uncertainty, confusion, and chaos. The group becomes dissatisfied with its performance, loses its sense of unity, and eventually turns out to be totally dysfunctional. Work produced by this type of group is usually of a poorer quality than with other leadership styles.

However, laisse-faire styles can be very effective when the group has a high degree of cooperation and maturity. "When all group members are highly self-directed, motivated, and able to coordinate their own activities with others, laisse-faire leadership can give them the freedom they need to be highly creative and productive" (Tappen, 1989). A good example of this is a research group composed of highly educated professionals.

Remember that no single style of leadership is suitable for every situation. Before selecting a style, assess the situation, the task, the group, and the leader (see p. 91). The multicratic leader combines styles from all categories and develops an effective array of leadership behaviors.

Also, recall that leadership is an art that requires practice, persistence, and patience. It may take some time to become adept at choosing which leadership style is best for a particular situation, but with effort, you will become skilled.

Formal and Informal Leaders

When Mary Morris graduated from nursing school and joined the staff of a large long-term care facility, she was assigned the task of supervising six nursing assistants who provided daily cares for 40 residents. As time passed, Mary became frustrated in her attempt to provide competent supervision because she felt the group was restricting most of her efforts. She discovered that each nursing assistant protected the other, which made it quite difficult to determine who was responsible for slipshod work. Even when Mary urged the group to improve, her assistants continued to provide the same substandard care. Although Mary was the appointed supervisor, she noticed that most of the time her assistants, instead of consulting her, took their problems to an older assistant in the unit.

Mary also observed that three of the assistants always had lunch together. Two others ate with nursing assistants from another unit. Mary usually ate with other supervisors, from whom she learned much about the facility. Before long, she began to realize that her assistants were more trusting of their informal leader and that she needed to work with this situation as well as the formal organizational process.

"Beneath the cloak of formal relationships in every organization there is a more complex system of social relationships consisting of many informal organizations [groups]" (Davis, Newstrom, 1989). These groups can have a powerful effect on work productivity and job satisfaction through their use of informal power.

Formal Leaders

In every organization, formal and informal leaders exist. The *formal* leader is the official leader who is appointed by the administration and given the authority or power to act. The responsibilities, rules, rewards, roles, and penalties of the position are established by the administration.

Formal leaders are able to exercise their power best when followers accept and trust their leader.

Informal leaders

Informal leaders have no official power. Members of the work group empower the informal leader; therefore, their power does not follow the authorized chain-of-command. Powers of informal leaders are usually more unstable and subjective than formal power. Since this type of power is influenced by the sentiments of people, it cannot be controlled by management in the same manner as formal authority.

"Members of work groups have identifiable characteristics that distinguish them from each other and give rise to status differences" (Davis, Newstrom, 1989). Based on the value given by the group, such factors as age, birthplace, competence, earnings, freedom to move about the workplace, personality, and seniority can provide status. Usually the worker with the most status becomes the informal leader and may procure a considerable amount of power. Informal leaders may socialize new workers, be called upon to perform intricate or complex tasks, or provide advice and recommendations for fellow workers. Frequently, it is the informal leader who communicates problems to the supervisors.

Informal leaders do not always make the best formal supervisors, however. They may fear the weight of official responsibilities or become arrogant once vested with official power. They may criticize management for not trying something new and then become even more conservative once they assume a management position. Some enjoy the power and lack of official responsibility that goes with an informal leadership position.

Both benefits and problems exist with informal leaders. If the goals, attitudes, and behaviors of the unofficial leader are in keeping with those encouraged by management, influences on other workers will be positive and in support of the organization. For a listing of other benefits, see the box on p. 104.

Problems associated with informal leaders can bring havoc to the organization's operations. Informal leaders are negatively influencing the group when they

- encourage negative attitudes;
- resist new ideas and support conformity;
- encourage the group to operate outside the formal system and seek sanctions from them for the group's activities;
- foster personal, role, or group conflict;
- spread undesirable rumors;
- reject, harass, or impede workers; or
- work to negatively affect workers' motivation or job satisfaction.

BENEFITS OF WORKING WITH INFORMAL LEADERS

- More effective working system
- Improved communications
- Lightened work load for management
- Enhanced cooperation between work groups and management
- Assistance with improving a manager's abilities
- Encouragement for leader to plan and act more carefully
- Provision of a 'safety valve' for workers' emotions
- Assistance with providing stability and satisfaction for the work group members

How should the nurse leader deal with informal leaders? First, **identify who the informal leaders are and accept them as leaders.** Second, **gain trust.** Find any common ground or shared interests, ideas, etc. Third, try to **integrate the interests** of the informal group or leader with those of the organization. Fourth, **consider all possible effects** *before* **making decisions** or taking actions. Last, **work with the informal leaders to keep work groups supportive** of the organization and its goals. Keep communication lines open. The ideal situation is one in which the group and its informal leaders are supportive of and willing to follow the officially sanctioned leader. Remember that each member of the staff is a person with individual and unique needs. Your respect and interest will go a long way toward promoting positive work interactions and your efficiency as a leader.

Development and Use of Power

Power is the ability to act — the force or energy required to accomplish a task, meet a goal, promote changes, or influence others. Because the majority of nurses are women (and the profession reflects this), nurses (women) have been taught to support power, not to develop and exercise it. If nursing is to truly evolve into an autonomous, respected profession, nurses must learn to develop and effectively utilize their power.

The concept of power can be divided into two parts: personal power and position power. Personal power comes from the internal qualities, capabilities, experiences, and wisdom of the individual. It includes one's sense of integrity, code of ethics, willingness to learn (even when it may be painful), and commitment to bringing out the best in others.

Personal power

Effective leadership requires your best personal power skills. Review Chapter 1 for a full discussion of psychosocial skills. Here, concentrate on the skills which convey competence and capabilities when interacting with and leading groups (LaBella, Leach, 1985).

Confidence. Remember to employ eye contact, facial expressions, and gestures that communicate assurance. As you practice projecting confidence, you will actually begin to *feel* confident. When you feel your confidence level starting to drop, remember the first rule for staying assured: "Fake it till you make it" (LaBella, Leach, 1985). Breathe deeply and use your voice to speak clearly and firmly. A strong, resonant speaking voice projects certainty and assertiveness.

Decisiveness. The ability to make sound decisions and speak with conviction is as valuable in group work as in other areas of management. "Decisiveness is made up of three basic elements:

1. The ability to analyze the costs and benefits of each option,
2. The freedom to allow ourselves the right to make a mistake, and
3. The freedom to allow ourselves not to be liked" (LaBella, Leach, 1985).

The decisions you make need to be based on a thorough consideration of all aspects of each option. Weighing the pros and cons and considering possible outcomes fosters competent decision making. Making mistakes and not being liked for the decisions you make is inherent. Learn to work with these, as the consequences of your decisions are not always popular with everyone. Decisive group members and leaders are willing to take these risks in order to make the best possible decisions.

Control. Two aspects of control important to the personal power of the nurse leader are **self-control** and **influence**. Self-control can be seen as the ability to limit self-expression appropriately. You do not have to suppress your feelings or opinions—only direct them in a manner that causes no discomfort to others. Self-control also includes your self-talk. Keep it upbeat. Consciously interrupt and redirect negative emotions and energies as soon as you become aware (see Chapter 1). Control also encompasses the ability to influence others. Because nurses are constantly interacting with people, they have influence. When two or more people interact, each has an effect on the other. This effect or influence can be a positive or negative type of control. When control (influence) is motivating and stimulating to others, it has a positive effect. A negative power style, demonstrated by manipulation and domineering behavior, invites problems. Influencing others by empowering people to do their best and stretch their limits is the only control a good nurse manager needs.

Skills. Practice the psychosocial and communication techniques discussed earlier. Management, leadership, and membership in groups all require practical people skills. Technical skills are also important. As a manager, leader, or supervisor, you will have two sets of technical skills: those relating to the nursing of people and those that relate to the management of people.

Awareness. Perhaps the most important aspect of personal power is awareness. Personal awareness of the physical, emotional, mental, and spiritual self is an everyday challenge. Your 'self' is shared with others and reflects your values and emotions. Spend time each day, even if only a short amount, empowering yourself. Find the power within yourself and use it.

Developing an awareness of your organization, its systems, methods, and dynamics helps to build political understanding. This awareness allows you, as a group member and leader, to work for positive, effective change.

Position power

Position power is granted by the administration with the manager or supervisor role. Although authority may be inherent in the position, power is needed to actually obtain results. Power of the position allows the nurse leader to make decisions, influence the behaviors of the work group, and change situations. However, position power must be used carefully if the nurse is to encourage and inspire others. True position power is derived from the respect of the group, and that *respect must be earned.* It does not come with the territory. Managers may be highly competent and functional, but without respect, the followers will not achieve all that they are capable of attaining.

To develop your position power, practice these five suggestions:

Directions. Give clear and concise directions. Make sure the employee understands. If necessary, have the employee repeat them back to you. Ask for feedback and be sure to provide simple and logical steps when explaining a procedure. Workers lose confidence in their leader when vague or incomplete instructions are given.

Involvement. Involve workers in decisions when possible. Certain problems must be solved by the supervisor alone. On the other hand, a wise nurse leader knows that many problems (especially those affecting the group) can be solved by the work group itself. Including workers in decision making promotes cooperation, confidence, and participation while reducing conflict and ambiguity.

Feedback. Provide feedback. Let staff members know how they are doing but be sure to correct the *behavior,* not the person, when providing negative feedback. Also remember to praise in public and correct in private. This allows the worker to focus on improvement while retaining personal dignity and self-worth. If you neglect this aspect, the frustration will grow.

Be approachable. Maintain an open-door policy. Create an environment that encourages a free exchange of ideas, suggestions, opinions, and even complaints. Remove both physical and psychological barriers. Sitting behind the large desk with the door to your office closed invites nothing but solitude. Psychological barriers include nonverbal behaviors and gestures (e.g., looking at your watch) while a worker is telling you something that is important or emotionally charged. Be mindful of your open-door behaviors. "Merely keeping the door to the office open and telling employees to drop by is not enough. You must work to create a non-threatening atmosphere of welcome that will cause employees to come to you. It's 95 percent attitude and 5 percent policy" (Chapman, 1975).

Qualities of leadership

Some of the most charismatic and creative leaders are found in unexpected times and places. 'Super leaders' share numerous characteristics. Levenstein (1985) lists 12 qualities of leadership:

Group advocacy. The nurse leader's ability and willingness to speak up for the work group directly influences his/her effectiveness as a leader.

Conflict resolution. Nurse leaders will always have conflicts. They are a part of the growth process for the individual, the group, and the organization. Creative leaders help provide order and stability by recognizing and resolving conflict in its early stages. Chapter 6 concentrates on conflict resolution skills.

Tolerance of uncertainty. Challenges, problems, and changes are full of uncertainties. Super leaders welcome this but realize that uncertainty and ambiguity are bound to exist. Anxiety and emotionalism in the face of uncertainty decrease the leader's effectiveness.

Persuasiveness. The ability to sell your ideas to others is important. When presented with enthusiasm and conviction, it is much easier to gain acceptance for your ideas.

Initiate structure. Former UCLA basketball coach, John Wooden, firmly believes, "In any group activity, there should be a different role for everyone. . . . If your people understand and accept their roles, they are people you can lead" (Rozek, 1991). Provide structure. Let your staff know their roles and your expectations.

Tolerance of freedom. Individuality and creativity are fostered by the leader who allows workers the freedom to be themselves while encouraging a high level of performance.

Role assumption. Even when permitting or encouraging autonomy for staff members, the leader remembers who has the ultimate responsibility. Leaders take the pats on the back when the group achieves success and, conversely, feel the heat when things go wrong. Right or wrong, the leader is ultimately responsible.

Consideration. "The duty to protect the comfort, well-being, and status interests of the individual is a continuing concern of an effective leader" (Levenstein, 1985).

Production emphasis. Good human relations are important, but they should enhance, not detract from, quality production (good patient care).

Predictive accuracy. Super leaders possess the ability to anticipate possible outcomes and any difficulties that may be present along the way. Practice considering the possible outcomes of decisions.

Integration. The ability to bring together people, meet the organizational goals, and promote harmony while working is a basic but important technique.

Consideration of superiors. Effective leaders consider their supervisor. They are people, too, deserving of the same respect and consideration as others.

Be aware of and cultivate these qualities. They are the foundation for effective leadership.

Your Leadership Potential

Although it may not be found in the job description, one of the nurse's functions is to nurture. To nurture is to provide sustenance — to promote development or growth. As caregivers, we practice the healing arts by nurturing our patients during times of illness or disability. Our profession has recently expanded to include client teaching in order to promote healthy growth, development, and high-level wellness. It is now time to generalize this function and begin nurturing ourselves and each other.

As a leader, you are setting an example for all with whom you come in contact. Leadership influences people; thus, workers reflect the philosophy and behaviors of their leaders. Skills needed for superior leadership include confidence, decisiveness, analytical abilities, technical and psychosocial skills, and awareness (LaBella, Leach, 1985). By nurturing these skills in yourself and others, you nurture and thus empower everyone with whom you work. Let us look at how your personal power skills can be applied to nurturing.

Confidence

By acting like a winner, projecting assurance and faith in your abilities and your group's abilities, you encourage others (and yourself) to grow.

Put your workers into situations in which they have a chance of succeeding. Once one has tasted success, no matter how small, confidence grows. Identify staff members' strengths and build on them. Help others to win.

Decisiveness

Leaders who are considered effective can make decisions, although they may not make the correct decision every time. Take the time to problem-solve. Consider the possible outcomes of each possibility, then *act.* "To be decisive and proactive we often need to act long before we're convinced we're doing the right thing" (LaBella, Leach, 1985). Encourage others to be decisive by providing information and resources. If the outcome is not quite what was expected, instead of pointing out the discrepancy, ask what other way the situation could have been handled. This approach encourages staff members to work with the problem-solving process while preserving their respect and dignity.

Analytical abilities

This is just a fancy way of saying to use the problem-solving method to assist in making decisions. For the leader, an important part of this process is the ability to analyze the costs, benefits, and amount of effort (work) related to each possible outcome. Learn to analyze the situation or problem, then encourage the process in others. Soon there will be the power of several good minds working together.

Technical and psychosocial skills

Review Chapter 1 to **brush up on your psychosocial skills.** Although effective leaders do not need to know how to do the job of the people they supervise, they need to be knowledgeable of each team member's job description. As a nurse, you supervise the delivery of patient care. If you are technically competent, the group will be more willing to consult you when problems arise. Good technical abilities also engender staff confidence and provide teaching opportunities, which improve the group's skill levels. If you are a nursing student, work as a nursing assistant on weekends or during vacations. The experience is invaluable, for you will learn about the realities of the job. Not only will you gain an insight of the job and its requirements, but you also will gain the experience of being a follower. If you are lucky, you will have super supervisors; identify their strengths and model them. If your supervisors are not very effective, at least you will learn what you do not want to do when *you* become a supervisor. Staff members are much more willing to be led by a nurse they know has 'been there.'

Awareness

First take some time each day to **become aware of your physical, mental, spiritual, and emotional self.** Your time, skills, and energies are your personal resources, and you are the only person who can effectively nurture, direct, and channel them. LaBella and Leach (1985, emphasis added) believe, "A structured awareness process also helps you to deal with your problems *as they arise.* When we try to ignore them — or are unaware — they surface months later in disease and burnout." Your personal awareness is important if you are to flourish and grow.

Awareness also includes sensitivity to the activities and problems of your work group. They are people, too, with all the needs and desires of any individual. Be alert to how the organization, your decisions, and your attitudes impact your staff. Sensitivity to the needs of others increases your effectiveness as a leader.

Practice these skills. As you become more adept with leadership power, you will feel a heightened confidence in your ability to empower yourself and those with whom you work.

Summary

Today's work force is changing. People demand more from the job than just a paycheck. Nurse leaders are in an excellent position to provide an environment that fosters growth and satisfaction of staff members. Leadership is the ability to get things done through others. It is a multidimensional process which encompasses consideration of the group, the organization, and the leadership theory. Theories of leadership include the great man, trait, situational, and interactional theories. Leadership styles refer to the manner in which the leader influences the group. When choosing a leadership style, the nurse should consider the organizational structure, the task, the people to be led, and the leader. Common styles include the autocratic, democratic, and laisse-faire (permissive) approach. Each has benefits and disadvantages, for no single leadership style is suitable for every situation.

Formal and informal leaders can have a strong influence on the work group. Informal leaders have a positive impact when goals, attitudes, and behaviors are in keeping with those promoted by the organization. Negative influences of informal leaders can bring about resistance to change, disorganization, and dissatisfaction. Power is the ability to act. Nurses and women have traditionally been taught to support, not develop or exercise, power. Personal power (the energy within) embodies the concepts of confidence, decisiveness, control, skills, and awareness. Position power (the authority to act) is derived from the administration but requires the respect of the followers if it is to be effective. Four suggestions for developing position power are offered. Highly competent leaders share certain characteristics. Super leaders are advocates, resolvers of conflict, communicators, and producers. Guidelines for reaching your leadership potential relate to the concept of nurturing. Through use of the nurturing role, the nurse manager empowers self as well as others and grows into a leader in whom workers have confidence and are inspired to develop to their fullest potential.

eL Key Concepts

- Every leadership situation consists of relationships between the nurse leader and the group, the organization, and the leadership theory.
- The 'Great Man' theory of leadership states that some people possess innate, or inherited, traits that make them destined to lead—the 'born leader.'
- The Trait theory identifies certain qualities or characteristics essential for leadership.
- The Situational theory states that the leader's behavior is determined by the situation. It is the first theory to explore the context (environment) in which leadership occurs.
- The Interactional theory contends that the basis for leadership is the interaction between the personalities and the situation.
- Leadership style is the manner used by the leader to influence the group to accomplish goals.
- Autocratic leadership and its variations provide a high-directive/low-supportive style in which the task is primary and worker support is minimal.
- Democratic leadership focuses on building an effective work group by stimulating and empowering workers to do their best.
- Laisse-faire leadership provides a permissive climate with no actual leadership direction.
- No single leadership style is suitable for every situation.
- Power is the energy required to act—to meet goals, promote change, or influence others.
- Formal leaders are those people who have been formally assigned power or authority by the administration.
- Informal leaders have no official power. They are empowered by members of the work group.
- Women have historically been taught to support, but not develop or exercise, power.
- Personal (internal) power is the energy we give to ourselves. It can be developed by practicing confidence, decisiveness, control, technical skills, and awareness.
- Position (external) power is the authority given by the administration. It is most effective when the leader is respected by the followers.
- Exceptional leaders share many of the same characteristics.
- Nurses have leadership potential that needs to be nurtured in order to grow.

eL Learning Activities

1. Divide the class into three groups. Elect one person from each group as the leader. Have each leader select one leadership style (autocratic,

democratic, laisse-faire) and role play the process of orienting a new employee to the unit using the assigned leadership style. After observing all three styles, have each group discuss their impressions.

2. Think about a job you once held. Discuss how the organization, the leader, and the work group helped or hindered your ability to do the job.
3. Discuss the concept of power. How does it differ between men and women? Identify how you feel about using power to get what you want.
4. Apply the 12 qualities of super leaders to two people you know who hold positions of leadership. Use no names.
5. Consider the following quotations and then describe their meaning to you:
   a. "Success is a result; it must not be a goal" (Flaubert).
   b. "To be what we are, and to become what we are capable of becoming is the only end of life" (Robert Louis Stevenson).
   c. "It's a psychological law that we tend to get what we expect" (Norman Vincent Peale).
   d. "I benefit myself by aiding him" (Sophocles).

References

Bernard L, Walsh M: *Leadership: the key to professionalism of nursing,* ed 2, St Louis, 1990, Mosby.

Campbell D: *If I'm in charge here why is everybody laughing?,* Allen, Tex, 1980, Argus Communications.

Chapman EN: *Supervisor's survival kit: a mid-management primer,* ed 2, Chicago, 1975, Science Research Associates.

Cribben JJ: *Effective managerial leadership,* New York, 1972, American Management Association.

Davis K, Newstrom J: *Human behavior at work: organizational behavior,* ed 7, New York, 1989, McGraw-Hill.

Douglas LM, Bevis EO: *Nursing management and leadership in action,* ed 4, St Louis, 1983, Mosby.

Hamilton JM: Personal power: your key to success, *Nursing 90* 20(10):146, 1990.

Heimann CG: Four theories of leadership, *Journal of Nursing Administration* 6(6):18, 1976.

Jung CG: *The development of personality, vol 117,* Collected Works, Bollingen Series XX, Princeton, NJ, 1964, University Press.

LaBella A, Leach D: *Personal power: the guide to power for today's working woman,* ed 2, Boulder, Colo, 1985, Career Track.

Levenstein A: So you want to be a leader?, *Nursing Management* 16(3):74, 1985.

McGregor D: *The human side of enterprise,* New York, 1960, McGraw-Hill.

O'Donovan TR: Leadership dynamics, *Journal of Nursing Administration* 5(9):32, 1975.

Rozek M: The winner's circle, *Entrepreneur* 19(6):119, 1991.

Tappen RM: *Nursing leadership and management: concepts and practice,* ed 2, Philadelphia, 1989, Davis.

Additional Readings

Autry JA: *Love and profit: the art of caring leadership*, New York, 1991, William Morrow. *A Fortune 500 executive manager shares his views on motivating others and coping with the intricacies of management.*

Chouvardas CA: Seven steps to asserting yourself, *Nursing 91* 21(11):126, 1991. *Describes seven techniques for assuming a more powerful role in nursing practice.*

Helgersen S: *The female advantage: women's ways of leadership*, New York, 1990, Bantam, Doubleday, Dell. *An exploration of the innovative organizational structures, strategies and theories of successful women leaders.*

Hendricks DE: The power problem, *Nursing Management* 13(10):23, 1982. *This article presents a consideration of the benefits of nurses becoming hospital administrators.*

Joel L, Patterson J: Nursing homes can't afford cheap nursing care, *RN* 53(6):57, 1990. *"An innovative experiment suggests that hiring more RNs and giving them greater autonomy can improve residents' health — and also save money."*

Layden M: Responsibility to self: first step to leadership, *Nursing Leadership* 2(3):26, 1979. *Nurses must be critically aware of themselves as individuals in order to foster growth and self-actualization in others.*

Ludeman K: *The worth ethic: how to profit from the changing values of the new work force*, New York, 1989, EP Dutton. *The author presents "Work Ethic managers who dedicate themselves to building self-esteem in themselves and others" and offers an eight-step changing process to empower managers.*

Manthey M: The nurse manager as leader, *Nursing Management* 21(6):18, 1990. *"Managers guide, direct and motivate. Leaders empower others. Therefore every manager should be a leader."*

Meissner J: Nurses: are we eating our young? *Nursing 86* 16(3):51, 1986. *One step in achieving professional status is the reexamination of interactions with novice nurses.*

Montisano-Marchi N: Power: from commanding turf to generating excellence, *Nursing Management* 21(11):72B, 1990. *This article offers a six-step process to become a leader of persons rather than a managing agent of systems.*

Nornold P: Power: it's changing hands and moving your way, *Nursing 86* 16(1): 40, 1986. *"Nurses can benefit mightily from changes in the health care system." The key is effective use of power.*

Porter K: Seven tips to make you a better leader, *Nursing 89* 19(12):90, 1989. *The author offers seven valuable suggestions for improving leadership skills.*

Smith RL, Kushel G, Korobow L: Think you're powerless: think again, *Nursing Life* 24:25, 1982. *Powerlessness is usually self-inflicted. This article debunks four myths concerning power and describes four principles for becoming a powerful person.*

Storlie FJ: Power — getting a piece of the action, *Nursing Management* 13(10):15, 1982. *This nurse believes that "getting a share of the power is the best prescription for Burnout."*

Straub JT, Attner RF: *Introduction to business*, ed 4, Boston, 1990, PWS-KENT. *This text provides an overview to the world of business and management.*

Zaleznik A: Managers and leaders: are they different? *Journal of Nursing Administration* 11(7):25, 1981. *Compares the similarities and differences of managers and leaders. Describes the personality, attitudes toward goals, and conceptions of work.*

MOTIVATIONAL 5

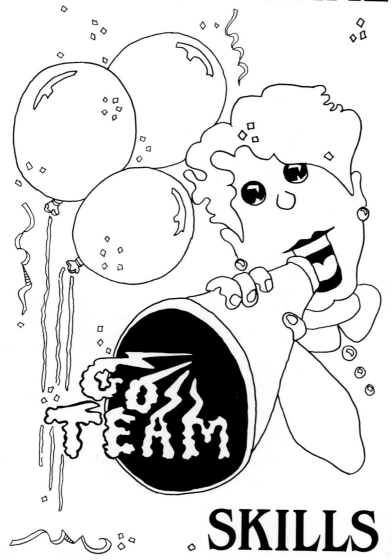

SKILLS

Upon completion of this chapter, the reader will be able to:

1. Define *motivation*.
2. Explain the differences between the words *motivation* and *manipulation*.
3. Compare internal motivators with external motivators.
4. Define Maslow's hierarchy of needs theory.
5. Describe how McClelland's basic needs theory differs from Maslow's theory.
6. Summarize Herzberg's two-factor theory.
7. Apply Skinner's reinforcement theory to the work setting.
8. Explain two basic components of the equity theory.
9. Develop your own theory of motivation based on the above concepts.
10. List three steps for replacing self-defeating attitudes.
11. Examine the following principle: "There are no failures, only outcomes."
12. Describe five steps for motivating yourself.
13. Discuss the value of praise and positive feedback.
14. List four methods to build trust and integrity with your co-workers.

Motivation or Manipulation

Motivation

One of the **most critical skills for effective leadership and management is the ability to motivate others.** A *motive* is a need, desire, emotion, or other impulse that brings about an action. Even the most basic animal, the amoeba, is motivated by the pain–pleasure principle. It moves away from any pain-inducing stimulus and toward food (pleasure). More complex animals, such as domesticated dogs or cats, are motivated to seek out the pleasure of being stroked or petted by humans. People, the most complex of creatures, are motivated by many complicated and subtle drives. Basic motivators are still related to the primary needs of all animals such as thirst, hunger, or fatigue. Man, however, has additional sets of drives. In the work environment, for example, people attempt to satisfy needs for security, socialization, adequate salary, or acceptable working conditions.

Motivation implies action. If the drive, need, or motive is strong enough, action will follow. Think of the last time you were caught in an unexpected rainstorm. The need to keep from becoming soaked provided you with the motivation to act. In this case, the action was to seek cover and remain dry. This example also illustrates the point that many motivators are outside the realm of consciousness. They are not cortically considered but automatically acted upon. All people are influenced to some degree by these underlying motives.

Manipulation

If leaders provide impetus for workers to act or behave in a certain manner, what is the difference, then, between motivation and manipulation? The answer is the *intent* of the leader. Managers who motivate stimulate action to improve patient care, working conditions, efficiency, or organizational goals. The intent is positive—focused toward achieving. Although the leader's needs may be considered, they are not the basis for motivating others. On the other hand, manipulation implies self-interest. By definition, **to manipulate means to influence or manage shrewdly or deviously,** especially for one's own advantage. Therefore, the difference lies with the intentions of the leader. Most people with highly developed motivational skills are willing to influence others only when they believe in their cause.

As you know, the first and primary rule for health care givers is, "Do no harm." If you suspect the patient has a broken hip, you certainly would not force him to walk. Similarly, you would not encourage your team members to complete their tasks in record time if the quality of care would suffer. To differentiate between motivating and manipulating, ask yourself one question, "What are *my* motivations?" If the answer involves a number of I's and me's, perhaps you should reconsider your viewpoint. This simple question, when answered truthfully, provides your basis for differentiating between motivation and manipulation.

Motivational Theories

Remember that a theory is a set of ideas developed to explain something. In this case, the theorists are attempting to explain what directs or motivates people. Knowledge of the more common theories of motivation encourages the nurse leader to think about people's behaviors and act with concern for staff members. (See box on p. 120 for summary.)

Maslow's hierarchy of needs

During the early 1930s, business and industrial leaders began to realize that something more than the paycheck was motivating workers. Early studies, such as the Hawthorne experiments, proved that the emotional climate of the worker was as great a motivator as the paycheck. This led to many ideas about motivating workers. One of the first scientists to consider human needs in relation to the workplace was Abraham Maslow.

MOTIVATIONAL THEORIES

Maslow's Hierarchy of Needs
Based on belief that human needs provide the motivation for individual behavior. These needs are: physical; safety and security; love, affection, and belonging; esteem and status; and self-actualization.

McClelland's Basic Needs Theory
Based on same belief as Maslow's hierarchy but added these needs: achievement, affiliation, and power.

Herzberg's Two-Factor Theory
Based on belief that the need to avoid discomfort and the need to seek out pleasure are the only two motivational factors for individual behavior.

Skinner's Reinforcement Theory
Based on belief that behavior is learned and is most affected by what immediately comes after it. Man instinctively moves toward positive stimuli and away from negative stimuli, hence the need for positive reinforcement.

Equity Theory
Belief that various intangible factors based on personal perceptions motivate individual behavior.

His model of **human needs was based on the thought that needs provide the motivation of the individual's behavior.** Maslow organized needs into five basic categories and placed them in an order (hierarchy) ranging from basic physical needs to the most esoteric psychological needs. The first two levels are referred to as lower-order needs because they involve survival. Higher-order needs include those in levels three, four, and five.

Level one needs. These are the physical needs that must be met in order to survive. These include the need for air, water, food, rest and sleep, temperature maintenance, and physical activity. When these needs are not fulfilled, the individual is in jeopardy of dying, and no other needs matter. For example, if one asks a starving child what his name is, more than likely he will reply, "I'm hungry." A client in the midst of an asthmatic attack is more concerned with breathing than being loved.

Usually, first-level needs are satisfied in workers, but not always. Consider the following example:

Mary Hart, CNA was observed twice in the past month eating the leftover food from patients' dinner trays. This was a direct violation of the rules. When Mary's supervisor, Teresa Nolan, LPN, was informed, she knew that something must be done. Instead of directly confronting Mary, however, she arranged time for a discussion over coffee. During the first 5 minutes of the conversation, Teresa discovered that Mary's husband had moved away 7 weeks ago, leaving three children for her to support on CNA wages. Then to make matters worse, her 10-year-old daughter became ill 4 weeks ago and required hospitalization. She was diagnosed with insulin-dependent diabetes mellitus and would require strict blood sugar monitoring and several daily insulin injections. Because Mary was attempting to cover the costs of the medications and monitoring equipment that were vital to her daughter's health, she decided that she could save money by only eating every other day. Teresa was shocked, but moved, by Mary's plan. She was also very relieved that, by taking the time to investigate the situation, she did not add to Mary's problems by confronting and chastising her.

The moral of the story? Do not assume that because employees show up for work that all their physiological (level one) needs are satisfied. It may prove to be a false assumption.

Level two needs. The needs for safety and security occupy the level two position. Once the basic needs (air, water, food, etc.) are fulfilled, attention will turn to satisfying physical and psychological needs for safety. To be safe is to remain free from the threat or danger of physical harm. It is not enough to *be* safe. One must actually *feel* safe, not only within the physical environment but also within important relationships. A wife who is continually told by her husband that he may become fed up and leave at any time does not feel safe within her relationship.

Once the basic physical needs have been met for today, attention turns toward assuring that these needs will be met tomorrow. To ensure security, our ancestors built cities surrounded by walls, granaries to store food for future use, and 'nest eggs' of valuables to see them through less secure times. Today, pension programs and Social Security are attempts to provide security for working people. Security needs are present in all people, but individuals vary in the amount of security they require. For some, work provides economic security, and a stable job ensures that future needs will be met. Others seek security in relationships. Religious affiliations provide a great deal of security for members. Because security needs are so individual, people will vary in the ways they try to provide security for themselves. One employee may try to become the model worker, while another may seek more education. Both are attempting to meet their need for security. The astute nurse manager is aware of these differences and considers security needs when working with staff members.

Level three needs. Although not imperative for life, the higher-order needs are essential for the well-being of the individual. None of these needs, however, will be recognized until level one and level two (the physical) needs are satisfactorily met. Third-level needs relate to affection, love, and belonging. "According to Maslow, the need for love encompasses both giving and receiving" (Kozier, Erb, 1987). People need love and affection. Without it, depression ensues. Notice how many Americans have pets, for example. Pets provide the focus for many needs, especially for our older citizens. They allow us to give unbridled affection. They are always accepting of our attentions. They give us the opportunity to feel that we are loved and that something belongs to us. Hopefully, needs for love and affection will be met by the relationships that are formed with people, but people will strive to compensate by meeting these needs in any possible way.

Love needs are also fulfilled by belonging to a group. Man is a gregarious animal. Unlike the bear or the polecat, man needs the group. Affiliation with the group provides people with acceptance, self-worth, and opportunities for socialization. Because man is a social animal, he eats, works, and plays in groups. People who are without a primary group (family) will try to meet their needs for love, affection, and belonging through secondary groups. (Refer to Chapter 3.) Many third-level needs are fulfilled by the work group. This is imperative for the nurse manager to recognize and support. The importance of this point is illustrated by the following example:

> Erma and Velda were two CNAs who worked together for years on the skilled wing of a very large and impersonal long-term care facility. They traveled, ate, and worked together. Sally Smart, their team leader, suspected that Erma was covering for Velda's slow pace by completing her work. She decided to separate the two by assigning Velda to a different unit. Within a week after the change, Erma was unable to complete her work assignment, and Velda was threatening to quit. Sally had not been so smart. She forgot the importance of the work group for meeting the belonging needs of both Erma and Velda. Although each still belonged to the work group, the separation brought about a feeling of loss within each worker.

Remember that the work group may be a very important factor in meeting needs for love, affection, and belonging.

Level four needs. After physical and affection needs are satisfied, attention turns to needs for esteem and status. Workers must feel that they have worth (self-esteem), and they want to feel that others think they are worthy (status). Most esteem and status needs are met in the work (or school) setting. In fact, many of today's managers of business and industry are beginning to acknowledge this and develop more appropriate management strategies.

Kate Ludeman, in her book, *The Worth Ethic,* has developed a philosophy for managers. She contends that

> Worth Ethic managers dedicate themselves to building SELF ESTEEM, their own and their employees. They replace political maneuvering with genuine support for risk, innovation, and growth. Worth Ethic employees, thriving in this environment, are free to put forth their best efforts. The result is a multitude of personal contributions that create broad corporate success (Ludeman, 1989).

The nurse manager who respects the value and dignity of each worker will be much more effective in motivating others toward success.

Level five needs. Maslow's highest level concerns self-actualization. Only when all previous needs have been satisfied will the individual focus on becoming self-actualized, and not all people will reach this level of need fulfillment. Just what is self-actualization? It is being the best you can be. It "means becoming all that one is capable of becoming, using one's skills to the fullest, and stretching talents to the maximum" (Davis, Newstrom, 1989). Even people who have achieved this level, though, will never be fully satisfied, for people always strive for more.

Three principles for the nurse manager and leader can be drawn from Maslow's theory. First, need satisfaction is continuous, and the work organization must consider this. Second, workers are "more enthusiastically motivated by what they are seeking than by what they already have" (Davis, Newstrom, 1989). In other words, employees will work to fulfill their needs. Last, no matter which level the worker has achieved, if any lower-order needs become unmet, the focus and energy of the worker will be redirected to meet the more basic need. For example, a staff member is unable to attend classes at the local college (higher-level needs of esteem and self-actualization) because she must work two jobs to support the family (lower-level physical and security needs). Figure 5-1 illustrates the interrelatedness of human needs.

McClelland's basic needs theory

David McClelland expanded Maslow's basic needs theory by adding the needs for *achievement, affiliation,* and *power* and finding that **each need corresponds to certain behaviors.**

Achievement. People trying to meet *achievement* needs usually assume responsibility, take risks, and ask for feedback. These people want to succeed, excel, and make a contribution. Projects with specific tasks and well-defined goals/objectives are suited for the achievement-oriented staff member.

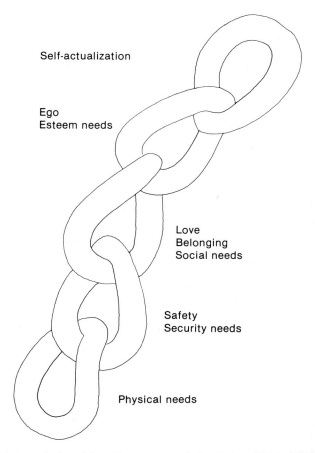

Self-actualization

Ego
Esteem needs

Love
Belonging
Social needs

Safety
Security needs

Physical needs

FIGURE 5-1   The interrelationship of human needs based on Maslow's hierarchy
of needs.

Affiliation. If the worker's need is for *affiliation,* he/she will be a people-
oriented person who needs to work in the human environment. Meaningful relationships with co-workers are important. Affiliation-oriented
workers will avoid making an unpopular decision, but they excel in fostering morale.

Power. Power people are oriented to achieving the objectives, gaining
control, and influencing others. Effective job performance may be secondary to the drive for personal power and prestige. They are appropriate
for unpleasant personnel tasks or when the decision, methods, or objectives chosen would alienate others. The nurse leader will want to consider
these three needs when matching tasks with people.

Herzberg's two-factor theory

An innovative theory of motivation was developed in the mid-1960s by Fredrick Herzberg. In his book, *Motivation and Personality* (1966), he states that workers are motivated by two distinct sets of needs — the **need to avoid discomfort** and the **need to seek out pleasure.** These needs make up a duality in man's nature, and he is continually moving toward pleasurable events and away from pain or discomfort.

This thought led Herzberg to study what daily motivates workers. He found two distinct sets of factors that determined job satisfaction: motivating factors and hygiene factors.

Motivating factors. Factors that satisfied workers were termed *motivators* because of the need to work toward personal growth and self-actualization. These factors provide the stimuli for achievement and gratification of needs. He further divided the factors into first-level and second-level factors. First-level motivators are related to

Achievement: the need to contribute and achieve.

Recognition: to know that one's efforts and abilities are noted and appreciated.

Work itself: a challenging environment that encourages creativity and self-expression.

Responsibility: to be accountable and responsible for performed or delegated responsibility.

Advancement: to improve one's position within the organization.

Possibility of growth: the need to know more than yesterday, to put new knowledge into context, and to maintain one's individuality even when under pressure.

Second-level motivators are important but more subjective. These factors do not promote a sense of growth because they do not provide significant meaning to the worker. They include the group feeling; job security; status; feelings about fairness, unfairness, pride, or shame; and salary. Both first-level and second-level motivators are necessary for workers to achieve their fullest possible potential. Nurse managers can promote an environment that fosters individual development as well as organizational goals by remembering Herzberg's motivators.

Hygiene factors. The dissatisfiers of job satisfaction are related to the work environment. Herzberg called them *hygiene,* or *maintenance,* factors because they are motivated by the need to avoid unpleasantness. He identified first-level hygiene factors as

Company policy and administration. If the organization supports its employees, they are satisfied — even motivated. The absence of supportive policies generates negative feelings toward the company.

Supervision. When supervision is positive and offers opportunities for improvement, workers are encouraged. Conversely, when supervision is task-oriented, workers become frustrated and perform minimally.

Working conditions. Adequate equipment and supplies in addition to a safe work environment are expected. Their absence is a strong dissatisfier.

Interpersonal relationships. If the employee dislikes peers, supervisors, or subordinates, motivation will be low and dissatisfaction high.

Salary. If workers feel they are being adequately paid, salary acts as a motivator. Needless to say, low salaries promote job dissatisfaction.

Personal life. Work has an effect at home, and home has an effect at work. When an employee's personal life is comfortable, he/she is usually motivated at work. The reverse is also true.

Status. Every employee needs status. When little or no status is granted, the employee feels unimportant.

Security. Retirement plans, health insurance, pay advances, and vacations provide no direct worker satisfaction, but without them, workers become strongly dissatisfied.

Hygiene/maintenance factors are incentives that satisfy only lower-level needs. They are short-lived, weak motivators. Workers, however, become dissatisfied when any hygiene factor is inadequate or missing.

Motivators are incentives that help to satisfy higher-level needs. By assessing each team member's motivators and hygiene needs, the nurse manager will be better able to encourage each member to give his/her best.

Skinner's reinforcement theory

B. F. Skinner was a social scientist whose work had a strong impact on many disciplines. His research led to the theory that **behavior is strongly affected by whatever immediately follows it.** Skinner felt that behavior was learned. Following the line of thought that man moves toward positive stimuli and works to avoid negative stimuli, he began to study *reinforcers* — those factors that strengthen or weaken behaviors.

Positive reinforcers. Skinner found that positive reinforcers strengthen a behavior, that a lack of positive enforcers weaken a behavior, and that negative reinforcers will reduce a behavior but teach nothing except how to avoid the reinforcer. Behaviors that are immediately and routinely positively reinforced tend to bring about a more lasting change. Intermittent reinforcers increase the resistance to change, while withholding positive reinforcers leads to a decrease in the behavior. By rewarding the desired behavior positively and frequently, scientists were able to encourage desired behaviors and decrease or even extinguish undesirable behaviors. Other names for Skinner's reinforcement theory are behavior modification and operant conditioning.

Organizational psychologists and other behavioral scientists recognized a powerful method of motivation, and Skinner's theory soon became a part of the people-oriented system for managers. "The major benefit of behavior modification is that is encourages managers to analyze employee behavior, explore why it occurs and how often, and identify specific consequences that will help change it when they are applied systematically" (Davis, Newstrom, 1989). Generalized praise and positive feedback recognizes the employee's worth and encourages better performance.

Techniques. To adapt positive reinforcement techniques to problems, the manager needs to do two things:

1. *Analyze the situation.* Look for anything within the working environment that may interfere with job performance. Consider equipment, supplies, time, pattern of traffic, methods, the system, and the like. If the source of the problem lies in this realm, make every attempt to erase the problem and improve environmental working conditions.
2. *Analyze the worker.* Are the worker's skills and abilities being properly utilized? Are all necessary skills and knowledge in place? Is the worker willing to learn, or would a reassignment be more feasible? What are his/her needs for growth? Once these factors have been identified, the source of the problem should surface. A positive reinforcement strategy can be appropriate when both the nurse manager and the staff member agree to work on a specific behavior, for example, late for work, swearing (see box on p. 128).

The equity theory

During the 1960s, motivational research began to focus on what psychological or intangible factors motivated workers. What did the *employee* feel was important?

Fairness. Jo Stacy Adams, along with other researchers, found that the worker's concept of fairness was an important motivator. The employee compares his/her energy input with the financial, social, and psychological rewards received. This is then compared with other workers. They analyze the *fairness* of their job, then compare the results to others. This process yields one of three results: equity, overreward, or underreward. If the employee feels that his/her energy output (e.g., education, experience, effort, seniority) is equal to the rewards received (e.g., salary, status, working conditions), then everything is equal, and he/she will work at the same level. Employees who feel underrewarded or overrewarded will sense an imbalance and act to restore the balance. Those who believe they are receiving rewards greater than their output may

---

✍ GUIDELINES FOR USING SKINNER'S POSITIVE REINFORCEMENT

1. **Describe the exact behavior to be modified.** E.g., T. C. arrives late for work (15 minutes or more) 4 out of 5 days.
2. **Describe the exact behavioral goal.** E.g., T. C. will arrive for work at 0700 5 out of 5 days (100 percent of the time).
3. **Decide on positive reinforcers.** E.g., Verbal praise, written praise, free lunch at the end of the week.
4. **Encourage steps made toward goal.** E.g., T. C. is 10 minutes late for the first week. Recognize her progress and effort.
5. **Ignore the undesirable behavior,** if possible. Frequently the unwanted behavior will *increase* before it begins to decrease and then fade. Ignoring unwanted behavior helps to decrease both its intensity and frequency. Behavior that is not rewarded becomes extinct. A word of caution here: Use good judgment when deciding which behaviors to ignore. The safety and comfort of the clients is always of first importance.
6. **Try to respond to the desired behavior soon after it occurs.** E.g., if verbal praise from the supervisor is T. C.'s reward for arriving for work on time, the supervisor needs to be there at least a minute early and prepared to greet T. C.
7. **Use positive reinforcers frequently.** Provide plenty of praise and recognition. Focus on the positive attributes of the staff member. It is important to be genuine. Praise that is hollow or given automatically is sensed as insincere and contributes to a loss of respect for the supervisor.
8. **Once the goal has been reached, frequently praise the desired behavior** to reinforce and strengthen it. To summarize Skinner's theory, a behavior is more likely to be repeated if it is followed by a positive (reward) reinforcement.

---

react by working harder, decreasing the value of the reward, or finding someone else for comparison. Employees who perceive they are being underrewarded for their efforts may work less, become less productive, increase the value of the reward, bargain with the administration for more actual rewards, find a new person for comparison, or as a last resort, quit the job.

Perception. A key component of the equity theory is the employee's *perception,* or viewpoint. Nurse managers need to talk with their team members and discover each person's feelings about fairness or equity. Assessing what rewards each worker feels are valuable helps the administration to plan for a high level of performance. The following example demonstrates this point: A large facility wanted to improve productivity, so they raised every staff member's salary. The staff, of which 92 percent were single parents, thought the raise was nice, but what they really wanted was assistance with child care. If the managers had been aware of the value of child care as a reward, they may have been able to provide a more highly valued reward and thus increase motivation. Be alert to employees' feelings of equity.

Commonalities

Thus far, we have surveyed five theories of motivation. Although each theory holds a unique point of view, common threads do exist. First, man is motivated to move toward pleasure and avoid discomfort. Second, employees are more motivated by higher-level needs. Third, people need to feel good about what they do. These are three simple points. Managers and leaders who remember them are better able to positively motivate others.

Self-Motivation Skills

To be a great motivator, one has to be motivated. People are influenced by other people's behavior. To prove this, stand on a busy street and look up. In 2 or 3 minutes, other people will stop what they are doing and look up. There may be nothing in the sky, but if people see one person looking intently, they will imitate or engage in the same behavior. Therefore, the nurse manager needs to feel and act motivated in order to stimulate or excite others.

Self-motivation is a growth process. It requires practice and effort to change one's thinking. Every person has the choice of how to interpret an event. To illustrate this point, a glass of water sits on the table. Two people see it. One views the glass as one-half full, while the other views the glass as one-half empty. Both are correct from their points of view. It is *how* we view the situation that differs, and it is this perception that motivates our behaviors. This is why self-motivation is an important component of effective leadership.

Several techniques to build self-motivation have been developed. Practice these techniques routinely and frequently. The rewards will enrich your personal as well as professional life.

Step one: develop positive thinking

Replace the negative or self-defeating emotions, attitudes, and opinions that have been nearly automatically established. Negative thoughts develop into negative behaviors. The first step toward positive thinking is to *recognize* each negative thought. If, for example, you were just informed that two CNAs called in sick and, therefore, the shift will be short-staffed, how would you view the situation? First reactions may include "Oh, no! How are we going to make it?", or "This is going to be a lousy day." STOP! Replace those self-defeating thoughts with something such as "This will be a challenge," or "Well, here is an opportunity to show our stuff." The shift may not be an easy one, but at least it will be approached with a more upbeat, 'can do' attitude. As Norman Vincent Peale, in his book, *The Power of Positive Thinking,* said, "It's a psychological law that we tend to get what we expect" (1987). Practice recognizing your 'negatives' and replacing them with 'positives.' At least this way, the glass is always one-half full.

Step two: break the low self-esteem cycle

This is another case of the 'glass is one-half empty' syndrome. First, recognize your positive abilities, talents, and attributes. You can afford to be modest with yourself when you are rich and famous, but for now, accept who you are and focus on all that is good about you. Second, picture success. Envision yourself as capable and competent. Give yourself pep talks and pat yourself on the back frequently. Third, take inventory of the day's successes. Perhaps you remained calm during the traffic jam or you finally got Ms. Jones to respond to you. Small successes also are important for a healthy self-esteem. Fourth, practice being successful. Give yourself (and your staff) praise for jobs well done. Reward yourself. Last, but very important, *smile.* When you smile, people smile back in return. Smiles generate positive feelings in every user and receiver.

Step three: conquer fear and anxiety

Remember one short sentence: There are no failures, only outcomes. We cannot learn, grow, or improve without failure. Failure is a component of growth. Watch the child who is learning to write or tie shoes. Adults show patience with the child because they recognize that it takes many failed attempts before an "A" is written or the bow is tied. Allow yourself (and others) this same patience by giving yourself permission to fail. Analyze the possible causes and cures, then move on. Guilt has no place when failure is believed to be a learning opportunity. "The way you cope with failure shapes you—not the failure itself" (Vestal, 1990).

Step four: find meaning in work

As health care workers, our patients, clients, or residents continually remind us of our purpose by their mere existence. We want to provide the best possible care, but often we become engulfed in the task or the goal and lose sight of the real meaning of our work. By giving special meaning to each task we undertake, we make the ordinary work of client care special for each person. This, in turn, increases the meaning in our work.

Step five: perform self-reviews

Identify your own needs, wants, and expectations. Using each of the five motivational theories, objectively assess yourself, both personally and professionally. Clarify your personal standards of integrity. Consider your code of ethics. Ask yourself, "Where do I draw the line between right and wrong behavior?" Knowing one's self offers opportunities for growth. Accepting one's self offers relief from guilt. Liking one's self offers opportunities for motivation.

Motivating Others

Once the nurse supervisor is confident and comfortable with the self, focus can be directed toward motivating others. The **enthusiasm and energy with which the goal, situation, or project is embraced has an important influence** on the employees' level of motivation.

Throughout this chapter, many techniques for motivating people have been presented. Here, six basic points for practicing a positive motivational style will be reviewed.

The winning attitude

Remind yourself every day that everyone wants to be a winner, not a loser. Practice recognizing the winning (positive) characteristics in every employee. Encourage everyone to do their best and be willing to do your best. "As a manager, never underestimate the power of your enthusiasm and example" (Wysenski, 1986).

Praise

Praise is defined as an expression of warm approval or admiration. It is perhaps one of our strongest motivators, as praise recognizes the worth of the worker's contribution. People feel valued when praised. This, in turn, fosters a desire to repeat or improve upon the behavior that was recognized.

Praise also involves respect. By recognizing a job well done, the nurse manager is acknowledging the effort and energy expended by the team member. When employees feel that their jobs are important and their efforts are recognized, respect (for self, others, and the organization) is fostered.

Begin by praising yourself. Look at how you coped with the situation. Then pat yourself on the back for every effective or positive thing. Now list the areas that you would like to improve, without guilt please. Last, praise yourself again for being willing to critically consider the ways in which you will focus for improvement.

In concert with self-praise is praise for others. Children and older folks accept praise with a gracious, matter-of-fact attitude, but most adults like to pretend they do not need it. Everyone from the janitor to the chief administrator of the organization needs praise. However, to be effective, praise must be genuine. Your words become empty if the praise is not sincere. Praise yourself. Praise others. Praise your workers. Praise your supervisors. Be genuine, though, with your expressions of appreciation.

Listen

Active listening is becoming a lost art. (For a more detailed discussion, see Chapter 2.) As a manager, daily communication with staff members is imperative. Just sitting and listening, if done every day, will yield a wealth of information. Staff members must first learn to trust the fact that you are truly interested in them and the problems they face. Then the workers will share their concerns, opinions, attitudes, and the like. Individual employees' needs can be assessed by listening. Possible or actual problems will be discovered, thus providing the nurse manager with opportunities for early interventions. Mutual respect will be engendered through the exchange of information, ideas, and opinions.

Problem-solve with the staff

Supervisors must solve problems. It is part of the job. Many problems that affect staff members require your solution. For example, CNAs working on Wing A usually run out of facecloths by early afternoon. A new shipment is backordered and will arrive in two weeks. What can be done in the meantime? The nurse manager has several options — instruct the laundry to wash an extra load of facecloths in the morning, rent the desired amount until the shipment arrives, instruct the CNAs to use the cloths only for washing faces and use other cloths for hands, etc. The point is that some decisions will be made by the nurse manager. However, whenever possible, all staff members should be encouraged to participate in planning and decision making. Workers who contribute to the decisions that solve their problems have a clearer understanding of the goals and become more motivated to support the changes brought about by implementing each goal. Besides, some of the best and most creative solutions are offered by the staff members most impacted by the problems. See Chapter 9 for a more inclusive discussion of the problem-solving process.

The process. For now, start working with team members to:

1. **Define the problem.** Work on only one problem at a time. Start with a relatively simple problem. Work with the group to clearly define the problem.
2. **List all possible solutions.** Use brainstorming and list any and all solutions offered. Consider no factors other than the problem.

3. **Determine the feasibility of each possible solution.** Now consider each factor that may influence the 'workability' of each solution. Time, money, amount of effort, available resources, and willingness of staff to become involved are examples of factors that need to be considered when weighing each solution.
4. **Choose one solution and try it out.**
5. **Evaluate the effectiveness of the solution.**

This sounds very much like the nursing process. Try this approach with team members next time a problem arises. You will be pleased with the results.

Set clear goals

Goal setting is both an organizational and a motivational tool. Goals allow employees to see where their work efforts are leading. They help focus energies by pointing everyone in the same direction. Attaining goals helps satisfy needs for achievement and esteem. **Goals also stimulate needs for further growth,** for success encourages employees to set even higher future goals.

Goals as motivators. Goal setting is most effective as a motivator when (Straub, Attner, 1991):

1. **The goal is clearly understood and** *accepted* by all staff members. People who were involved in the goal-setting process are more likely to accept and support the goal.
2. **The goal is specific.** Use simple, clear terms to encourage understanding. Goals must be stated in measurable terms and provide targets for measuring progress.
3. **The goal is challenging.** People seem to strive harder to reach a difficult goal, perhaps to fulfill achievement and self-actualization needs. The astute nurse manager ensures that the goal is challenging but achievable. We all want challenge, but we all need success.
4. **Feedback is provided.** Team members need to know how well they are progressing. By applying the specific measurements already determined, workers can judge their performance. This kind of self-generated feedback is a powerful motivational tool.

Build trust and integrity

Integrity is being true to yourself and others. No matter what the title — manager, team leader, or supervisor — your integrity is the basis of genuine leadership. Your staff needs to know that you can be trusted and relied upon to act in their best interests. Trust and integrity are not established overnight. The process takes time and patience. To help guide you, the following suggestions should be frequently reviewed (Husted, Miller, Wilczynski, 1990):

> *Always tell the truth.* People are basically honest, but it sometimes becomes easier or more advantageous to tell a 'little white lie' or break your word. The problem is that people who are not always honest are sabotaging themselves by becoming caught up in their own untruths. The *Wall Street Journal* of July 14, 1992, reported that, according to a recent poll, "about 38% of young adults up to age 30 say corruption and deceit are vital for getting ahead." The only way to reverse this type of thinking is to practice honesty, even with the smallest things. By example, the nurse manager will communicate that honesty is expected and encouraged.
>
> *Keep your word.* Patients and workers remember what is promised. Do what you say you will do. It is the primary rule for building integrity. If you have to break a promise, speak with the persons involved as soon as possible. Putting people off or covering up compromises your integrity.
>
> *Encourage others.* Be willing for others to prosper. Foster growth in others by recognizing each person's positive traits and attributes Envy has no place in people with integrity. It is a destructive (negative), self-defeating emotion which only serves to diminish your own successes. Wish everyone well.
>
> *Practice excellence.* The strongest motivator in the work group is the behavioral example set by the supervisor. **Work to create a climate that encourages excellence** (see Chapter 12). If you set the standards high, your team members will follow your example. If you set your standards low, you will never know what you are capable of doing.

Trust and integrity are the basic ingredients of great managers. Remember: leaders inspire and motivate others by what they *say* and what they *do* more than anything else.

Summary

Motivation is a drive or need to act. People are motivated by many complex needs and drives, including the pain–pleasure principle and the drive to fulfill primary physical needs, as well as more complex security, social, and achievement needs. In the work setting, the nurse manager motivates workers toward achievement. The intent is focused in a positive, rewarding direction. Conversely, manipulation implies influencing people shrewdly for one's own purposes.

Motivational theories are ideas developed to explain what drives or motivates people. Early theories include Maslow's hierarchy, which ordered human needs into five categories, ranging from lower-order survival needs to higher-order needs for self-actualization.

Theorist David McClelland expanded Maslow's work by adding the needs for achievement, affiliation, and power. People attempting to fulfill these needs exhibit specific behaviors and function best when presented with tasks that match their needs.

Fredrick Herzberg's two-factor theory looked at motivation in terms of job satisfaction and found two distinct sets of drives — motivating factors, which stimulate needs for growth and achievement, and hygiene or maintenance factors, which are motivated by the need to avoid unpleasantness or discomfort.

Following this line of thought, B. F. Skinner researched what factors strengthened and weakened a behavior. Positive (reward) reinforcers, when applied immediately and routinely after the desired behavior, tend to strengthen the behavior; few or no positive reinforcers tend to weaken a behavior; and negative (punishment) reinforcers teach avoidance. Skinner's reinforcement theory is also referred to as behavioral modification or operant conditioning theories.

The work of J. S. Adams and others focused on what was important to the employee and found that the employee's concept of fairness, as compared to others, was an important motivator. The equity theory states that employees analyze the fairness of the job, compare it with other jobs, and feel overrewarded, equal (in equity), or underrewarded. If an imbalance is perceived, the employee will attempt to restore balance by engaging in certain behaviors.

All five theories share several commonalities. Knowledge of motivational theories is useful for creating a climate that fosters employees to do their best.

To be a great motivator, one has to be self-motivated. People are drawn toward an upbeat, enthusiastic person. Self-motivation can be developed by practicing techniques that encourage positive thinking, break the low self-esteem cycle, cope with fear of failure, seek out the meaning of work, and encourage self-review.

Motivating others requires energy and enthusiasm. To develop a positive motivational style, leaders and managers need a winning (positive) attitude, trust, and integrity. They also need to praise, to listen, to share clearly defined goals, and to include staff in decision making. One of the most important motivators in any work group is the example set by the leader.

ꙮ Key Concepts

- Motivation is the drive, need, or stimulation to act.
- The equity theory of motivation — workers assess 'fairness' by comparing their work output and rewards with other workers.
- Herzberg's motivation–hygiene theory — five main factors determine job satisfaction and thus become motivators for personal growth. Five main dissatisfiers of the job become hygiene or maintenance factors because of the need to avoid unpleasantness.
- Maslow's hierarchy of needs theory — motivation is the drive to satisfy five basic levels of human needs.
- McClelland's basic needs theory — motivation is the drive to satisfy three basic work needs of achievement, power, and affiliation.
- Skinner's reinforcement theory states that a behavior is more likely to be repeated if it is followed by rewards or positive reinforcement.
- Revising self-defeating (negative) attitudes breaks the cycle of low self-esteem.
- The fundamental principle for overcoming fear is, "There are no failures, only outcomes."
- Identifying personal needs and expectations will help clarify your standards of integrity and develop a personal code of ethics.
- One must be able to motivate the self before motivating others.
- People want to be winners, not losers.
- Respect for the value and dignity of each worker is essential for motivation.
- Leaders motivate others by example.

ꙮ Learning Activities

1. Divide the class into two groups. One group will defend, and one group will challenge the following statement: There are times when manipulation of others is justifiable.
2. For *each* of the five theories of motivation:
   a. List what you think are the advantages and disadvantages.
   b. Describe three ways in which you would apply the theory to the work setting.
3. Discuss what the following statements mean to you:
   a. Find the meaning in work.
   b. There are no failures, only outcomes.
4. Listen to a talk given by a motivational speaker (e.g., Barbara Jordan, Jesse Jackson, Leo Buscaglia, ministers, politicians, salespeople). What techniques did the speaker use to motivate the audience?
5. Assume that you have accepted the position of afternoon nurse at XYZ care facility. You are in charge of a staff of two nurses, seven

nursing assistants, and one housekeeper. Productivity (quality of care) and morale are extremely low when you become the supervisor. Outline a detailed plan to motivate your staff and improve productivity.

References

Davis K, Newstrom J: *Human behavior at work: organizational behavior,* ed 7, New York, 1989, McGraw-Hill.

Herzberg F: *Motivation and personality,* New York, 1966, World Books.

Husted G, Miller M, Wilczynski E: Five ways to build your self-esteem, *Nursing 90* 20(3):152, 1990.

Kozier B, Erb G: *Fundamentals of nursing concepts and procedures,* ed 3, Menlo Park, NJ, 1987, Addison-Wesley.

Ludeman K: *The worth ethic: how to profit from the changing values of the new work force,* New York, 1989, EP Dutton.

Peale NV: *The power of positive thinking,* ed 2, New York, 1987, Prentice-Hall.

Straub JT, Attner RF: *Introduction to business,* ed 4, Boston, 1991, PWS-KENT.

Vestal KW: Failure: making it a positive experience, *AORN Journal* 12(3):111, 1990.

Wall Street Journal, July 14, 1992.

Wysenski NJ: Motivating your staff to do their best, *Nursing Life* 6:52, 1986.

Additional Readings

Barrett GJ: Are you a winner?, *Nursing 90* 20(9):120, 1990. *A short article in which the author describes 10 winning qualities of confident and optimistic people.*

Baur M: Setting goals for success, *Nursing 91* 21(9):88, 1991. *This article describes an easy method for establishing personal and professional goals.*

Chopra A: Motivation in task-oriented groups, *Journal of Nursing Administration* 3:55, 1973. *In an attempt to learn what makes some groups more successful in achieving goals, the author found that motivation and task accomplishment are strongly influenced by the manner in which group members listen, react, and respond to each other.*

Durald MM: Toward positive attitudes and feelings, *Nursing Management* 20(10):64A, 1989. *Ms. Durald offers a formula for channeling negative thoughts, feelings, and self-talk in a positive direction.*

Galarowicz LR: Six steps for keeping your spirit strong, *Nursing 91* 21(1):94, 1991. *Six suggestions for developing energy, optimism, and enthusiasm for your work are discussed.*

Grainger RD: Are you overreacting?, *American Journal of Nursing* 92(3):11, 1992. *Using the theory that thinking can interrupt habitual or automatic behavior, Ms. Grainger offers three techniques for coping with the self-perpetuating behavior of overreacting.*

Hamilton JM, Keiffer ME: Personal power: your key to success, *Nursing 90* 20(10):146, 1990. *The authors offer several hints for fostering the power within yourself to work effectively with others.*

Karshmer JF: Just say yes, *Nursing 90* 20(11):124, 1990. *To build team spirit and accomplish tasks adopt an upbeat, 'can do' attitude.*

Kaye BL: Six paths for development, *Nursing Management* 13(5):18, 1982. *Describes six career options for nurses to consider when planning multiple career goals.*

Kenwood NJ, Martens LC: Morale problems, *Nursing Management* 13(7):37, 1982. *The authors discuss a structured, open-system approach for coping with the internal problems of a nursing unit by channeling individual feelings into group planning and action.*

Migut PJ: Self-care for nurses: assertiveness, *Nursing Management* 13(2):13, 1982. *One of the first steps in motivating others is learning to show confidence in your behavior and decision making.*

Reishstein J: Let's make nursing the visible profession, *Nursing 91* 21(11):148, 1991. *The author strongly feels nurses need to take credit for what they do by sending the message that they are competent, responsible, and helpful.*

Smith J: Managing employee performance, *Nursing Management* 13(8):14, 1982. *Supervisors can increase their effectiveness through the self-examination process.*

Sossong A: Motivating others, *Nursing Management* 13(6):26, 1982. *Identifying and solving attitude problems at the beginning of a task are important tactics for fostering employee motivation.*

CONFLICT RESOLUTION

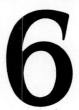

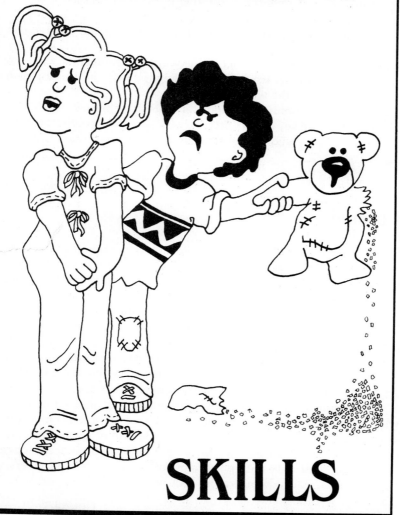

SKILLS

✐ Learning Objectives

Upon completion of this chapter, the reader will be able to:

1. Define *conflict*.
2. Discuss two nursing situations in which conflict occurs.
3. List three disadvantages of applying values or emotions to conflict.
4. Identify five characteristics of a conflict situation.
5. Describe four categories of conflict.
6. Differentiate between intrapersonal and interpersonal conflict.
7. Name 10 guidelines for preventing intragroup conflict.
8. Identify the five phases of a conflict situation.
9. Examine the importance of intervening during the early stages of conflict.
10. List five sources of conflict in the work environment.
11. Describe how the work flow or design affects the development of conflict within the work group.
12. Explain five common methods for resolving conflict.
13. Identify three key factors necessary for successful conflict resolution.
14. Discuss 10 techniques for improving conflict resolution skills.

Conflict Defined

Conflict is a struggle or clash between two or more opposing forces. When an individual or group appears to be benefiting at the expense of others, conflict results. When ideas, values, or interests that seem to be incompatible exist, conflict usually arises. Whenever two or more people work together, the potential for conflict exists. Conflict is an element of life. Every day, each of us copes with conflict. It is an inevitable part of the personal growth and development process.

Because conflict is an unavoidable component of human relationships, it is always found in every work environment. Within most health care organizations, a substantial amount of conflict exists. Complex organizational structures require health care providers to assume numerous roles which can lead to conflict. For example, the nurse's role as employee requires him/her to conserve supplies, but the role of client advocate requires the nurse to provide the necessary supplies to meet needs for care. Nurses also must cope with physicians, other health care providers, clients, families, and administrators. All provide ample opportunity for conflict.

Conflict in itself has no value. Although usually viewed as negative, conflict can be beneficial to organizations. It can be a powerful motivator for positive, innovative change. The key to successfully managing conflict is to analyze the value given to the conflict situation. It is only when people assign an emotion or value to conflict that it becomes a negative experience. When emotions are mixed with the conflict situation, the nurse manager loses perspective and then becomes guided by emotional responses rather than logical thinking. Loss of perspective also colors the interpersonal relationships with those people involved in the conflict. Last, giving values or emotions to conflict stifles creativity and innovation in both workers and managers. Changing your values in relation to conflict is the first and most important step in successfully managing conflict.

Characteristics of Conflict

Conflict creates feelings of tension within the people experiencing it. Because they wish to move away from or relieve the discomfort produced by the conflict, people will engage in various types of behaviors.

Elements of conflict

Not every interaction in which a disagreement exists is a conflict. Diverse points of view and opinions can coexist without discord. Conflict situations have certain characteristics (see box below). Disagreements do not include the 'I win; you lose' component that is present in conflict. The

---

 CHARACTERISTICS OF CONFLICT

1. At least two parties are involved in some form of interaction
2. Differences in goals and/or values either exists or is perceived to exist by the parties involved
3. The interaction involves behavior that will defeat, reduce or suppress the opponent or gain a victory
4. The parties come together with opposing actions and counteractions
5. Each party attempts to create an imbalance or favored power position

From Filley AC: *Interpersonal conflict resolution*, Glenview, Ill, 1975, Scott, Foresman.

---

nurse manager who recognizes the characteristics of conflict can assess the situation and intervene in the early stages.

Categories of conflict

Progressing from simple to complex, four categories of conflict can be identified (Schmidt, Tannenbaum, 1960):

Facts. Differences in the amount, type, or accuracy of information can lead to conflict. In the highly structured settings of the health care profession, factual differences are a common source of conflict. To illustrate, the nurse received information during the change-of-shift report that Mr. Brown was scheduled for an upper GI series at 0800, so she planned to have his morning care completed by 0745. When the x-ray orderly arrived for Mr. Brown at 0700, he was informed that the client was scheduled at 0800. His information, however, showed that the appointment was for 0700. The nurse and the orderly disagreed about the facts. Conflict due to inadequate or inaccurate information can easily be managed by **seeking information from reliable sources.**

Methods. When no one standard or absolute way of doing things exists, conflict can arise from differences in methods. All parties involved in the conflict agree that there is more than one way (method) to meet the goal. It is deciding on the method or procedure to be used that produces the conflict. For example, two nursing assistants are assigned to work together to provide morning care for a group of clients. Assistant A wants one aide to do all the hands and face washing, while the other does all the oral care. The other aide believes that each assistant should provide all the care for half of the clients. The conflict here is between two valid methods of meeting the same goal. **Conflicts involving methods can be minimized by setting guidelines for selecting procedures.**

Goals. Staff members frequently have different goals. When each pursues his/her own goal at the expense of the other, conflict occurs. When a supervisor works hard to contain costs and physicians or staff demand that every possibly needed supply be readily available, conflict results. The supervisor's goal is to control costs; the physician's goal is maximum use of time. Although these goals are in conflict, both the supervisor and the physician share the concern for quality of care. **Identifying the commonalities of each goal helps to provide greater opportunities for managing goal-related conflict.**

Values. Conflict that arises from different values or belief systems is complex and requires a high level of motivation to solve. Agreement is seldom achieved, but rigid positions (right or wrong) should be avoided. The goal in managing values conflict is to **develop an un-**

derstanding and acceptance of the other's beliefs. For instance, a value conflict occurs when the nurse works with a noncompliant client. The client is terminally ill, in obvious pain, and refuses pain medication. The client's value (to be alert throughout the dying process) is in conflict with the nurse's value (to keep the client as comfortable and pain-free as possible). Because conflicts relating to values are complicated and sometimes emotional, nurse managers need to provide support for staff members during conflict situations that involve values.

An important intervention in managing values conflict is 'agreeing to disagree.' This conveys acceptance of the other's viewpoint and paves the way for the next step, finding compatible goals. To return to the example, the nurse could discuss his/her concerns and negotiate with the client to accept pain medication only during the night in order to rest comfortably and still be alert during the day. By considering the categories of conflict, the nurse manager is better able to tailor interventions to each unique situation.

Types of Conflict

Conflict occurs in many areas of life and on several levels. In the work situation nurse managers can experience conflict on vertical, horizontal, or interdepartmental levels (Marriner-Tomey, 1992).

Vertical conflict

Unresolved differences between managers and one or more members of a work group lead to vertical conflict. The perceptions, interests, or values of the individual or group differ to the point where the manager attempts to control staff behavior through the use of position power and bureaucratic rules. Vertical conflict also occurs when the nurse manager clashes with his/her supervisors.

Horizontal conflict

Disputes among staff members over territory, methods, assignments, and the like are considered as horizontal conflict. Because this level of conflict can adversely affect the quality of client care, the nurse supervisor needs to closely monitor horizontal conflict.

Interdepartmental conflict

Health care organizations have wide ranges of specialized personnel all gathered together in one large work group focused on providing client

---

〰️ INTRAPERSONAL CONFLICT CLASSIFICATION

1. **Motivation.** Discord relating to motivation arises from conflicting goals. The staff nurse who wants to become a supervisor but is threatened by the associated responsibility is an example of a motivational conflict.
2. **Choice.** "Choice conflict arises out of a lack of the information necessary to make a decision" (Lewis, 1976). Without adequate data, uncertainty about the consequences of each choice occurs. The staff nurse who is considering a new position does not know what to expect in the new role (lack of information) and is, therefore, uncertain of which choice to make illustrates the idea of an intrapersonal conflict relating to choice.
3. **Allegiances.** Conflicting allegiances arise from loyalty to two or more groups. The newly appointed nurse manager who feels loyalty to the work group now has new allegiances to the administration. Differences between groups may test loyalties and produce conflict.

From Adams RH, Applegeet CJ: Managing conflict: techniques managers can use, *AORN Journal* 46(6):116, 1987.

---

care. The interdependence among departments demands cooperation and collaboration. If attitudes, values, or goals differ sufficiently, conflict occurs. Also, the personalities and status of the involved individuals have an impact on the conflict situation.

Intrapersonal conflict

Discord or dissention within an individual occurs when one is faced with two or more incompatible demands. There are three classifications of intrapersonal conflict: motivation, choice, and allegiances (see box above).

Interpersonal conflict

Interpersonal conflict, the most frequent type of conflict, occurs between two or more individuals. Health care facilities are dynamic, intense, and complex environments. People are constantly interacting and, in many instances, disagreeing. Interaction can lead to two kinds of interpersonal conflict: issues conflict and personal conflict (Schulz, Johnson, 1990).

Issues conflict. When people disagree on the issues (e.g., facts, methods, goals, policies, etc.) the conflict is usually not personal but the result of each individual acting as an advocate for his/her work group.

Personal conflict. Differences in values, attitudes, and personalities can result in personal antagonisms. Because they deal with emotions, personal conflict can escalate if left unattended.

Intragroup conflict

Discord within an established group occurs regularly. "Conflict is necessary to assist teams [groups] in considering new ideas, approaches, contemplating moves forward, growth and change. Conflict needs to be managed and resolved to the team's advantage" (Neuhaus, 1990). Common causes of intragroup conflict are included in the box below.

Group leaders should not avoid or stifle conflicts within the group but should manage and focus them in productive directions.

Prevention guides. One of the best methods for **managing intragroup conflict is preventing the group from polarizing around such unproductive issues as personalities, philosophies, or styles** (see box on p. 146).

✐ CAUSES OF INTRAGROUP CONFLICT

1. **New Problems.** Changes in roles and relationships within the group are often required to solve new problems.
2. **Lack of Support.** If group members are not respected and recognized for their efforts, group cohesiveness fades. The group then becomes unable to accomplish its objectives.
3. **Imposed Values.** When outside values are imposed upon the group, conflict results. To illustrate, most nurses value the quality of care, while most administrators value the timeliness of care. This fosters conflict within work group members. Some team members will pursue the administration's value and strive to reduce the time required to perform client care tasks, while other group members will ignore time frames and focus on meeting as many client care needs as possible.
4. **Role Conflict.** Intragroup conflict can be the result of a member's intrapersonal discord. When an individual's role outside the group disagrees with his/her role inside the group, the impact is felt by all group members.
5. **Negative Emotions.** Feelings of dislike, competition, and jealousy can foster serious intragroup conflicts. Incompatible hidden agendas and self-serving roles also cultivate strife.

GUIDELINES TO PREVENT CONFLICT

1. The group should work hard to keep open its internal channels of communication.
2. Dissent must be depersonalized. The ground rule is that members of the group are allowed and even encouraged to address the issue but not to attack other members.
3. Each member needs to try to "look inside" the other's frame of reference, to understand his point of view.
4. The door must be left open for creative and meaningful participation by every member of the group.
5. Members of the group must have new opportunities to invest themselves in the goals.
6. The group should seek agreement on specific short-term goals.
7. Diversity must be recognized and accepted.
8. A sense of mutual trust must be cultivated.
9. Grievance mechanisms need to be established.
10. Events that have a paralyzing effect — real roadblocks — need to be recognized and dealt with.

From Schaller LE: *The change agent*, New York, 1972, Abingdon Press.

Intergroup conflict

Health care organizations are comprised of many interdependent, specialized, and diverse groups. Levels of authority and power differ with each group, which, along with other differences, lead to conflict between groups. Intergroup conflict exists when one group achieves its goals at the expense of the other group. In the health care setting, conflict can occur among groups within a unit or department or among departments. Nurse and physician groups have historically disagreed on many issues.

Sources. Conflict among groups usually arises from differences in role expectations, value systems, and communications (Douglas, Bevis, 1983). Competition for resources, time, recognition, and the like can produce intense conflict.

Management. Intergroup management of conflict usually resolves in one of three ways:

1. Dominance of one group over another.
2. Compromise, which is frequently unsatisfying for either group.

3. Integration of goals, which occurs when each group recognizes the other's role within the system.

Intergroup conflict does not have to be negative. On the contrary, it **"can stimulate creativity, innovation, and progress** [emphasis added]. A conflict-free organization suggests stasis, a situation that offers little challenge for group members" (Marriner-Tomey, 1992).

Health care providers commonly experience several types of conflict at one time. Conflicts relating to internal issues, clients, staff members, or superiors can challenge or demoralize an individual. It is important for you, the nurse manager, to identify the type of conflict that is being experienced. This knowledge will assist you in solving the problems that are at the source of the conflict.

Phases of Conflict

The process of conflict moves through several phases. A. C. Filley (1975) developed a model for explaining how conflict develops and resolves. Filley's five stages of conflict are anticipation, perceived conflict, manifest conflict, conflict resolution, and conflict aftermath.

Anticipation

The group or individual begins to develop an awareness of discomfort. Emotions such as unfocused anxiety, tension, hostility, or anger begin to surface. These sentiments are often described as a 'hunch,' or a feeling, that something is not right. The anticipation phase is also referred to as the latent stage of conflict.

Reactions. At this stage of conflict, the group or individual can cope with the discomfort by

- ignoring the emotions generated in relation to the conflict,
- gathering more information, or
- preparing to do battle.

The discomforts associated with this stage also involve stress. Because the source of anxiety can not yet be identified, the fight-or-flight response is triggered in the individual. This has an effect on the group's interactions. Managers who recognize these emotions and their resulting behaviors in staff members are better equipped to provide early and, thus, more effective interventions.

Perceived conflict

When the anxieties and emotions are strong enough to reach the cognitive or thinking level, an awareness of a stressful situation exists. Each involved person experiences the problem and is able to identify it, but no one will talk about it. These unexpressed differences affect the morale and productivity of the group.

Reactions. Defense mechanisms are sets of behaviors used to cope with unpleasant situations. Because the conflict situation is not acknowledged, the person or group experiencing the discord may react in the following ways:

> **Increase work efforts.** Throwing one's self into work provides temporary relief and increases productivity, but it does not solve the problem. This defense is called 'flight into activity.'
> **Rationalize.** Providing acceptable explanations for undesirable behaviors allows the user of this defense mechanism to continue engaging in the behavior without guilt because it has been justified. The nursing assistant who does not record the client's oral intake because "no one else does it" is an example of rationalization.
> **Displace.** Displacement moves the emotions and behaviors from the source of the conflict to a more acceptable outlet. To illustrate, the staff had a hectic day. The weather was bad, and the patients seemed cranky. During the afternoon staff meeting, a group of members became argumentative and hostile. Because staff members had experienced conflict earlier in the day and it was unacceptable to argue with the patients, they displaced their feelings to their peers during the meeting.
> **Physical symptoms.** If the group or individual perceiving the conflict remains in this stage long enough, physical manifestations such as tension headaches, GI disturbances, or hypertension may result.

The most important intervention at this phase is to move those involved in the conflict toward the next stage of open discussion.

Manifest conflict

Overt behaviors characterize this stage. People begin to openly discuss and react, either constructively or destructively. Perceptions may be accurate or inaccurate, and individuals may personalize the situation. Feelings and attitudes also affect the conflict situation.

Reactions. People react individually to conflict situations, but their general reactions progress as follows:

Discussion. The individuals or groups begin to openly talk about their differences. The discussion can be depersonalized and focused on the problem or focused on individuals, personalized, and emotionally charged.

Open dispute. This is the 'battle preparations' stage. Those experiencing the conflict now openly acknowledge its existence, choose sides, and take positions on the issues. Each side works to amass power by attempting to convince others that their point of view is the 'right' one.

Open conflict. By now, the individual or group has assumed rigid positions relating to the issues. Negotiation is not an option. Taking sides is completed, and the battle begins. A win-lose situation is established if constructive intervention is not immediately undertaken.

Conflict resolution

The conflict resolution process will follow one of three paths: win-lose, lose-lose, or win-win.

Win-lose. In this situation, one side 'wins' by dominating the other side through the use of superior power. One group or person is satisfied, while the others are not. Members of the 'losing' side may feel hostility and resentment. Future interactions may also be affected. The solution may resolve the conflict temporarily, for those who lost may become frustrated and unwilling to make the solution work.

Lose-lose. With a lose-lose resolution, neither side is willing to objectively consider the other's ideas. The conflict is resolved through the use of avoidance, bribery, coercion, threats, or withdrawal. The conflict remains basically unresolved, and neither side is satisfied with the outcome. Members of both groups are likely to feel frustrated and angry.

Win-win. An outcome that satisfies both sides is the main characteristic of a win-win process. Conflict becomes constructive through the use of "open and honest dialogue to examine ideas until decisions are produced that are satisfying to all participants" (Douglas, Bevis, 1983). All involved individuals collaborate to mutually set goals or develop solutions that are satisfying and supported by everyone. Although the decision may take longer to implement, the potential for success is much greater because all sides are enthusiastic and willing to work.

Conflict aftermath

Once the conflict appears to be on the road to resolution, the emotional level drops, and participants are more able to **examine the conflict situation.** To use conflict aftermath as a tool, consider the following:

Sources. Identify the basic causes of the conflict. Develop strategies or methods for eliminating or reducing the sources.

Process. Ascertain if the conflict was handled in a constructive or disruptive manner. Devise possible ways to cope with personalities whose behaviors influence the group negatively.

Outcome. Was the conflict managed to everyone's satisfaction? If not, assess the strategies used be each side to resolve the conflict. Identify what affect the group's or individual's behavior may have had on the outcome of the situation.

After an analysis of these three factors, use the data to formulate new attitudes and approaches for managing future conflicts. Each successfully managed conflict experience builds confidence and abilities and prepares you for the next situation.

Sources of Conflict

Conflict can arise from any source. Because each person defines a situation differently, **conflict occurs when a person or group** *perceives* **or believes a conflict exists.** In health care settings, many opportunities for disagreement exist. Nurse managers can often track the source of the conflict to one or more of the following.

Resources

Resources include everything necessary to do the job. They relate to work space, equipment, supplies, salaries, budget allocations, and recognition for work. Too many or too few staff members or inadequate or improper equipment or supplies all serve to create tension within staff members that may eventually progress to conflict.

Competition

Competition is a form of conflict that follows definite rules. Our society generally values competitive behaviors. However, true competition is characterized by an impersonal struggle. Athletes, for example, will be fierce competitors during the event and close friends afterward.

Competition is power-oriented, aggressive, and uncooperative. It implies struggle, winners, and losers. "It is argued that competition strengthens performance and increases cohesiveness within each individual group, and this does happen. After the competition is over, however, only one person or group is the winner and likely to remain satisfied and cohesive. The defeated individual or group may seek an opportunity for retaliation" (Douglas, Bevis, 1983).

Differences

Genuine disparities exist because of the unique nature of each individual. Some differences may be incompatible and, therefore, lead to conflict. Cultural differences, for example, influence one's concept of work, change, and interpersonal interactions. Revealing personal feelings is easy for some people. Others, because of their cultural heritage, may view the demonstration of emotions as a sign of weakness or lack of control. Other incompatible differences may be due to values, beliefs, experience, education, or unresolved prior conflicts. When differences appear to be legitimately incompatible and unresolvable, persons involved in the conflict usually agree to accept and live with each other's dissimilarities. Good listening skills are especially important here.

Roles

When the expectations of two or more roles clash, role conflict occurs. Every mother has experienced role conflict when she must work while her child is ill. In the work setting, both staff members and supervisors experience role conflicts. Nurses continually cope with the conflict of providing individualized, high-quality client cares within the time and resource limits of the organization.

Types of role conflict. Within the work environment, several types of role conflict exist. The box on p. 152 describes six types of role conflict.

Work design and flow

The structure of the work environment as well as the way work is organized can have a strong impact on relationships. When people get in each other's way, the opportunity for conflict increases. Watch the flow of traffic in and out of commonly used spaces (e.g., utility rooms, nursing station, chart area). Assess the use of work spaces. Small improvements in traffic flow can reduce the potential for conflict.

Observe the daily routine. Are there times when the staff members are running hectically one minute then sitting with nothing to do the next minute? Are several departments' staff requiring time with the patient simultaneously? For example, do the diet trays arrive during bath time? Changes in procedures or routines should involve those who actually do the work. Involving all parties can minimize conflict and improve performance.

Miscommunication

Perhaps the most common source of both personal and professional conflict, miscommunication results when messages are not clearly received or understood. Remember that communication is what is received, not what is sent. Messages can be clearly and succinctly sent, but the communication is incomplete until the message is received and understood.

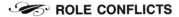 **ROLE CONFLICTS**

1. ***Intrasender*** conflict occurs when the sender gives conflicting messages or expects contradicting behaviors. The manager who demands a higher quality of nursing care and then refuses to provide sufficient personnel exemplifies intrasender conflict.
2. ***Intersender*** conflict arises when the person receives conflicting messages from two or more sources. This frequently occurs when one nurse instructs a CNA to do one thing, and then, moments later, another nurse wants the CNA to follow his/her instructions.
3. ***Interrole*** conflicts commonly occur when people belong to more than one group. Personal roles such as spouse, parent, child, and relative often conflict with professional and work roles. Nurse managers assume multiple roles within the work organization. Here, interrole conflicts can arise from loyalties to the work group, responsibilities, time requirements, and role expectations. Learn to develop a system of trade-offs. It will help to decrease the impact of interrole conflicts.
4. ***Person–role*** conflict results from differences between one's internal perceptions and expectations and the external role. This is the source of conflict responsible for many 'burned out' nurses. The health care provider who highly values psychosocial care will surely suffer person–role conflict when working in a large, impersonal clinic with a high patient turnover. Expectations that exceed the individual's current knowledge or skill level also foster person–role conflict. Leaving a CNA in charge of a unit while the nurses go to dinner together illustrates this point.
5. ***Role ambiguity*** results from unclear, or ambiguous, expectations. When an individual does not know what is expected in order to do the job, role ambiguity develops. "Inadequate job descriptions, incomplete explanations of assigned tasks, rapid technological change, and the increasing complexity of organizations contribute to role ambiguity and produce uncertainty and frustration."
6. ***Role overload*** results when the individual or group is simply unable to meet all the expectations of various roles.

Modified from Marriner-Tomey A: *Guide to nursing management,* ed 4, St Louis, 1992, Mosby.

Communication barriers are those factors that limit or impede understanding. Cultural, social, educational, and language differences all affect communications. Generalists, such as nurses, can disagree with specialists, such as dieticians.

Miscommunications can lead to a perceived threat. When a group or individual has an inadequate understanding, the uncertainty becomes a threat to the status quo, and conflict is the inevitable result. Review Chapter 2 for techniques to decrease miscommunications and reduce this source of conflict.

Conflict Management

Objectives

Conflict can be a positive experience if it leads to growth and understanding. When individuals or groups are able to **consider various alternative solutions to the conflict situation and select a mutually acceptable course of action, conflict is constructive.** If, however, an excess of dysfunctional energy is being expended, strategies to manage disruptive, interpersonal conflict must be implemented. Managers, supervisors, and team leaders who perceive conflict as a naturally occurring challenge will be more effective with its management. The experienced nurse manager will intervene early in the conflict and encourage the mature expression of differences and resolution of problems before the conflict situation becomes uncontrollable and does irreparable damage. According to Neuhaus (1990), "The object of any conflict resolution technique should be to enable all members to feel that they have emerged from the conflict situation successful." Every person involved should have a role in resolving the conflict.

Consequences

Conflict situations can result in both positive or negative outcomes, depending on the communication process and behaviors of the involved individuals. Possible consequences of conflict within the work environment are as follows (Douglas, 1992):

Recognition of issues. By fostering open and honest communications, the nurse manager is openly identifying and discussing issues that may later become a source of conflict.

Improved group cohesion. When intergroup conflict faces a group, its members tend to ignore former disagreements and close ranks to present a united front. This cohesion can result in positive or negative group behaviors.

Changes in performance. Conflict can improve productivity when the worker feels challenged and respected for his/her opinions. Conversely, extremely passive individuals who are afraid to 'rock the boat' may repress the conflict and accept the status quo. Eventually these repressed feelings will evolve into less productivity and a lower work performance.

Leadership changes. During the conflict situation, a new leader may emerge from the group. Possibly the conflict brought to light the talents and abilities of an individual who may not otherwise have been recognized.

Understanding. Successfully experiencing conflict promotes a deeper understanding of other people's beliefs, values, attitudes, and viewpoints. This understanding can provide personal enrichment as well as foster an acceptance of the validity of individual differences.

The process

Effective conflict management follows an orderly process which is much like the nursing process. Procedures used by the nurse manager to manage conflict include prevention, assessment, diagnosis, interventions, and evaluation (Tappen, 1989).

Prevention. By taking steps to **prevent conflict,** the manager is able to reduce the number of possible situations that may lead to conflict. Especially helpful preventative techniques focus on creating a work environment that respects individual differences and encourages a free exchange of various ideas. Meeting the needs of individual staff members before a conflict develops also helps to reduce the potential for discord.

Assessment. The first step in **assessing a conflict** situation is to recognize and accept its existence. The nurse manager then gathers data in order to establish a conflict diagnosis (Cushnie, 1988). To define the conflict situation, the nurse manager assesses the following:

- **Category of conflict** — facts, methods, goals, and values associated with the situation
- **Type of conflict** — intrapersonal, interpersonal, intragroup, intergroup, horizontal, or vertical
- **Phase of the conflict** — anticipation, perception, overt conflict, resolution, aftermath
- **Sources** — resources, differences, competition, miscommunication, work organization, and design

Diagnosis. The data obtained from assessing each element of the situation allow the nurse manager to identify and define the problems which lie at the source of the discord. This **'conflict diagnosis'** can be used as a basis for specific interventions, which can be tailored to a certain element of the conflict.

Interventions. Several methods or strategies are utilized to manage conflict. Seeking areas of agreement and generating acceptable solutions are effective resolution strategies for many conflicts.

Evaluation. The aftermath phase of the conflict process provides an opportunity to assess the effectiveness of the interventions and identify areas and methods that could be improved. Learning to assess the elements of a situation and formulate a conflict diagnosis requires practice, but it is well worth the energy. Actually, the supervisor with effective conflict management skills saves time and energy by diagnosing conflict and intervening during the early stages.

Interventions

The emotions generated by conflict produce tension and a sense of imbalance within the individual or group. If the stimuli is sufficiently intense, the 'fight–flight' (stress) reaction will be triggered. As a result, the person(s) involved in the conflict will attempt to manage or resolve the conflict situation by using one of the following strategies, approaches, or interventions.

Avoidance. Behaviors relating to avoidance include denial of the conflict, ignoring it, repression, and withdrawal. Avoidance methods are unassertive and uncooperative and commonly lead to a lose-lose outcome. "This approach may be appropriate when the other party is more powerful, the issue is unimportant, one has no chance of meeting his/her goals, or the cost of dealing with the conflict is higher than the benefits of the resolution. It may also be used when it is more appropriate for others to solve a problem, when more information is needed, or when one wishes to reduce tension and gain composure" (Marriner-Tomey, 1992).

Accommodation. Commonly referred to as "smoothing things over," accommodation focuses on areas of agreement while downplaying differences. Behaviors include complimenting, finding small similarities, and acting as though little disagreement exists. Accommodation is an unassertive, self-sacrificing technique that usually results in a win-lose outcome. It is an appropriate conflict resolution style when the issue is of greater importance to someone else, the other side is more powerful, or preserving harmony or networking is a more significant issue. Although the conflict may be soothed, accommodation tactics seldom address or solve the underlying problems.

Competition. Most competitive situations are assertive, uncooperative, and orientated toward the use of power to gain at the expense of others. A win-lose situation is created. Emotions frequently run high when competition is used to manage conflict, and the 'loser' is likely to be permanently alienated. However, in some situations, competition can be an effective approach. When a quick resolution is needed, an unpopular decision must be made, or neither side is willing to concede anything, competition is useful. When the other side is determined to make you lose or protection from other aggressive people is needed, competition is employed. Competition strategies may resolve the conflict, but not everyone is satisfied. The nurse manager who uses this method too frequently will find staff members unwilling to admit mistakes or offer new ideas or opinions.

Compromise. Bargaining is the behavior that characterizes this approach to conflict management. Compromise involves assertiveness and cooperation. All involved parties are willing to work for mutually acceptable solutions by giving and taking a little. Making concessions may reduce the conflict, but it produces a lose-lose result because each side must 'lose' on one point to 'win' on another. As a result, neither side 'wins.' Compromise usually requires time, for the give-and-take process is specific for each issue. It is a useful approach in long-term situations where both sides desire resolution but cannot find a way to win. In situations where both parties have an equal amount of power or a decision must be immediately made, compromise is appropriate. "From a management point of view, compromise is a weak resolution method because the process usually fails to reach a solution that will best help the organization to reach its goals" (Douglas, 1992). Hopefully, compromise can be used as the first step toward collaboration and problem solving.

Collaboration. One of the most difficult but effective approaches to managing conflict is cooperative problem solving. It is an assertive, cooperative, and constructive method which results in a win-win situation. Individuals on both sides of the conflict agree to problem-solve in order to arrive at mutually satisfying outcomes. All involved individuals identify the problems, explore alternatives and consider the ramifications of each possible option until solutions are reached and difficulties resolved. People must work to establish an environment that promotes a sense of trust and commitment. Open and honest discussions of facts and feelings as well as clear definitions of problems, values, purposes, and goals are necessary for collaboration to be effective. The one disadvantage of this conflict resolution technique is that it takes time, sometimes more than the results are worth. Collaboration is most effective when both parties have equal power, time to work through the process and wait for an agreeable resolution, a strong commitment, and trust.

Managing group conflict

The nurse manager as group leader can keep conflicts productive by remembering the **three tasks for resolving group conflict productively: support, clarify, and negotiate** (Sampson, Martha, 1977).

Support. Support the group during the process of disagreeing. Keep the group focused on the task. Do not allow emotional comments to dominate the interactions. When group members feel that they can disagree openly and freely, problem solving is encouraged, integrity remains intact, and members have the opportunity to discover different ideas. Let the group know you feel disagreements are healthy. As the leader, you set the tone or create the atmosphere. By supporting different points of view, you are facilitating healthy group interactions and respecting the worth of each individual member.

Clarify. Second, the leader helps to define the source of the conflict in clear, objective terms. This is a great tool for keeping the conflict focused on the topic and removing emotional overtones. For example, the nurses on two different shifts are clashing over which shift should be responsible for totaling intake and output records. By asking each party to present their definition of the problem and reasons for their positions, the basis for the conflict can be discovered. In this case, the group discovered that one shift had recently assumed responsibility for reviewing all the documentation in the client's record for the past 24 hours. Adding a new chore seemed unfair. Upon learning this, the group was able to discuss the situation and negotiate for an acceptable solution.

Negotiate. The last task of the group leader when dealing with conflict is negotiation. A good collaborator is able to move the group from opposing sides to the middle. The middle is the compromise solution. Where should one start when people are in opposition of each other? The first and most important technique is to *focus* on *what they have in common.* By emphasizing what is shared rather than the differences, the group has a starting point for discussion. Concentrate on the goal and creatively explore all possible options. As the group works, positions or points of view will change, and solutions will be found.

Key factors

Each conflict situation evolves under a unique set of circumstances and, thus, requires a uniquely tailored solution. To successfully manage conflict, certain elements must be present (or established) in the situation, regardless of the conflict diagnosis. These include commitment, communication, and trust.

Commitment. Every individual must be resolved to work toward a mutually acceptable solution, behave responsibly when emotionally affected by the conflict situation, and actively participate in problem-solving processes. When people are committed, they are more willing to recognize and confront the issues relating to the conflict.

Communication. During a conflict situation, it is especially important to maintain open communication lines. Encourage a thorough discussion of both positive and negative emotions and opinions, but keep the talk focused on and limited to the topic. Do not allow personal attacks. Find the similarities and concentrate on moving both sides toward the middle ground.

Trust. If all sides are committed to resolving the conflict and open communications are well established, trust will be fostered. Those involved in the conflict must also trust the premises that

1. a mutually acceptable solution exists,
2. a mutually acceptable solution is desirable,
3. statements made by others are truthful and legitimate, and
4. differences of opinions are helpful (Douglas, Bevis, 1983).

Include the elements of commitment, communication, and trust in the conflict assessment. Work to establish these within the environment before and during the conflict situation because a positive environment facilitates effective conflict resolution.

Helpful hints

Because each conflict is a dynamic and unique situation, no single method or strategy is best for every situation. The nurse manager's approach to conflict creates a climate for resolution that affects all other staff members. To practice effective conflict management skills, consider the following suggestions:

Identify the conflict. Make sure that all parties recognize that conflict exists. Have each side define the problem from their point of view. Clarify the issues.

Find the balance of power. Ascertain if one party holds an unequal amount of power. When both sides share power equally, collaboration is encouraged. Promote an equal balance of power by meeting in a neutral location or having representatives meet in lieu of the entire group.

Force communications. Use the communication technique of paraphrasing (see Chapter 2) to ensure understanding. Have the receiver repeat the sender's message until the sender is satisfied that his/her message (feelings, opinions) have been heard and understood. Promote clarification. Many times people actually agree and find that conflict does not really exist. The problem was with the communication.

Recognize human needs. Each person needs to be treated with respect and dignity. Treating others as you would like to be treated fosters many more opportunities for productive conflict management.

Handle your emotions. It is the viewpoint or perception you choose that determines your emotional reactions. Do not react; respond. If anxiety or anger develops, deal with it by recognizing and taking responsibility for your feelings. Use the suggestions in Chapter 1 to positively cope with emotions.

Problem-solve. Create a problem-solving situation out of a conflict situation. Work with all involved persons to identify the problems and their solutions. Prevent each side from threatening, attacking, or coercing the other.

Strengthen self-respect. Focus on specific behaviors, not personal motives. Use a positive approach when dealing with individual feelings and ideas. Use gentle humor to break the tension.

Allow experiments. Encourage each party to propose experimental solutions, then consider the ramifications of each proposal and try it. Some of the most creative solutions to conflict started as experiments.

Project into the future. Use role playing to consider the consequences of each proposed solution. To gain an understanding of the other viewpoint, have those involved in the conflict role play the opposite position.

Follow through. Keep your word and do what you say you will do. Follow-up provides the people involved in the conflict with information and feedback that may prove useful for evaluating resolution methods or planning new strategies.

Be patient with yourself. As with any skill, conflict management improves with practice. Use the conflict management checklist in Figure 6-1 to practice applying the nursing process to conflict situations. Nurse managers with highly developed conflict resolution abilities contribute to more satisfying, effective work relationships. As Filley (1975) so aptly reminds us, "The opposite of conflict is problem solving."

I. Assessment

Type of Conflict

_____ intrapersonal
_____ interpersonal
_____ intragroup
_____ intergroup
_____ vertical
_____ horizontal
_____ interdepartmental

Phase of Conflict

_____ anticipation
_____ perceived conflict
_____ open conflict
_____ resolution
_____ aftermath

Source of Conflict

_____ resources
_____ miscommunications
_____ competition
_____ roles
_____ differences
_____ facts
_____ methods
_____ goals
_____ values

Level of Trust

_____ commitment
_____ communications

II. Planning

Conflict Diagnosis: (define problem) _____

_____

Expected Outcome: _____

_____

III. Intervention
(circle one or more) Avoidance
                     Accommodation
                     Competition
                     Compromise
                     Collaboration

IV. Evaluation   Causes: _____

_____

                        Process: constructive, destructive
                        Outcome: satisfactory, unsatisfactory
                        Resolution: win-win, lose-lose, win-lose
                        New Strategies: _____

_____

Comments: _____

_____

FIGURE 6-1   The nursing process applied to conflict situations.

ℐ Key Concepts

- Conflict is a struggle or disagreement between two or more opposing forces.
- Conflict is an inherent part of daily life.
- It is the value we give to conflict that determines our behaviors.
- Conflict is an inescapable component of the nursing profession.
- Five characteristics of a conflict situation are the interaction, the differences, a win-lose situation, opposing actions, and struggle for power.
- Conflict among health care workers can arise from differences in facts, methods, goals, values, and roles.
- Conflict can occur within one's self (intrapersonal), between people (interpersonal), within a group (intragroup), or among groups (intergroup).
- The best method for coping with intragroup conflict is prevention.
- The process of conflict proceeds through the phases or stages of anticipation, perceived conflict, open conflict, resolution, and aftermath.
- It is important for the nurse manager to recognize and intervene during the early stages of the conflict process.
- Sources of conflict within the work environment are related to miscommunications, roles, differences among people, work flow or design, and resources.
- Common conflict management techniques include avoidance, accommodation, competition, compromise, and collaboration.
- Application of the nursing process to the conflict situation results in a 'conflict diagnosis,' which is useful for planning management resolution strategies.
- Successful resolution of conflict requires communication, commitment, and trust.

ℐ Learning Activities

1. Discuss your opinion of the following statement: "Conflict in itself has no value." Do you agree or disagree? Why?
2. List three conflicts you have experienced. For each experience (conflict situation):
   a. identify the type.
   b. review how the process moved through each phase of the conflict.
   c. identify the source.
   d. describe the management technique you used to resolve the conflict.
   e. evaluate the effectiveness of the technique.
   f. list one way in which you would handle the situation differently as a result of reading this chapter.

3. Scenario: You are working as a team leader for ABC facility. The administration has decided to computerize its payroll system and has a choice of programming the system for weekly or bimonthly paychecks. The decision will be made by the staff. Divide the group into two sides. One group feels strongly about weekly paydays. The other group feels just as committed to bimonthly paydays. Allow 5 minutes for each side to convince the other that their way is best. After 10 minutes, stop the action and examine your emotions (feelings) about the conflict situation.

4. Divide the group into five sections. Using the scenario described in activity #3, resolve the conflict (solve the payday problem). Group 1 will use avoidance. Group 2 will use accommodation. Group 3 will compete. Group 4 will compromise. Group 5 will use collaboration. Each group is limited to 5 minutes. After each method has been applied, describe:
   a. what you felt while using the technique.
   b. what was most and least effective about the technique.
   c. which technique you found most effective.

5. Apply the nursing process, including a conflict diagnosis, to the scenario described in activity #3. Is it a more effective method? Why?

References

Adams RH, Applegeet CJ: Managing conflict: techniques managers can use, *AORN Journal* 46(6):116, 1987.

Cushnie P: Conflict: developing resolution skills, *AORN Journal* 47(3):734, 1988.

Douglas LM: *The effective nurse leader and manager*, St Louis, 1992, Mosby.

Douglas LM, Bevis OE: *Nursing management and leadership in action*, ed 4, St Louis, 1983, Mosby.

Filley AC: *Interpersonal conflict resolution*, Glenview, Ill, 1975, Scott, Foresman.

Lewis JH: Conflict management, *Journal of Nursing Administration* 6(12):18, 1976.

Marriner-Tomey A: *Guide to nursing management*, ed 4, St Louis, 1992, Mosby.

Neuhaus RH: *Long-term care administration:teamwork and effective management*, Lanham, Md, 1990, University Press.

Sampson EE, Marthas MS: *Group process for health professions*, New York, 1977, John Wiley & Sons.

Schaller LE: *The change agent*, New York, 1972, Abingdon Press.

Schmidt W, Tannenbaum R: The management of differences, *Harvard Business Review* 38(11):108, 1960.

Schulz R, Johnson AC: *Management of hospitals and health services: strategic issues and performance*, St Louis, 1990, Mosby.

Tappen RM: *Nursing leadership and management:concepts and practice*, ed 2, Philadelphia, 1989, Davis.

Additional Readings

Barton A: Conflict resolution by nurse managers, *Nursing Management* 22(5):83, 1991. *The author suggests that collaborative modes of conflict management should be encouraged.*

Bernard LA, Walsh M: *Leadership: the key to professionalization of nursing,* St Louis, 1990, Mosby. *Chapter 10, "The Nurse–Leader and Conflict Management," offers a thorough discussion relating to conflict.*

Bruha SM: You can conquer conflict, *Nursing 86* 16(1):81, 1986. *Ms. Bruha describes four personality conflicts.*

Burleson EJ: Creative tension: problem solving in conflict, *Nursing Management* 18(5):64J, 1988. *Conflict, when creatively managed, can promote growth.*

Collyer ME: Resolving conflicts: leadership style sets the strategy, *Nursing Management* 20(9):77, 1989. *Solving conflicts depends on managers' priorities as much as on their power.*

Curtin LL: Conflict avoidus: the humming birds of prey, *Nursing Management* 20(9):7, 1989. *The author offers several suggestions for avoiding 'conflictus avoidus,' fear of conflict, confrontation, and decision making.*

Danford K: I knew more than Ardie, but she was my manager, *Nursing 91* 29(5): 106, 1991. *Mr. Danford shares his interpersonal conflict situation and learns that a willingness to work through the conflict can really turn things around.*

Grainger RD: Are you overreacting?, *American Journal of Nursing* 92(3):11, 1992. *Responding, instead of reacting, to situations helps to creatively control how we think, feel, and behave.*

Guttenberg RM: How to stay cool in a conflict and turn it into cooperation, *Nursing Life* 3:25, 1983. *The author suggests an approach to resolving differences without a power struggle.*

Hibbert J, Craven R, Balinski, J: Instant problem solving, *Nursing Management* 12(12):37, 1981. *A quick fix on frustration to keep peace within the staff.*

Issac S: Ways to resolve conflict, *Nursing 86* 15(3):89, 1986. *Ms. Issacs describes the games people play and discusses five techniques for resolving inevitable conflicts.*

Mallory GA: Turn conflict into cooperation, *Nursing 85* 14(3):81, 1985. *The author identifies the causes of conflict and describes three conflict resolution techniques.*

Marriner A: Managing conflict, *Nursing Management* 13(6):29, 1982. *This article compares five conflict resolution strategies and their frequency of use in a clinical nursing setting.*

MANAGEMENT 7

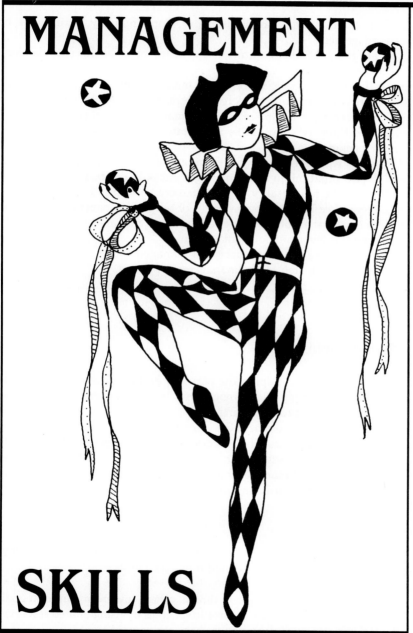

SKILLS

♪ Learning Objectives

Upon completion of this chapter, the reader will be able to:

1. List three main characteristics of contemporary definitions of management.
2. State the general organizational goal for most health care delivery facilities.
3. Define the five basic functions of management.
4. Identify at least four tasks for each management function.
5. List seven components of effective management practice.
6. Name three types of skills important for successful management performance.
7. Discuss four reasons for developing effective management skills.
8. List two situations in which management skills can be used effectively.
9. Explain the universality of management concept.
10. Differentiate between management of self and management of others.
11. Discuss 15 attributes of an effective nurse manager.
12. Name the seven sins of management.
13. Identify seven hints for successful management.
14. Describe each step of the management process.

What is Management?

Now that you are developing the personal and group skills so essential for dynamic leadership and management, let us focus on how your new skills can be applied to managing.

Management is one of the most often used but least defined words in business today. Some use the word as a noun to describe those people with the authority to set policy, establish standards, and define goals. Others use the word manage as a verb to define the process of making things happen. The word can also be used to refer to a body of specific knowledge.

Management defined

At least six contemporary definitions of management have evolved. Briefly, each group of theorists has defined management as

1. a process by which a group directs others toward a common goal,
2. a process of achieving organizational goals by using limited resources and the efforts of others in a changing environment,

MANAGEMENT CHARACTERISTICS

1. Management is a process or series of continuing and related activities.
2. It involves and concentrates on reaching organizational goals.
3. It reaches these goals by working with and through people and other organizational resources.

Reprinted, with permission, from Certo SC: *Principles of modern management: functions and systems,* ed 4, Needham Heights, Mass, 1989, Allyn & Bacon.

3. the coordination of resources in order to achieve the goal,
4. establishing an effective 'people' environment within a formal organization,
5. activities that coordinate others to meet goals that cannot be achieved by one person alone (Certo, 1989).

Characteristics. Although each definition focuses on a specific aspect of management, basic areas of agreement exist. All definitions share three characteristics (see box above). To simply sum it up, managers are people who accomplish through the efforts of others.

Health care goals. Organizational goals will be more fully discussed in Chapter 8. Most health care delivery facilities (organizations) share the overall goal of providing the highest possible quality patient care for the lowest cost. In addition, most long-term care facilities include the goal of providing for the psychological, emotional, and social needs of the residents. Organizational goals are an important component of any business. Thus, nurse managers need to be aware of their facility's particular goals.

Management functions

Managers achieve goals by working through other people. Actions or activities that bring about goal achievement are referred to as management functions. No matter what the business, the five basic functions of managers are to plan, organize, coordinate, direct, and evaluate.

Plan. "Planning is the process of setting goals and deciding on the methods of achieving them" (Reinecke, Dessler, Schoell, 1989). The planning process consists of four main steps (see box on p. 168).

Many managers are involved in two kinds of planning. **Strategic plan-**

✎ PLANNING PROCESS

1. **Develop forecasts and basic planning assumptions.** For example, do you foresee any changes in the number of occupied beds or staff members? Are there any plans for increasing or changing services? What are the new federal and state regulations that may affect your facility's operations?
2. **Define specific objectives.** Establish a goal for each plan. Serious planning cannot take place without defining goals and listing the steps necessary to meet each goal.
3. **Develop alternatives.** Assess all available resources as well as the strengths and weaknesses of the plan and then decide how to meet each goal. List all possible courses of action.
4. **Choose a course of action.** After evaluating all possible actions, make a choice and implement the plan.

---

ning is broad-based and includes planning of long-term goals, strategies for coping with competition or increasing market share, policies, and future plans. **Operational planning** relates to the short-term plans for implementing the facility's strategic plan. Most nurse managers use operational planning daily. Managers help to establish goals, identify resources, set priorities, and develop action plans. They choose tasks that will best meet the goal, outlining how and when the tasks are to be performed, and they consider both the short-term and long-term goals of each plan. Effective planning is a critical management skill, for all other management functions depend on it.

Organize. The manager who is well organized creates the mechanism for putting each plan into action. "Organizing involves establishing a formal structure that provides the coordination of resources to accomplish objectives, establish policies and procedures, and determine position qualifications and descriptions" (Marriner-Tomey, 1992).

This function also includes a knowledge of the organizational structure which delineates each position (job) and describes the responsibilities, relationships, and authority for each position in the structure. Organizational charts are one way to illustrate a facility's structure. Each organization also has a culture, the customary way of thinking and doing. All members share in the culture and transmit it to all newcomers. Organizational culture is a "combination of assumptions, values, symbols, language, and behaviors that manifest the organization's norms and values" (Marriner-Tomey, 1992). A facility's policies and procedures reflect its organizational culture.

Last, organization encompasses the use of personal skills and abilities such as time management, job analysis, effective communications, and team building. Successful organizing abilities contribute strongly to the overall success of the facility and rank second in importance only to planning.

Coordinate. Nurse managers routinely coordinate people's work efforts with available resources in order to get the job done (meet the goal). Commonly referred to as *staffing*, this management function includes such activities as recruitment of new staff members, screening and selection of personnel, orientation of new workers, ongoing staff development, composing staffing schedules, and providing technical direction. Nurse managers also assist in coordination strategies to minimize absenteeism, decrease staff turnover, and determine appropriate staffing levels. Patient classification systems, which document the acuity or severity of clients' conditions and their care needs, are used by the manager to determine staffing schedules appropriate to the work load. The ability to coordinate resources, both human and otherwise, is a crucial management function.

Direct. The function of directing is primarily concerned with people. Directing is also referred to as motivating, leading, monitoring, actuating, or influencing. In its broadest sense (influencing), directing can be defined as "the process of guiding the activities of organization members in appropriate directions" (Certo, 1989). The appropriate direction is the one that meets the organization's goal. Managers who function in the 'director' role use power, problem solving, conflict management, and leadership skills to make appropriate decisions and affect positive changes. The amount of direction needed by staff members varies from continual, direct observation to little monitoring at all. Assessment of the situation's requirements as well as the initiative, knowledge, and experience of the group members will guide the manager in determining the amount of direction needed.

Directing also includes monitoring—overseeing the progress made toward goal achievement. Nurse managers also monitor individual staff members' work performances, the performance of the unit as a whole, the level of patient care received, relationships with staff from other departments, and staff satisfaction. Monitoring can be a formal process through the use of peer review procedures, chart audits, or employee performance appraisals. Informal monitoring methods include direct observation, questioning, and on-the-spot suggestions. Monitoring is an important process, for it identifies problems and trends early. Solving small problems early prevents them from becoming much larger problems later.

To direct is to get work done through others. To do this, the manager's communication skills and assertive behaviors will assist him/her to motivate, lead, work with conflict, and keep the group focused on the goal. Managers who are proficient directors enjoy higher productivity and a more satisfied work group.

Evaluate. This last, but important, step is also referred to as 'controlling.' When nurse managers function as evaluators, they

1. gather information that measures recent performance within the organization;
2. compare present performance to preestablished performance standards; and
3. from this comparison, determine if the plan should be modified to meet preestablished standards (Certo, 1989).

Evaluation is an ongoing process. Managers continually monitor and evaluate group and individual effectiveness. The purpose of evaluation or controlling is to identify problems early, take preventative or corrective actions, and plan more effective future actions.

Controlling responsibilities of the nurse manager include evaluation of personnel, reward and discipline of personnel, counseling problem employees, assisting with program evaluations, and labor relations. Several specialized methods of evaluation are used in the health care profession. **Quality assurance committees monitor and evaluate the quality and appropriateness of patient care** by identifying problems, developing solutions, taking action, and monitoring each action for effectiveness. Quality assurance programs focus on quality management and health care delivery.

Programs that focus on liability control are called risk management. "Risk management involves the development and implementation of strategies to prevent patient injury, minimize financial loss, and preserve agency assets" (Marriner-Tomey, 1992). Committees involved in risk management routinely review incident reports and other data in order to identify potential or actual risks to the patient. The situation (risk) is analyzed, and an action plan is then implemented and evaluated, with follow-up provided when necessary. Programs relating to safety and security, plant management, quality management, and patient and family relations are included in the risk-management category.

In 1972, Public Law 92-603 was passed by Congress. In an attempt **to control the costs and quality of health care, a monitoring system called the Professional Standards Review Organization (PSRO) was created.** The PSRO made local health care professionals responsible for reviewing and evaluating the appropriateness and quality of health care services in their area. In 1973, the American Nurses' Association (ANA) developed the ANA Standards of Nursing Practice based on the nursing process.

These standards serve as a model for evaluation of patient care and nursing performance.

A less formal, but very effective, tool is **peer review,** which is "the evaluation of an individual's practice by colleagues [peers] who have similar education, experience, and occupational status" (Tappen, 1989). The purpose of peer review is to provide constructive feedback about the quality of a health care professional's performance. Observations are compared with preestablished standards and then shared with the individual in a nonjudgmental manner. Although sometimes perceived as threatening, effective peer review reinforces high-quality performance, stimulates staff members to analyze their own levels of performance, and encourages learning in order to improve levels of health care delivery.

Patient care audits also provide the nurse supervisor with an efficient evaluation tool. Client records are analyzed and evaluated for the type, frequency, amount, and quality of nursing care. Chart audits may be *concurrent*, that is, the record is evaluated during the patient's stay; or they may be *retrospective*, with the evaluation occurring after the patient has been discharged. The purpose of care audits is to assure documentation of patient care received as well as compliance with state and federal regulations.

Last, supervisors involved with the evaluation function participate in the utilization review processes. The **purpose of utilization review is to evaluate the use of resources and provide justification for expenditures related to patient care.** Originally mandated by the federal government for Medicare reimbursement, utilization review programs essentially ask the question, "Does the patient need to be here and, if so, for how long?" The physician must document the client's needs and reasons for admission, while all health care providers must document the care provided as well as the client's responses to treatment. Utilization reviews limit the number of days in the facility allowed each client according to the guidelines for each diagnostically related group (DRG). Facilities that do not implement utilization review programs are subject to losing federal and state reimbursements for Medicare clients.

As one can see, the manager has many devices and methods available to assist with the functions of evaluation and control.

Management roles

J. S. Ninomiya, in his clever article, *Wagon Masters and Lesser Managers* (1988), believes that the most "basic requirements for effective management are an understanding of the human condition and an appreciation of people." He contends that the wagon masters of the old West were some of this country's most effective managers by explaining:

> A wagon master had two jobs. He had to keep the wagons moving toward
> their destination day after day despite all obstacles. He also had to maintain

harmony and a spirit of teamwork among the members of his party and to resolve daily problems before they became divisive. A wagon master's worth was measured by his ability to reach the destination safely and to keep spirits high along the way. He had to do both in order to do either (Ninomiya, 1988).

Nurse managers are like wagon masters, balancing productivity and quality with harmony and team spirit. To achieve this worthy goal, **managers assume various roles.** Astute managers work to improve their effectiveness in the following roles (Ninomiya, 1988):

Decision maker. By far, the most important tool for managers is the ability to make decisions. An inability to make decisions leads to a very brief career in management. By allowing employees to participate in the decision-making process, the manager elicits support and, possibly, solutions. Work with team members to solve problems but be prepared to make the final decision, if necessary.

Listener and communicator. Managers who are in touch with their staff members are sensitive to their moods, opinions, and attitudes. Although it requires serious effort to get to know staff members individually, good wagon masters recognize and appreciate each individual employee. See Chapter 2 for a more complete discussion of communication skills.

Teacher. Nurse managers fill the role of teacher in two ways. First, as client teacher, nurse managers develop teaching plans for patients. Second, they stimulate staff members to improve their skills and abilities by training everyone who has potential (and we all have some potential). Last, nurse managers train and encourage some subordinates to become managers. Building positive self-images in employees through training allows the manager to trust in the team members' abilities and delegate appropriately. Effective teachers constantly challenge their workers' creativity and strive to improve their knowledge.

Visionary. Just as wagon masters pushed the group toward their destination, managers who set specific, meaningful goals move the organization toward achievement. When goals are specific, well defined, and understood by all team members, enormous amounts of time and energy are saved. Dynamic managers never allow themselves or their team members to lose sight of collective and individual goals.

Team captain. Decisions that affect the whole work team, unit, department, or organization should be made through teamwork. When employees whose voices are not usually heard participate in the decision-making process, satisfaction increases and mistakes are minimized. "Consensus decision making is one of the most powerful tools at a manager's disposal" (Ninomiya, 1988). As team captain, it is your responsibility to coach the best possible decisions from your work group.

Leader. The best wagon masters genuinely enjoy working with people. They lead with such qualities as understanding, trust, politeness, and sensitivity. Respect for each individual's dignity and worth provide their philosophical framework for leadership. To brush up on your leadership skills, review Chapter 4.

Peacemaker. Facing day-to-day problems as they occur helps to minimize conflict. Managers in the peacemaker role confront problem situations early and encourage others to minimize conflict through mutual collaboration and problem solving.

Self-critic. Managers with self-confidence admit their mistakes. When workers feel that "the boss is always right," they tend to withhold information that could minimize or even prevent problems that result from the decision. Workers lose respect for managers who cannot admit they made a mistake. Effective self-critics are quick to assume responsibility for their errors, assess the causes, and control any damage generated by the decision. The major focus is to learn from their mistakes and use that knowledge to improve future decisions. Assigning blame is unimportant when managers consider errors as an inherent element of human behavior.

Three basic abilities

Managers, administrators, and supervisors are judged by their productivity, but "a manager's ability to perform is a result of the **managerial skills** [emphasis added] possessed" (Katz, 1955). Three basic sets of abilities are important to the growth and development of effective management performance: conceptual skills, technical skills, and human skills.

Conceptual skills. The ability to see the 'big picture,' the organization as a whole, is vital for a manager. "A manager with conceptual skills is able to understand how various functions of the organization complement one another, how the organization relates to its environment, and how changes in one part of the organization affect the rest of the organization" (Certo, 1989). Conceptual skills are the ability to see the interrelatedness of several different and dynamic parts of your facility.

Technical skills. Knowledge of the jobs you are supervising is essential. Technical skills are the "knowledge of and ability to use the processes, practices, techniques, and tools of a specialty responsibility area" (Straub, Attner, 1991). Managers need enough technical skills to do the jobs of those workers they supervise. Credibility with technical skills is based on ability.

Human skills. Perhaps the most important of the three, psychosocial abilities allow you to interact with other people successfully. Managers who nurture their workers achieve the group's goals faster and more harmoniously.

A manager's job description

The five basic functions of management, planning, organizing, coordinating, direction, and evaluation (controlling) can be summed up in the following job description: **The health care manager is a person with good conceptual, human, and technical skills** (see box on p. 175). It sounds like a tall order, but you are already halfway there. Practice, patience, and experience, when added to your present abilities, will foster your evolution into the competent, humanistic manager that you are capable of becoming.

Why Develop Management Skills?

Before the advent of the Industrial Age, people would usually work alone. Artisans would craft or build an item from start to finish without assistance, and most tradesmen worked in one-person or two-person shops. Managers simply were not needed.

The invention of the steam engine in the mid-1800s heralded the Industrial Age and, shortly thereafter, dramatically changed the way people worked. Machines were invented and people were needed to operate them. Work groups were formed. The task became the focus. Production lines and specifically trained workers would repeat one task in the overall assembly of an item. The worker became removed from the finished product and, thus, was denied the rewards of creativity and pride in workmanship. People who could understand the overall process of production and direct the workers' energies were now needed. New jobs such as overseer, leadman, team boss, and supervisor were born. When people began to work in groups, someone had to provide direction. That someone became the manager. Today, managers are an essential part of every successful business.

Nurses traditionally spent most of their time at the bedside, delivering care to the individual patient. However, complex social and technological changes have redefined the nurse's role. Although the nurse's primary concern remains patient care, much of that care is delivered through the hands of others. The nurse has now also become a manager.

The need for management skills

Ensure success. To meet an organization's goals, its members must work together as a cohesive unit. Managers (supervisors) are needed to provide

---

✎ BASIC MANAGER FUNCTIONS

1. Gathers data by assessing each situation.
2. Actively engages in organizational (short-term) and strategic (long-term) planning. Considers the current and future work of the team.
3. Actively assumes leadership of the work team.
4. Organizes work efficiently by comparing the task requirements with the workers' abilities.
5. Coordinates staff with work requirements. Fosters the development of each staff member.
6. Directs and monitors the work done by staff members to maintain quality and productivity.
7. Recognizes and rewards quality and productivity.
8. Represents both administration and staff members as needed.
9. Participates in evaluating individual and group productivity.
10. Uses psychosocial skills to meet individual and group needs.

Adapted from Tappen RM: *Nursing leadership and management: concepts and practice*, ed 2, 1989, Philadelphia, Davis.

---

the work group with the direction, coordination, and resources necessary to meet the facility's goals. Managers are catalysts that link the goals of the administration to the productivity of the workers. In short, managers are "needed to ensure the success of an organization" (Straub, Attner, 1991).

Monitor quality. The overall goal of health care organizations is to provide the client with high-quality health and illness care. Each care facility, aided by the state and federal government, defines its services, plans, and methods for delivering its services and evaluates the effectiveness of the health care services provided. Managers, supervisors, team leaders, and department directors all monitor and improve upon their services continually. Health care workers with strong management skills can have a powerful impact on the quality of client care.

Work with others. Employees need to know where their organization is heading, how it will get there, and, perhaps most importantly, what it all means to them. Workers know that their well-being is intricately tied to the success of their organization. They want to contribute, and they need to be informed. Managers are the communication links between the planners and the producers. They are the flesh-and-blood representatives of the administrators who can understand and express the worker's viewpoint.

Effective management skills are also used to provide an organized work flow and design. When the work flows smoothly because the needed resources are readily available and employees can move freely within their work areas, relationships among staff members tend to be more upbeat and positive. Managers set the flow and tone of work relationships among staff members. You can empower and encourage your workers through effective use of your management skills.

Live effectively. Skills in organizing and managing bring order and focus into our sometimes chaotic, never idle lives. Time is like the family bank account — it is always limited in amount, and its effectiveness is determined by how it is spent. A day is only 24 hours long. Much must be accomplished within this time. How you 'spend' your minutes and hours determines how effective you will be in meeting your goals. Good management skills also allow you to spend more time doing what you would *like* to do rather than what you *have* to do.

Positions in management also offer other personal benefits. "Managerial positions can yield high salaries, status, interesting work, personal growth, and intense feelings of accomplishment" (Certo, 1989).

Where Are Management Skills Used?

Broadly speaking, management skills are used in two situations: personal situations and group situations.

Personal situations

When you need to accomplish tasks, achieve goals, or improve upon something, applying the steps of the management process can decrease extra steps and produce greater results. Effective management begins with self-direction. By ably managing personal situations, you are developing the skills to manage professional situations.

Group situations

Wherever people come together with a common purpose (goal) in mind, management skills are needed. Groups who have no goals other than to socialize or work on hobbies usually do not require management beyond agreeing upon when to schedule the next meeting. However, if group members meet with specific purposes or needs to accomplish something, planning and organizing skills will be required. Groups increase in their effectiveness and achieve goals more smoothly when management techniques are applied. Effective management skills can be successfully used for any situation in which a group needs to achieve a goal.

When Are Management Skills Used?

Management is a process, a series of related activities that brings about a desired result. It is a dynamic process with the manager actively using several skills concurrently.

The universality of management

The **principles of management are universal.** This means that "all managers do the same job regardless of title, position, or management level. They all execute the five management functions" (Straub, Attner, 1991). Different levels of management will emphasize specific functions, and differing amounts of time will be spent for each function. All managers do the same job, though; they produce work through others. Skills in management are needed whenever people work.

A repeating process

The competent nurse uses management skills continuously. Work loads and tasks must be planned, time frames coordinated, and progress monitored and evaluated. The list goes on. Fortunately, developing effective management skills is also a process. Practice applying the five management functions. Work with one technique or skill at a time. Growth is a process, too.

Who Manages?

The best supervisors possess certain characteristics. Some of these characteristics are innate, while others can be developed. Most workers are content to remain nonmanagers. Many people do not have the temperament or personality for successful leadership or management. Those who do, however, will find a dynamic, exciting experience awaiting.

Should I be a manager?

Ask yourself these questions to start you thinking about becoming a supervisor:

- Do I sincerely like, respect, and enjoy working with people?
- Would I rather work with problems involving human relationships or mechanical, clerical, or mathematical relationships?

- Do I like working as a member of a team?
- Do I like having the responsibility for decisions?
- Can I effectively make decisions, solve problems, and assume responsibility?
- How important is money, ambition, and recognition?
- Do I want the freedom to do planning rather than being told what to do?
- Can I feel satisfaction by achieving work goals through the efforts of others?
- Would I prefer to actually do the job or see that the job is done?

Think about these questions to discover your attitudes about work, people, and supervision. The answers will help you decide if you want to be one of those who manages rather than being managed.

Whom do I manage?

The two basic who's of management are self and others. **The first and most important person to manage is yourself.** Your attitude, confidence, time, and image all require active management. The psychosocial skills discussed in Chapter 1, when practiced, will assist in developing effective self-management.

Second, using the abilities developed through self-management, the nurse guides, supervises, and coordinates patients, work teams, special interest groups, meetings, assorted professionals, and personnel from other departments. All these people interact within the management process.

How Do I Manage?

Fortunately, developing good management skills is a conscious growth process. As you become comfortable with using the five basic management tools, your particular style will evolve. Remember to routinely evaluate yourself for areas that could use improvement.

Basic ingredients

The most successful managers share many similar qualities, attributes, and skills which provide the matrix, or framework, for their effectiveness (see box on p. 179).

The seven sins

The 1990s have ushered in revisions in workplace thinking. The days of "grab the profit dollars" are passed, especially in relation to the health care delivery systems.

BASIC INGREDIENTS FOR A SUCCESSFUL MANAGER

1. A *commitment* to becoming an effective manager
2. A belief that people are of worth and that all workers can contribute positively to the organization
3. A positive, professional self-image
4. Learning to take pride in getting the job done through others
5. Effective and therapeutic communication skills
6. Working effectively with groups
7. Competent leadership skills and use of power
8. Motivating and inspiring skills
9. Skills that help to resolve conflict
10. Time-management skills
11. Techniques for problem solving, critical thinking, and use of the nursing process applied to management
12. Negotiation and team-building skills
13. Delegation skills
14. Planning, organizing, and evaluation skills
15. Positive energy

According to Owen Edwards (1992), the result of this rethinking is a redefinition of what managers "can and cannot get away with. Following are the **Seven Deadly Sins of Management in the New Age** [emphasis added]."

1. Blind ambition. The struggle to succeed sometimes resulted in the fittest rising to the top, but it also resulted in elevating the meanest and most selfish people. The way to "get ahead" was to constantly move upward, regardless of the cost. This fierce competitiveness lowered the productivity and decreased the effectiveness of many organizations. Fortunately, many companies have 'flattened' their hierarchies, thus reducing the number of management positions. Others encourage managers to move laterally by offering more responsibility and higher pay. Blind ambition is no longer a viable technique for getting ahead.

2. Flabby ethics. "Clearly, ethics took some time off during the '80s" (Edwards, 1992). Any observer of recent history can attest to that. However, ethics are now becoming a strong component of many companies. In business, ethics programs are becoming very popular. In fact, "According to one study, 45 percent of the 1,000 largest U.S. companies currently have some sort of ethics programs" (Edwards, 1992). Flabby ethics have no place in business. Health care organizations have a special ethical responsibility, for our product is the quality of our patients' lives.

3. Greed. "Greed is what makes the world go round" was an acceptable mode of thought prior to the 1990s. Executives with seven- or eight-figure salaries were leading companies to bankruptcy. Hostile takeovers were motivated by projected profits, and productivity was little considered. Managers who 'played rough' may have improved their pocketbooks, but they did little to improve the organization's productivity. Today, greed is considered very outdated. Companies are becoming sensitive to the fact that some people are very overpaid. In fact, several studies show little correlation between the company's productivity and executive manager's income.

4. Perk-elation. Perks are the extra benefits enjoyed by the organization's elite. Lavish offices, cars, and entertainment allowances were common benefits of management positions. "Perks are more than amenities or even material recognition of our worth to an employer; they are expressions of power, of the superiority of the perked to the non-perked" (Edwards, 1992). Companies that emphasize teamwork and collaboration downplay status symbols, and as a result, perks are rapidly losing their appeal.

5. Success stress. Constant 12-hour days, giving more than 100 percent, and total devotion to the job will exhaust you both physically and emotionally. Every job has its own special demands. It is up to each of us to find the balance between work and the rest of our lives. True professionals learn to handle responsibility calmly, quietly, and gracefully.

6. Toady tolerance. "Toadies" are those people who waltz into the facility and immediately lavish you (the manager) with praise about your brilliance, abilities, and outstanding personality. As Owen Edwards (1992) describes them:

> Toadies are a loathsome species, unerring in their ability to locate powerful people who will put up with them. And they're not harmless. Toadies cloud the air with flattery and cheery tidings, getting in the way of people who have something important to offer, like the truth.

Today's leaner and more productive organizations cannot afford to keep toadies on the payroll solely for the purpose of massaging managers' egos.

7. The Mother Teresa syndrome. Self-righteousness may not be the sin that makes the headlines, but it can become a problem. The manager who exudes a smug sense of superiority may manage (things) but will seldom lead (people). Work to be the best you can be but never think that others are inferior.

Temper your ambition with strong ethics. Strive to be successful but learn to balance work with other activities. Forget the perks. Do not get greedy or superior. Work with toadies to make them productive team members; and remember your own needs for improvement.

Seven hints

Richard Sloma, an international manager with 25 years' experience, believes that the world of management belongs to the bold — those people who have the commitment, skill, and motivation to succeed. In his book, *No-Nonsense Management* (1977), Sloma describes numerous principles for managers to follow in order to become highly effective achievers. Seven of these principles are discussed here.

Act the part. If you want to be a manager, begin to behave like a manager. Demonstrate that you can make the transition from worker to supervisor by accepting responsibility. The more you visualize, think, and act like a manager, the more you will be recognized as one.

Never tolerate mediocrity. A manager's job is to achieve results. Your superiors expect it, and your staff wishes it. "Your people must identify you with an expectation of high levels of performance" (Sloma, 1977). Workers strive to achieve the performance levels expected of them. Once mediocrity is accepted, the productivity of the entire organization will be affected. It is better to set your standards high and fall a bit short than to settle for inferiority.

Line up problems. "Never try to solve all of the problems all at once — make them line up one-by-one" (Sloma, 1977). Solving all the problems at hand at the same time is a recipe for failure. Learn to tackle one problem at a time. Prioritize them, then summon your resources and conquer (solve) each problem one at a time.

Be effective, then efficient. Managers who are effective achieve results because they know that there are numerous courses of action that will achieve the same goal. *Effectiveness* relates to meeting the goals. *Efficiency* is mainly concerned with the technique used to achieve the goal. Unfortunately, efficiency requires time for measuring and evaluating each alternative. If too much time is spent being efficient, the opportunity to be effective may be lost. Learn to balance efficiency with effectiveness.

No one gives 100 percent. No worker (yourself included) gives 100 percent all of the time. Managers who consistently motivate employees to *want* to reach their potential have elevated motivation to an art form.

One of the most effective methods of motivating employees "is to push the limits of your own imagination and innovation so that you generate a stream of ever-expanding challenges for subordinates. As they move from one achievement to another, they will realize that they are growing and developing" (Sloma, 1977). By reinforcing each success, you will encourage the employee's desire to perform at high levels of excellence.

Planning is not complicated. The management function of planning is not complicated at all, but it is tedious, time consuming, and important. Planning involves the examination of all probable alternatives, weighing of the pros and cons of each course of action, and the consideration of every possible scenario. Only then is the manager prepared to attain the goal. The 'doer' who makes everything flow so smoothly usually has spent hours and hours in preparatory planning. On-the-spot decisions can easily be made when you have previously considered the alternatives. Planning requires perseverance, patience, and time; but without it, your effectiveness as a manager, doer, or achiever is severely limited.

Managers are jugglers. A highly effective manager is an accomplished juggler who can successfully balance the interests, pressures, goals, situations, and priorities of the organization with those of the workers and clients. Many internal and external forces constantly influence an organization. It is the manager who must juggle to successfully rank and realign priorities in order to serve the best long-term interests of the organization and its employees.

Summary

Remember the suggestions in the box on p. 183. They will serve you well, especially in complex or confusing situations. Keep in mind that the process on management is the use of skills and techniques. Because they are skills, each can be developed, practiced, and improved. All journeys begin with a single step. Let us go for a walk.

SUMMARY OF MANAGEMENT FUNCTIONS AND TASKS

Plan
Gather data and identify resources
Assess the situation
Establish specific goals
Develop objectives, policies, standards
Set up a budget
Establish priorities
Determine procedures
Develop alternative plans of action
Choose an action plan
Communicate with all involved people

Organize
Know organizational structure, culture
Fit action plan into formal structure of facility
Determine job descriptions and evaluation criteria
Collect resources
Build support (team-building skills)

Coordinate
Recruit new staff
Screen and select personnel
Orient new staff
Plan for staff development
Determine staffing needs
Devise staffing schedules
Develop retention, absenteeism strategies
Provide technical direction

Direct
Guide group toward goal
Problem-solve to make decisions
Manage conflict
Lead positively
Determine need for direction
Review job performances
Monitor progress toward goal

Evaluate
Compare performance with standards
Identify problems
Take corrective and preventative actions
Employee evaluation, discipline, counseling
Program evaluation: Quality Assurance committee
      Professional Standards Review Organization
       (PSRO)
      Risk management
      Peer review
      Patient care audits
      Utilization review

✍ Key Concepts

- Though several different definitions of management currently exist, each explanation shares three characteristics:

  1. Management is a process of related activities.
  2. Management concentrates on meeting the goals of the organization.
  3. Management meets its goals through its resources and the efforts of its workers.

- The general goal of most health care delivery systems is to provide the highest quality patient care for the lowest possible cost.
- The five basic functions of management are planning, organizing, co-ordinating, directing, and evaluating.
- Managers play several roles simultaneously, including the roles of decision maker, listener and communicator, teacher, peacemaker, visionary, team captain, leader, and self-critic.
- Components of effective nursing management practice are leadership, planning, directing work, staff development, monitoring productivity, recognition, reward, and representation.
- Three types of skills important for successful management are technical skills, human skills, and conceptual skills.
- Effective management skills are useful in both personal and professional areas of life.
- Management skills can be applied to any situation in which people need to achieve a goal.
- The universality of management concept states that all managers do the same job—the five management functions.
- Management of 'self' is prerequisite to managing others.
- Outstanding managers work to develop their skills through a conscious growth process.
- Practice of communication, leadership, conflict resolution, motivation, time-management, and problem-solving skills improve managerial effectiveness.
- Seven deadly sins of management are blind ambition, flabby ethics, greed, perk-elation, success stress, toady tolerance, and the Mother Teresa syndrome.
- Seven suggestions to guide the manager in becoming effective and identified with high performance levels relate to the manager's behavior, mediocrity, problems, effectiveness, motivation, planning, and prioritizing.
- The process of management includes five basic steps: assess the situation and set goals, organize to meet goal, guide and stimulate progress, measure progress, and evaluate effectiveness.

☙ Learning Activities

1. Have each class member interview two employees and ask, "What are the most (and least) effective activities of your manager?" Compare answers and suggest improvements. Use no names.
2. Discuss the impact of each management function on the quality of patient care.
3. Outline the relationships of the five functions of management.
4. Scenario: The administrator of your facility, in cooperation with members of the Quality Assurance committee, has decided that all patients will be monitored for Intake and Output (I&O) for a one-week time period. You, as team leader, are in charge of making this happen. Using the management process summary, develop a management plan for meeting this goal.
5. Describe the difference between effectiveness and efficiency.

References

Certo SC: *Principles of modern management: functions and systems*, ed 4, Needham Heights, Mass, 1989, Allyn & Bacon.

Edwards O: The seven deadly sins (of management), *Working Woman*, March:81, 1992.

Katz RL: Skills of an effective administrator, *Harvard Business Review* 33:33, 1955.

Marriner-Tomey A: *Guide to nursing management*, ed 4, St Louis, 1992, Mosby.

Ninomiya JS: Wagon masters and lesser managers, *Harvard Business Review* 66:84, 1988.

Reinecke JA, Dessler G, Schoell W: *Introduction to business: a contemporary view*, ed 6, Needham Heights, Mass, 1989, Allyn & Bacon.

Sloma RS: *No-nonsense management: a general manager's primer*, New York, 1977, Macmillan.

Straub J, Attner R: *Introduction to business*, ed 4, Boston, 1991, PWS-KENT.

Tappen RM: *Nursing leadership and management: concepts and practice*, ed 2, Philadelphia, 1989, Davis.

Additional Readings

Armstrong N: How to assess your unit before you take report, *American Journal of Nursing* 91(2):57, 1991. *Ms. Armstrong offers suggestions for interpreting the subtle cues of the unit's functioning before receiving the change-of-shift report.*

Beaman AL: What do first-line managers do?, *Journal of Nursing Administration* 16(5):6, 1986. *Specific descriptions of the actual tasks performed by first-line nursing managers are needed to provide the information necessary to design a clear role description for the development of nurse managers.*

Blank W: It's hard to work with strangers, *Supervisory Management* 31(5):12, 1986. *To improve your managerial effectiveness, use the "strangeness audit" to overcome the feeling that you and your workers are strangers.*

Curtin LL: Attitude: the new posture for the nineties, *Nursing Management* 23(11):7, 1990. *Ms. Curtin discusses the attitudes of the three generations in today's work force — the Transition Generation, the Baby Boomers, and the Cornucopia Generation.*

Douglas LM: *The effective nurse leader and manager,* St Louis, 1992, Mosby. *Chapters 6 and 7 offer excellent information about planning and directing.*

Flarey DL: Redesigning management roles, *Journal of Nursing Administration* 21(2):40, 1991. *"To confront future change and developments in nursing and management practice, the role of the first-line nurse manager must take on new dimensions."*

Forbes BJ: Let your actions do the talking, *Nursing 84* 13(3):112, 1984. *The author shares a personal experience to remind us that small actions can be powerful examples.*

Hansen MR: To-do list for managers, *Supervisory Management* 31(5):37, 1986. *An excellent article that offers numerous guidelines for those managers who are new at the job.*

Hensey M: Consulting patterns of successful managers, *Supervisory Management* 31(5):32, 1986. *The author describes two consulting patterns that can be successfully applied in problem situations.*

Mlynczak BA: Improving management, *Nursing Management* 13(7):45, 1982. *A formal communication system, devised by the staff, fostered group decision making and a more cohesive work team.*

Sullivan MP: *Nursing leadership and management: a study and learning tool,* Springhouse, Pa, 1990, Springhouse. *This book provides an overview of basic theories, concepts, methods, and processes of nursing management.*

Tucker NJ, Smith LM: All through the night, *Geriatric Nursing* Sept/Oct:256, 1987. *The authors describe how application of the nursing process and positive strategies brought about administrative changes in a long-term care facility.*

Wiley L: Juggling patients on the head of a pin or how much can a mere mortal do?, *Nursing 75* 5(12):55, 1975. *Ms. Wiley suggests six rules of thumb to guide the charge nurse in planning when there is more work than one can possibly do. Suggestions for turning the fight–flight reaction into the reflect–direct response.*

UNIT TWO: APPLICATION OF LEADERSHIP AND MANAGEMENT SKILLS

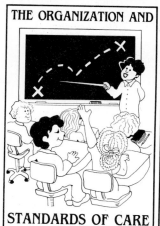

THE ORGANIZATION AND

STANDARDS OF CARE

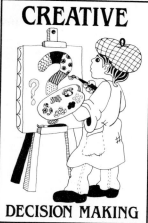

CREATIVE

DECISION MAKING

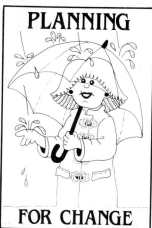

PLANNING

FOR CHANGE

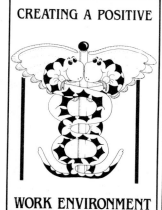

CREATING A POSITIVE

WORK ENVIRONMENT

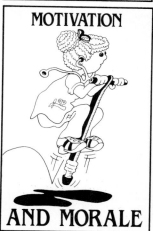

MOTIVATION

AND MORALE

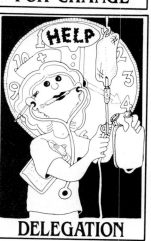

DELEGATION

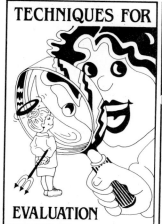

TECHNIQUES FOR

EVALUATION

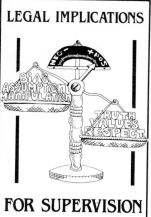

LEGAL IMPLICATIONS

FOR SUPERVISION

THE ORGANIZATION AND

8

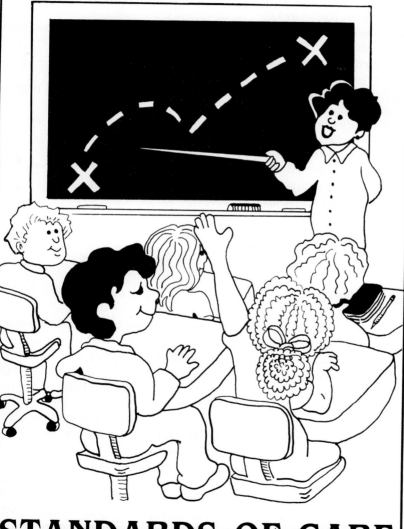

STANDARDS OF CARE

✒ Learning Objectives

Upon completion of this chapter, the reader will be able to:

1. List two definitions of *organization*.
2. Describe two characteristics of the classical organizational theory.
3. Define the basis for the humanistic organizational theory.
4. Identify two research approaches of modern organizational theory (systems framework).
5. Differentiate between formal and informal organizational structures.
6. Identify the four elements of a formal structure.
7. Describe four types of formal organizational structures.
8. List eight guidelines for assessing organizational culture.
9. Explain the difference between centralized and decentralized organizational authority.
10. Name two types of authority the nurse manager may exercise.
11. Define *client care delivery system*.
12. Describe four types of client care delivery systems.
13. Recognize one advantage and one disadvantage for each client care delivery system.
14. Explain the importance of standards of care.

Organization Defined

Organization has several meanings when applied to the work situation. One definition of an organization is "a group of two or more persons that exists and operates to achieve clearly stated, commonly held objectives" (Straub, Attner, 1991). Organizations can be situated within a single building or scattered in numerous locations throughout the world. They range in size from two persons to thousands of people.

When organization is used to describe a structure, it refers to the lines of authority, communication, and delegation, as well as the philosophy and policies of the group. Organizations may also be referred to as a company, business, facility, institution, or corporation. When used to describe a process, organization relates to the methods or ways in which the goals of the group are achieved. Supervisors, for example, use the management process to accomplish organizational goals. Thus, organization refers to both a structure and a process in which the manager uses human, material, and financial resources to achieve goals.

Organizational Theory

An organizational theory is a set of related statements that describe what an institution (company, facility) is, how it functions, its parameters or limits, and the setting in which the health care manager works. **A knowledge of organizational theories helps to provide the basis for effective management and leadership,** enables the nurse to contribute meaningfully to the facility, and assists in clarifying roles and functions. Health care institutions are major industries in today's society. They are structured on many principles found in organizational theories. Nurses and other health care providers need to become well versed in organizational theories if they are to have a part in directing the future of nursing and related health care issues.

Three basic categories or organizational theories have evolved since the late 1800s. Each group of theories has its unique characteristics. Modern health care institutions use principles or elements from all three schools of thought.

Classical organizational theory

The advent of the Industrial Age during the mid-1800s changed the pattern of work. Because of increasing complexity of design, products were no longer made by one person. Specialists (people with detailed knowledge of one area) became more and more important, and, thus, the need for people to oversee the work began to evolve. As soon as workers and supervisors came into being, so followed the theorists with their attempts to scientifically study the work organization.

One of the earliest studies of organizations was conducted by Max Weber, who developed an 'ideal' form of organization called the bureaucracy. Theoretically, the bureaucratic organization was based on rational decision making and definitions of the 'one best way' of doing things.

The bureaucracy. Bureaucratic organizations focus primarily on individual productivity — the amount of work done by one person in a specified time. Rational, critical, and well-thought-out approaches and techniques were viewed as essential for meeting goals effectively in a bureaucracy. The primary focus of the bureaucracy was "the proper allocation of work to people and machines" (Magula, 1982). Workers were rigidly controlled to promote high levels of production. The bureaucracy is the oldest form of organizational structure and serves as an example of the classical organizational theory.

Basic premises. Theorists of the classical school believed that productivity could be improved by rationally defining the *one best way* of doing any-

CLASSICAL ORGANIZATIONAL THEORY

1. **Division of labor.** Each worker performed a specialized task for which he was properly trained. Managers were also trained in task performance. Their responsibility, however, was not to actually execute the task but to make sure the work was completed. "The proper division of labor has been called the most important economic concept ever devised" (Kimball, 1925). Each of the other three premises are based on the division of labor pillar.

2. **Vertical and horizontal processes.** Classical theory states that as an organization expands (horizontal growth) it will add more levels of supervision (vertical growth). The basis is, again, a division of labor.

3. **Structure.** The classical structure is the bureaucracy, which resembles a pyramid. Control is held by the few at the top. A chain-of-command, or hierarchy, defines each supervisor's responsibilities, communication lines, and span of control. Classicists believed that defined patterns of authority and responsibilities provide coordination for the work of the organization.

4. **Span of control.** Each supervisor/manager in a bureaucratic organization occupies a specific position in the chain-of-command. Rigid rules and regulations define the pattern of authority as well as the number and type of workers supervised. The manager's span of control refers to the number of workers (subordinates) supervised. Because the question of how many workers a manager could effectively supervise was of primary importance to the classical theory, studies were done. A major contribution to the span of control concept was made in 1937 by V. A. Graicus. He contended that a manager's span of control is limited by the nature of the work as well as the abilities of both the workers and the supervisor.

thing. By studying each part of an organization as well as how each component interacted or coordinated with others, the classical theorists founded their theory on four basic premises (see box above).

Thus, the structure of an organization is comprised of the collective spans of control. The classical bureaucracy is tall and narrow with few workers reporting to a given supervisor.

Scientific management. Because a primary concern of the classical theory was the one best way of doing things, the study of this process became known as the scientific method. The title "father of scientific management" was given to Frederick W. Taylor, a shop worker of the steel industry. "His primary goal was to increase worker efficiency by scientifically designing jobs" (Certo, 1989). He believed that any worker's job could be scientifically analyzed by considering the exact amount of time and effort needed to do the job to certain standards. To prove his theory, he analyzed the jobs of shovelers at Bethlehem Steel. After considering such factors as the materials to be shoveled, the kinds of shovels, the time required to swing a shovel and throw a load a certain distance at a certain height, the size of the worker, and the weight of the load, Taylor implemented his efficiency plan. Three years later, records indicated the need for shovelers was reduced from 600 to 140, each worker's output increased from 16 to 59 tons, and costs fell by two thirds. This was impressive research that spurred many further studies.

Frank and Lillian Gilbrath developed time–motion techniques for analyzing each step of a task. Henry Gantt theorized that the manner in which tasks are scheduled and workers are rewarded determines the effectiveness of the organization. The Gantt chart for scheduling is still widely used today. "Basically, the chart provides managers with an understanding of what work was scheduled for specific time periods, how much of the work was completed, and by whom it was done" (Certo, 1989). The ideas of many theorists have contributed to the classical theory of scientific management.

Analysis of management. While proponents of scientific management focused on studying the structure and design of the job, other theorists became concerned with analyzing managerial performance. An outstanding contributor to this area of study was Henri Fayol, whose efforts were concentrated on explaining how an organization's administrative levels work. He believed it was possible to construct a set of principles that could be applied to any administration to improve its management practices. Fayol then developed 14 principles of management that could be applied to any organization (see box on p. 194). The 'universality of management' theory was born.

Regarded as a pioneer of administrative theory, Fayol also outlined five key elements of management—planning, organizing, command, coordination, and control. Today's managerial functions are still based on Fayol's work. Fayol's theories and principles, when added to the work of earlier theorists, provided the foundation for classical school of organizational theory.

Humanistic organizational theory

The humanistic theory, also referred to as the **behavioral school or neoclassical theory, is composed of theories from psychology, sociology, and the social sciences.** The behavioral school accepted the classical

FAYOL'S PRINCIPLES OF MANAGEMENT

1. **Division of work.** Specialization is the best way to use resources.
2. **Authority.** The power to give orders and expect obedience is authority. Without authority, specialization and division of labor could not be coordinated or monitored.
3. **Discipline.** Fayol felt that, although discipline was necessary to keep the workers focused on the common effort, it should be carefully applied in order to encourage the common effort.
4. **Unity of command.** This is an important principle (especially for health care workers) that states an employee should receive orders from only one manager.
5. **Unity of direction.** One person at the top has one plan, and the entire organization should be moving in a common direction — toward the goals stated in the plan.
6. **Subordination of individual interests.** The interests of one person do not take priority over the organization's interests. Institutional activities and goals always come first.
7. **Remuneration.** Salaries should be viewed as fair by both workers and employers.
8. **Centralization.** All communications flow from the top down and are received from the bottom up. Each manager exchanges information with his/her workers and supervisor.
9. **Scalar chain.** Each manager is linked to the organization in a hierarchy, or chain-of-command, and, thus, yields a certain amount of authority. The president or CEO has the greatest amount of authority, while the first-line supervisor has the least.
10. **Order.** In an efficient organization, there is a place for everything (and everyone), and everything (and everyone) should be in its place.
11. **Equity.** All people will be treated as equally or alike as possible.
12. **Stability of tenure.** A high priority of management is the retention of stable, productive workers. Hiring new workers increases costs and decreases productivity.
13. **Initiative.** Managers should encourage workers to use initiative (self-directed, new, or additional work).
14. **Esprit de corps.** Managers who encourage harmony and cohesiveness build commitment to the work group and organization.

From Fayol H: *General and industrial management,* London, 1949, Pitman & Sons.

organizational theory but modified it to place emphasis on increasing productivity through an understanding of the worker and his social group. Whereas the emphasis of the classicists was on the task or job, the behaviorists emphasized people.

History of the humanistic movement. Working conditions in the early 1900s were poor. People worked 12 to 14 hours a day in poorly lit, unsafe conditions. Children were employed for work requiring nimble hands. The death and injury statistics for workers were appalling.

This lack of concern for workers' welfare led to the development of a new organizational theory based on studies done between 1924 and 1932 by Harvard University Researchers (Roethlisberger, Dickenson, 1939). These studies focused on workers' attitudes, behaviors, and productivity under different working conditions at the Hawthorne Works of the Western Electric Company in Chicago.

The first set of experiments was designed to find the working conditions that maximized production. To their surprise, the researchers found that the human (social) factors influenced workers' productivity more than the physical environment (i.e., lighting, temperature, etc.).

Further studies were done to analyze the social relationships of the work group. Researchers were again surprised when they found that the influence of the social (work) group was stronger than the drive to make money. The results of these experiments are known as the Hawthorne effect. In short, the Hawthorne effect states social and psychological factors influence workers' productivity more than physical conditions.

Later, the research of Roethlisberger and Dickenson (1939) identified two main functions of an organization: maintaining the economic or external balance (classical theory) and maintaining the social needs of workers or internal balance (humanistic theory). These two equally important functions provide the basis for the humanistic theory.

Encouraged by the results of these earlier works, the behaviorists began to concentrate on the study of group dynamics, motivation, role performance, leadership, and the informal organization.

Theories X and Y. In 1960, Douglas McGregor published a set of assumptions about the nature of people in the workplace. He referred to these as Theory X and Theory Y.

According to Theory X, the average worker:

1. Is inherently lazy and prefers to avoid work.
2. Associates no pleasure with work.
3. Avoids responsibility and prefers to be directed.
4. Is motivated by fear of being demoted or fired.

5. Must be "controlled, threatened, and coerced to put forth sufficient effort to meet the organizations objectives" (Gillies, 1989).
6. Believes adults resist change and remain static.

Theory Y views the worker as growing, dynamic, and adaptable. According to Theory Y, the average worker:

1. Finds work itself can be rewarding and motivating.
2. If personally committed, will exercise self-direction and assume responsibility.
3. Is motivated by needs for personal pride, self-fulfillment, responsibility, and the need to grow.
4. Is capable of applying creativity and imagination to solving organizational problems.
5. Believes adults are dynamic and capable of learning and accepting responsibilities.

McGregor drew upon Maslow's needs theory to propose that the role of managers is to provide an environment and opportunities for employees to meet their needs and grow.

Theory Z. A more recent theory, referred to as Theory Z, emerged during the 1980s. It expanded upon Theory Y and added the democratic approach to leadership. The philosophy of Theory Z "is based on the idea that organizations can significantly benefit from facilitating the creative ideas and input of the members of that organization" (Adair, Nygard, 1982). Believing that better-motivated employees were more productive and satisfied, researchers based this theory on six key elements (see box on p. 197).

Many articles have been written that adapt Theory Z to nursing management. Administrators that have applied Theory Z principles to nursing have found:

1. A decrease in turnover rates.
2. Increased autonomy.
3. Decreased feelings of alienation.
4. Improved skills and commitment to nursing careers.
5. Fewer interdepartmental conflicts.
6. Improved integration of home and career demands.
7. Improved quality assurance and risk management (Adair, Nygard, 1982).

Critics of Theory Z dismiss it as trendy and inappropriate for our short-term, goal-oriented society, but researchers such as R. Likert and his

---

〜 ELEMENTS OF THEORY Z

1. **Holistic concern.** Concern for each worker as a whole, his/her well-being, physical and mental health, and performance are important. Workers are treated with respect, trust, and fairness. Loyalty and commitment to the organization and work group improve when managers are concerned with the whole person.
2. **Consensus decision making.** Every worker participates in the decision-making process through the use of quality circles—weekly meetings devoted to analyzing problems, developing solutions, and evaluating results. Quality circles keep employees informed, encourage participation, and help them commit to decisions.
3. **Staff development.** Improving the skills and abilities of each worker is considered an important investment in the company's future.
4. **Long-term employment.** Employees are expected to spend many years with the organization. Movement within the organization is encouraged, but moving from one company to another is not.
5. **Slower promotions.** Allowing time for group relationships to develop and workers to thoroughly learn the job improved productivity. Slower promotions also discouraged game playing and competition while allowing management the time to evaluate a worker's long-term contribution to the organization.
6. **Indirect supervision.** Workers who believe in the organization's philosophy, embrace its values and goals, and are involved in making decisions that affect them need little direct supervision. Another source of indirect supervision is the work group's influence. The desire for peer approval motivates group productivity.

---

colleagues found that, in general, the more worker participation was encouraged, "the greater the likelihood of superior performance and job satisfaction" (Likert, 1967).

Modern organizational theory

During the early 1960s, researchers began to recognize that, in both the classical and the humanistic theories, something was still missing. **Modern organizational theory was an attempt to integrate research from various disciplines** such as sociology, economics, administration, mathematics, and engineering into a single unifying strand—total human systems.

A system is comprised of a number of dynamic, interacting, interdependent parts functioning as a whole. To illustrate, consider the human body. The respiratory system, like the other body systems, performs its specialized function, which, in this case, is taking oxygen from the air to the blood and releasing carbon dioxide from the blood to the air. It is a complex, dynamic (always working) system. However, the respiratory system is also interacting and dependent upon the circulatory system to transport the oxygen molecules via the blood to the tissues. Each system requires the other (interdependence) to fulfill its own functions. Without the cooperative interactions of each system, the whole body will eventually fail. Organizations are similar to bodies. Each interdependent system contributes to the success or failure of the entire organization. Following this line of thought, researchers adopted two main approaches to analyzing organizations: systems and contingency.

Systems. The hallmark of the modern organizational theory is a systems framework. This allows us to view organizations as an open system—one that interacts with the environment by receiving input (materials and ideas received from the environment), moving materials or information through the organization (throughput), generating output, and evaluating. This focus on the organizational process differed from earlier theories which focused on structure.

The concept of 'wholeness' is the basis for the systems framework. All parts of an organization are interrelated, and change in one area will affect the whole organization in one way or another. Emphasis is placed on the need for communication and cooperation among all members of the organization.

The role of management is to coordinate and monitor communications as well as the flow of energy (work) throughout the system. Although few health care organizations are based on modern organizational theory principles, nurses who work within this system "are directly responsible for planning, implementing, and evaluating all the functions of input, throughput, and output for their clients" (Sullivan, 1990).

Contingency. The contingency approach emphasizes the "relationship between the organization and its environment" (Sullivan, 1990). The context or situation determines which methods of management will be most successful. Contingency theories consider the realities of a specific organization by stressing an 'if-then' approach. *If* a certain situation (environment) exists, *then* a specific managerial action will be most effective.

Researchers found that many factors can influence the outcome of a situation. Studies done by F. Fiedler (contingency theory), R. House (path–goal theory), and other researchers found that several factors can influence and, thus, determine the outcome of a situation. Some of these factors are (Tappen, 1989):

1. The nature and scope of the task.
2. The employee's perceptions and expectations of the task.

〜〜 MBO PRINCIPLES

1. It is a result-oriented system.
2. It relates to concepts of human motivation.
3. It emphasizes participation from all levels of employees.

---

   3. Role ambiguity.
   4. The favorableness (or unfavorableness) of the situation.
   5. The power and effectiveness of the leader.
   6. Group size.
   7. Communication networks.
   8. Organizational structure.
   9. Social status and position in group.
  10. Stress, especially interpersonal or interdepartmental.

Managers who consider the impact of various factors on the situation are better able to understand the dynamics of each situation and its influences on the whole organizational system.

Management by objectives. Introduced in the 1950s by Peter Drucker, the **management by objectives (MBO)** approach to organizational theory incorporated principles from the classical, humanistic, and modern schools of thought (see box above).

    MBO uses a four-step process, which includes setting goals, action planning, developing tools for periodic reviews of progress, and performance appraisal (evaluating). The manager's role in this system is to assist with common goal setting and planning in addition to conducting periodic reviews. Application of the MBO system is discussed in Chapter 10.

The importance of theories

So why, you ask, are these theories important to me? The answer: A knowledge of organizational theories helps you to:

- Assess the organizational theory used by a specific health care facility. The facility's philosophy, structures, functions, and treatment of employees is based on its organizational theory.
- Develop a basis for more effective management and leadership.
- View the 'big picture' and, thus, contribute to the organization.
- Clarify individual roles and functions within the organization.
- Foster group loyalty, cohesion, and productivity.
- Improve morale and productivity through staff participation in decision making and planning.

- Improve your communication effectiveness and role flexibility.
- Communicate to society about nursing—who we are, what we do, why clients need our services, and why our costs are justified.
- Understand the business of health care delivery.

Organizational Structure and Functions

In order to work effectively and, thereby, achieve goals, people require a framework within which to work. This framework, or matrix, is called a structure.

Definitions

Organizational *structure* is the framework for the working relationships of all its resources. *Resources*, in this case, include both human and material assets. Structure within an organization arranges work systematically, thereby allowing managers to use and coordinate resources in order to achieve goals. Without an organizational structure, work could not be efficiently done.

An organization's overall *function* is to achieve its goals and, thus, profit in some manner. The goal of health care organizations, for example, is to provide high-quality, preventative and restorative client care for the lowest possible cost.

Organizational *process* refers to the manner or methods used to achieve the company's goals. In short, an organization's structure and function defines what the company *is* and what it *does*, while organizational process defines *how* it is done.

All organizations (companies, facilities) have specific lines of authority, patterns of communication, and policies that define its structure. Basically two types of structure exist within an organization: formal and informal. Managers who are aware of and work within each structure can be more effective.

Formal organizational structure

The formal structure of an organization is the pattern of defined relationships and duties. This pattern is visually represented by the organizational chart—a blueprint that specifies lines of formal authority and communication. Figure 8-1 illustrates an organizational chart for a long-term care facility. Titles such as charge nurse or supervisor broadly describe job activities. Status is indicated by the job's position on the chart and its distance from the top. Written job descriptions assist in defining formal relationships. Formal structure also includes the rules, policies, and procedures used by managers to guide employee behaviors toward goal

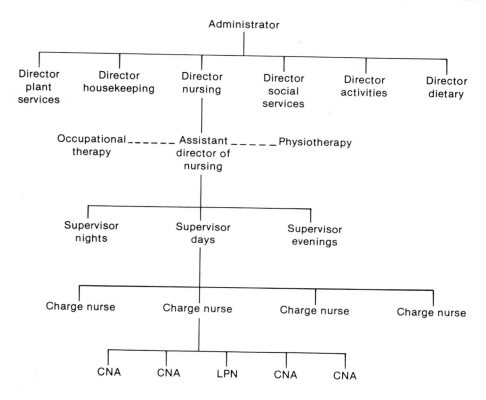

FIGURE 8-1 An organizational chart for a long-term care facility.

achievement. Within the nursing profession, an "institution's organizational chart depicts how the nursing department fits into the organizational structure and indicates the status and accountability of nurses within the organization" (Sullivan, 1990).

Elements. All formal organizational structures consist of four basic elements (see box on p. 202). Although formal structures may differ in size and scope, they all consist of these four elements.

Types. Formal organizational structures may also be classified by type. Most health care facilities (and nursing departments) use one or more of the following:

1. **Bureaucratic structure.** As discussed earlier, the bureaucracy is structured on a simple, direct chain-of-command pattern which defines the authority, responsibility, and span of control for each position. Work-

ELEMENTS OF ORGANIZATIONAL STRUCTURES

1. A mission statement or philosophy, which describes the facility's purpose and goals. This mission statement (philosophy) is the basis or foundation of the organization's formal structure.
2. An organizational chart, which serves as a visual reminder of the organization's patterns of authority, responsibility, and communication. Health care facilities typically use a pyramidal or bureaucratic structure.
3. Designated levels of management that define the authority and responsibility (in writing) for each position within the structure.
4. Written policies and procedures, which provide the basis for the organization's standards and methods of work.

ers are accountable to only one supervisor and are expected to place the organization's goals ahead of their own. Nursing departments using this approach refer to it as a 'line' or 'pure line' structure, for relationships and responsibilities are defined in a line from the top down. The bureaucratic structure has many specialized positions and hierarchical levels. It is the most widely used structure in health care institutions.

2. **Functionalized structure.** When an organization becomes large or contains a number of specialties, help is usually needed to assist with the management process. In a hierarchical organization, the line functions are control and command. 'Staff' functions are separated from the chain-of-command and rely on the expert's (specialist's) knowledge to increase effectiveness. If, for example, the director of nurses becomes too busy to effectively carry out all the duties of the position, he/she may share the work load with a specialist who remains subordinate and does no supervision. Specialists serving in staff roles serve one of three functions: they provide a service, offer advice, or control a specialized function. People in staff roles serve and support the line (authority) structure by providing information and expertise; however, they have no authority to enforce decisions.

In a long-term care facility, line positions are exemplified by such titles as director of nursing, head nurse, and team leader. Specialty (staff) positions have such titles as in-service educator, activities director, and occupational therapist. Specialists may inform, advise, and exercise certain control, but they are not allowed to "usurp command responsibilities of line managers" (Gillies, 1989). Functionalized structure is also called 'line and staff' organization.

3. **Ad hoc structure.** An open, flexible mode of operation characterizes the ad hoc structure. Based on the premise that most workers are motivated, self-sufficient, and enjoy solving problems, the ad hoc structure consists of teams that are created by top managers for a specific task, goal, or purpose. These teams are temporary and usually are composed of workers from different levels in the hierarchy with diverse backgrounds. Ad hoc teams study specific problems, attain specific goals, or perform complex, important nonroutine tasks. Once the objectives have been achieved, the team disbands. In short, ad hoc teams help advise, solve problems, and coordinate work. The goals, guidelines, and amounts of authority are determined by the top level of management.

4. **Matrix structure.** When project teams or task forces are built into the hierarchical organization (listed on the organizational chart [see Figure 8-1]), a matrix structure results. Efforts of various specialists are coordinated through the chain of command and integrated by the manager who supervises them all. Matrix structures have fewer hierarchical levels and fewer rigid formal rules, procedures, and regulations. Decision making is more decentralized, and employees are expected to integrate the efforts of others to meet goals. In the health care setting, for example, a nurse is responsible for the full range of nursing care provided for the client. He/she will integrate and coordinate the efforts of such specialists as a dietitian, pharmacist, and various therapists. Decisions are formally made and reinforced by the care team, but the nurse uses his/her influence and expert knowledge to coordinate all client care.

Modern health care institutions are usually structured bureaucratically, but many facilities are assessing and implementing other, less rigid, organizational structures.

Functions. Regardless of the type, an efficient formal organizational structure accomplishes four purposes. An organizational structure:

1. Coordinates effort
2. Defines common goals
3. Saves labor
4. Identifies the authority hierarchy (chain-of-command)

Informal organizational structure

While an organization's formal structure is a well-planned, deliberate attempt to establish relationship patterns, another interwoven structure exists—the informal organization. Magula (1982) defines the informal organizational structure as a pattern of "relationships and interactions which

CHARACTERISTICS OF AN INFORMAL ORGANIZATION

1. Interactions, associations, and friendships that cross formal authority lines. The janitor, for example, may be the administrator's golf partner.
2. Relationships, lines of authority, and communications are unspoken, often covert, and not recorded in the organizational chart.
3. Informal lines of communication referred to as 'the grapevine' (see Chapter 2).
4. Inevitable formation. Management can choose to change any part of the formal structure, but they have no power over the informal organization. As long as there are people, there will be an informal structure.
5. Small groups whose members exert a strong on influence behavior and performance.
6. Positive and negative consequences for the company.

occur spontaneously out of the activities and interactions of members of the organization, but which are not set forth in the formal structure." In other words, informal structure refers to the groups and relationships that naturally develop as people interact.

Although classical theorists concentrated on the formal organizational structure and the behaviorists (humanists) focused on the informal structure, both structures are inseparable and intricately entwined.

Characteristics. The informal organization has a powerful impact on the company. In fact, it is the combination of both the formal and informal structure that makes the organizational setting where work is carried out to meet goals (see box above). Learn to become aware of the informal structure of your facility. By working with it (rather than ignoring it), you will succeed where others may fail.

Types. Informal structures are comprised of people who have formed groups. Informal groups are generally viewed as two types:

1. *Interest groups.* Formed because each group member is concerned about a specific issue. Once the issue has been resolved, the group tends to disband. Interest groups share issues of common concern.
2. *Friendship groups based on social relationships.* These groups de-

---
FUNCTIONS OF AN INFORMAL ORGANIZATION

1. They meet an individual's needs for friendship, belonging, status, and power.
2. They perpetuate social and cultural values that are important to group members.
3. They increase the ease of communication among group members.
4. They stabilize and increase the desirability of the work environment.
5. They act to modify the formal structure when members are not satisfied.
---

velop because of personal affiliations of members. Simply stated, people who like each other tend to want to be together. Membership in friendship groups, like interest groups, tends to change over time as old friendships dissolve or new friendships begin.

Functions. Informal structures serve several functions for group members (see box above). To maximize effectiveness when working with informal groups, the nurse manager needs to consider the group's size, degree of cohesiveness, norms (values), and status. Support from the informal group is important if the manager is to be effective.

Organizational Culture

According to social psychologist, Kurt Lewin, employee behavior (B) "is a function of the interaction between personal characteristics (P) and the environment (E) around the person," or $B = P + E$ (Davis, Newstrom, 1989). An important part of the environment is the social culture of the organization.

Culture defined

Organizations, like fingerprints, are unique. Each has its own set of culture values and norms. Organizational culture, then, is the combination of symbols, language, assumptions, beliefs, values, and norms that are shared among the company's members (Davis, Newstrom, 1989; del Bueno, Vincent, 1986). The organization's culture provides the human environment in which employees work.

CHARACTERISTICS OF ORGANIZATIONAL CULTURE

- The elements (the values, norms, patterns) are compatible with each other. Each aspect of the company's culture fits with and complements the other, similar to puzzle pieces fitting together.
- Most workers accept or embrace the company's culture.
- Although employees seldom talk about the culture, it is always present and influential.
- Most company culture evolves from the examples set by the top managers and administrators. These examples powerfully influence employees.
- Cultures can have a relatively strong or weak influence on employee behaviors.
- The organization communicates key elements of its culture to the employees through the process of formal (training) and informal (role modeling) socialization (also known as the process of 'learning the ropes').
- A single employee can exert influence on the company's culture (referred to as individualization).

From Davis K, Newstrom J: *Human behavior at work: organizational behavior,* ed 8, New York, 1989, McGraw-Hill.

Characteristics

Culture consists of an organization's unique history, philosophy, systems and procedures, patterns of communication, stories, and myths. For example, some organizations have a fast-paced atmosphere, while others may be easygoing.

Self-preservation. As time passes, a company's culture becomes known to the public and tends to perpetuate itself. The first characteristic of an organization's culture, then, is that it tends to sustain and preserve itself by attracting employees who are compatible with its values and beliefs.

Other aspects. Other characteristics of organizational culture that are noteworthy are listed in the box above.

Levels of culture

Within an organization, three levels of culture exist (del Bueno, Vincent, 1986):

Visible level. The visible level is seen in the use of physical space as well as the social environment. To illustrate, if the director of nurses' desk is situated to remove it as a barrier and the office door is usually open, a causal, comfortable atmosphere is encouraged. The visible level of a company's culture can be assessed by observing the environment, practices related to dress and personal appearance, and status symbols.

Values level. Values constitute the second level. They relate to what *should be* rather than *what is* and are seen in the organization's philosophy, customs, expectations, rituals, and myths. The phrase, "We've always done it this way," is indicative of the values level of culture.

Basic assumptions. The basic assumptions that guide behavior reflect the third cultural level. These are the sacrosanct (sacred), undebatable, not-open-to-question, underlying assumptions of the organization. They include beliefs about the nature of man, human relationships, and the community served by the company. Are people or profit more important? Are all employees interdependent or are some more important? Are people (customers, clients) able to make decisions, or are they basically ignorant and need to be led? Such questions illustrate the focus of the third level of culture.

Managers and supervisors need to take the time to learn about the facility's culture. It is an important part of the employee's social environment.

Assessing culture

Dorothy del Bueno (1987) believes that nurse managers can better understand an organization's culture by assessing the following areas:

Communications. Ascertain how important communications are handled, written or verbal. If written, is the style formal or informal? Learn the language or jargon used. Observe how information flows (from top down or bottom up) and is distributed (verbal, rumor, memo, bulletin board, newsletter). Find which reports are considered important, which are filed in the wastebasket, and, perhaps most importantly, determine where the important communications take place (the meeting room, hallways, social functions, the rest rooms, away from the business). Many important decisions may be made in unexpected places.

Deportment. Assess the appearance and presentation of the employees (e.g., dress codes and their enforcement, status related to dress, use of makeup and jewelry, facial hair, issues relating to hair length and style, use of first or last names, acceptance of jokes, and any off-limits places for employees). Determine what kind of relationships are acceptable off the job, between sexes, and among different authority levels. Is touching or affection acceptable? Do sexist behaviors exist? Do workers 'let themselves go' during social events? The behaviors demonstrated by employees reveal much about an organization's culture.

Environment. Observe the use of public space. Is it cold and sterile or warm and inviting? Consider the employees' spaces, the lounge, dining area, individual touches in work areas, and who eats with whom. Get the feel of the environment — the ambiance.

Image. Observe how the organization wishes to be perceived. What image is presented to the public? Is there money being spent to create or sustain the image? Find how the public gains access to the facility, how visitors are treated, and if employees are expected to be involved in off-duty community activities.

Meetings. Assessment of meetings can be very helpful. Look for the following: time frames (strictly enforced or casual), agenda (predetermined, able to adjust), unwritten rules, amount of discussion, refreshments. Ascertain which meetings can be skipped without reprisal or loss of important information.

Rituals, ceremonies, rites. Evaluate the orientation process for new employees: who greets, who orients, how the process is done, special orientations for different levels. Know which established rituals must be attended (e.g., the head nurses' breakfast, the Friday afternoon get-together, the annual Christmas party or picnic). Find out how the organization recognizes employees' length of service, births, marriages, retirements, and achievements. If sport teams or other groups exist, how important is participation? How many years does one have to work before he/she is considered an insider?

Sacred cows. "A sacred cow is a person, place, thing, or belief that cannot be discussed, attacked, or ignored. Sacred cows are revered and protected" (del Bueno, 1987). Their existence cannot be denied or ignored. Analyze which myths, subjects, rules, or policies are off limits, or taboo. What relationships or behavioral differences cannot be challenged or questioned? How are relationships with the media handled? Are there any heroes in the organization, and, if so, how did they become heroes? Be alert. Every organization has at least one sacred cow.

Status and rewards. Determine: if titles are true reflections of status and authority; what the bases for promotion are (e.g., performance, loyalty, longevity); how status symbols (i.e., title, office space, restricted areas) and privileges are used; and what elitist committees or social groups exist.

Carefully assessing these eight areas will assist you in gaining an overview of organizational culture, an important part of a manager's environment.

Organizational Authority

To be effective as a manager, it is imperative to use authority appropriately. Terms such as power, respect, responsibility, and authority must first be clarified.

Definitions

Authority is the *right* to make decisions, take action, direct, and evaluate the work of others. In short, it is the right to command or perform. Authority is the legitimate power inherent in the position. Employees at the top of the organizational chart have more authority than those at the bottom. To be effective, authority must be accepted by those existing under it.

Power is the *capacity* or *ability* to influence others. See Chapter 4 for a more complete discussion of power.

"Responsibility is the *obligation* [italics added] to perform assigned activities" (Certo, 1989). In other words, managers who are responsible do what they say they will do. A manager's attitudes, values, and behaviors all reflect his/her feelings about responsibility.

Respect may be one of the most important concepts when using authority. *Respect* is a feeling of deference, esteem, honor, or regard for an individual. It is important to remember that authority is *granted*, but respect must be *earned*.

Authority structures

Organizational authority follows the facility's structure. Usually, health care organizations follow a centralized or decentralized authority structure.

Centralization. Facilities that use centralization are usually bureaucratic. The decision-making power is held and exercised by the few individuals at the top. Minimal authority is delegated. All major decisions are coordinated and integrated from one point. Centralization has the advantages of better coordinated resources, which avoids duplication and permits pooling of resources when necessary.

Decentralization. In decentralized facilities, employees participate in making decisions, but control over company-wide matters remains with those in top management positions. Much authority is delegated, and motivation at the facility's lower levels is enhanced. Decentralization can lead to quicker decisions, improved performance, and lightened work loads for overworked managers. It can, however, also lead to uncoordinated efforts if not adequately monitored.

Types of authority

Within the organization, the supervisors and managers may exercise two types of authority: **line and/or expert authority.**

Line authority. As stated earlier, *line* refers to the hierarchy or chain-of-command. Thus, line authority is the formal authorization to issue orders, direct, monitor, and evaluate the work of others. Assigning CNA staff members to care for certain clients is an example of the use of line authority.

Expert authority. People with specialized knowledge have expert authority. Nurses have a broad range of knowledge and skills relating to the care and rehabilitation of other human beings, thereby possessing expert authority. Teaching a client to monitor his blood sugar or recommending a new client feeding method to the physician illustrates the use of expert authority. Nurses and their managers need to become comfortable with (and learn to effectively exercise) their expert authority.

Staff authority. Because health care workers are commonly referred to as 'the nursing staff,' some confusion exists. When referring to the organization, staff authority is defined as "the right to advise or assist those who possess line authority" (Certo, 1989). People with staff authority provide the support, advice, and services to help achieve the facility's goals. Although staff authority may involve the use of suggestions, recommendations, and action plans, the actual decisions are made by those employees with line authority. Examples of staff authority are diet changes recommended by the dietitian, exercises planned by the physiotherapist, or recreational outings encouraged by the Activities Department director.

Span of control

The concept of span of control is an important consideration for nurse managers. Span of control is the number of persons that a manager can effectively supervise. Bureaucratic, centralized companies have a tall structure (many levels of supervision) with each manager having a short span of control (few employees to supervise). Companies using the humanistic or modern organizational theories have a flatter structure with fewer levels of supervision. Each manager supervises a larger number of workers and, therefore, has a wide span of control. Figure 8-2 compares centralized and decentralized organizational spans of control.

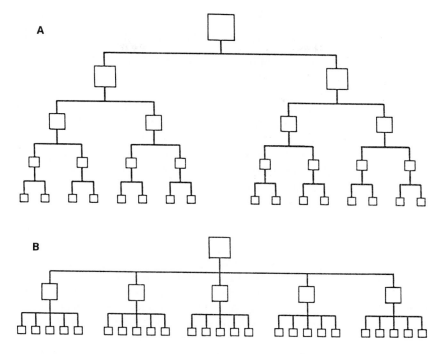

FIGURE 8-2 A comparison of **(A)** centralized and **(B)** decentralized spans of control. *(From Bernhard LA, Walsh M: Leadership: the key to professionalism of nursing, St Louis, 1990, Mosby.)*

Within the nursing profession the study of the span of control has been largely neglected. One study (Alidina, Funke-Furber, 1988), however, found that the nurse manager's span of control was influenced by several factors. Remember to consider these when assessing your own span of control.

Influencing factors. The average team leader or unit or department supervisor of nursing has nine key factors affecting his/her span of control (see box on p. 212). By considering how each of these factors affects your particular situation, you will be better able to identify the strengths and weaknesses inherent in your span of control.

Levels of management

Remember the 'universality of management' concept which states that all managers perform the same functions? (See Chapter 7.) Regardless of title, position, or level, managers all execute the five management functions

FACTORS AFFECTING SPAN OF CONTROL

1. **Patient profile** — client characteristics such as age, illness, degree of dependence, complexity and duration of care
2. **Nursing care program** — the nursing department's philosophy, goals, objectives, and policies
3. **Physical layout** — arrangements of client units, locations of supplies, equipment, and departments
4. **Manager profile** — skills, training, experience, clinical and management knowledge
5. **Employee profile** — staff mix (CNA, LPN, RN), training and competence levels
6. **Job-related factors** — the amount of similarity and interdependence of tasks, number of nonsupervisory tasks
7. **Support systems** — resources available, patient care policies, procedural systems, unit secretary
8. **Organizational factors** — company size and complexity, its developmental stage, management philosophy
9. **Environment factors** — social, technological, political, economic, the 'greying of America'

(plan, organize, coordinate, direct, and evaluate). However, various levels of management require different skills and emphasis. Most of today's companies, following the pyramid structure, have three levels of management: top, middle, and first-line.

Top management. The fewest managers are at the top. Most of their time is spent in developing plans and making the decisions that guide the organization. Processing and transmitting information are key elements of top management positions. Administrators and directors of nursing are examples of top-level managers.

Middle management. Middle managers have a wide range of jobs. Much of their time is spent in "translating the goals and plans of top managers into specific projects" (Reinecke, Dessler, Schoell, 1989). Department directors and shift supervisors are usually middle managers.

First-line management. The first-line supervisors and their workers are the people who actually implement the projects devised by top managers and organized by the middle managers. Nurses in first-line management positions have two basic responsibilities. The first is to ensure the delivery of safe and effective care to a usually large number of patients. Good management skills are imperative here. Second, the nurse manager is responsible for providing for the "physical, emotional, and economic welfare of a defined group of employees" (Gillies, 1989). As one can tell, first-line manager responsibilities are broad in scope and challenging in nature.

Standards of Care

In order to measure and evaluate quality, standards are necessary. Nurses are responsible for ensuring high standards of practice and devising methods for achieving these standards. Let us take a closer look at standards.

Standards defined

A standard is a defined level of excellence. **Standards are statements that describe a desired level of performance.** Every standard contains components that can be judged. For example, "The CNA will accurately count pulse rates" has no component for evaluation or judgment. "The CNA will count pulse rates with a deviation of less than 2 beats/minute, 100 percent of the time" is a much more accurate standard, for it defines a certain level of performance and allows for a judgment to be made.

Nursing care standards. A nursing care standard is "a descriptive statement of desired quality against which to evaluate nursing care given to a patient" (Gillies, 1989). Standards of nursing care serve as the basis for evaluating the quality and effectiveness of care received by clients.

Purposes

Standards can be used as planning tools or control devices. When a standard is used as a goal (e.g., all RNs will be able to identify and list two client problems within 1 hour after admission), it becomes a planning tool. However, when a nurse is reviewing client records and tallying the number of times the RNs listed two client problems, the standard is being used as a control or monitoring device.

In the profession of nursing, standards serve several purposes. The use of standards can:

1. Monitor and improve the quality of nursing care (quality assurance).
2. Help to decrease the costs of nursing care by eliminating nonessential nursing tasks.
3. Be used as a framework or basis for determining nursing negligence.
4. Motivate nurses to achieve excellence.

To be effective, however, standards must be well known by the staff and routinely reviewed.

Types of standards

Several types of standards are used to coordinate and direct nursing actions. They are commonly classified as **structural, process, and outcome standards.**

Structural. Structural standards are group- or 'thing'-oriented. They are the policies that "define conditions and mechanisms that facilitate desired staff functioning, systems operation, and patient care delivery" (Rutkowski, 1987). Examples of structural standards involve such topics as the patient population, code–no code policies, the environment, staffing, equipment and supplies, infection control, safety, and health.

Process. Process standards are action-oriented. They describe the specific methods used for nursing care delivery and specify expected nursing actions or behaviors. Process standards are described in a variety of formats. Job descriptions, protocols, procedures, guidelines, and performance standards all describe process standards.

Outcome. Standards relating to outcomes are results-oriented. They are statements describing the desired patient care results (hopefully in measurable terms). Outcome standards can also be applied to the nurse (e.g., Teach Mr. B. to inject insulin, using correct technique, prior to discharge.). Because outcome standards describe results, they are often used as goals. When utilized as goals, the process used to reach the goal (outcome standard) should be described.

These three types of standards, along with monitoring and corrective action procedures, constitute the core of quality assurance programs and assist nurse managers in ensuring a high level of nursing care delivery.

ANA's standards of practice

Standards formulated and based on valid and sound principles protect the client, the caregiver, and the institution. Although standards can be developed by state, local, or institutional groups, the national standards of practice developed by the American Nurses' Association have become most influential and widely accepted. The ANA originally developed one set of standards for all areas of nursing practice, but as the profession evolved into specialty areas, standards have been developed for such specialties as maternity, pediatric, psychiatric, medical/surgical, and geriatric nursing.

Geriatric care standards. As an example, the box on pp. 215 and 216 lists the 11 standards of gerontological nursing practice.

✎ STANDARDS OF GERONTOLOGICAL NURSING PRACTICE[1]

Standard I. Organization of gerontological nursing services
All gerontological nursing services are planned, organized, and directed by a nurse executive. The nurse executive has a baccalaureate or master's preparation and has experience in gerontological nursing and administration of long-term care services or acute care services for older clients.

Standard II. Theory
The nurse participates in the generation and testing of theory as a basis for clinical decisions. The nurse uses theoretical concepts to guide the effective practice of gerontological nursing.

Standard III. Data collection
The health status of the older person is regularly assessed in a comprehensive, accurate, and systematic manner. The information obtained during the health assessment is accessible to and shared with appropriate members of the interdisciplinary health care team, including the older person and the family.

Standard IV. Nursing diagnosis
The nurse uses health assessment data to determine nursing diagnoses.

Standard V. Plannning and continuity of care
The nurse develops the plan of care in conjunction with the older person and appropriate others. Mutual goals, priorities, nursing approaches, and measures in the care plan address the therapeutic, preventive, restorative, and rehabilitative needs of the older person. The care plan helps the older person attain and maintain the highest level of health, well-being, and quality of life achievable, as well as a peaceful death. The plan of care facilitates continuity of care over time as the client moves to various care settings and is revised as necessary.

Standard VI. Intervention
The nurse, guided by the plan of care, intervenes to provide care to restore the older person's functional capabilities and to prevent complications and excess disability. Nursing interventions are derived from nursing diagnoses and are based on gerontological nursing theory.

Standard VII. Evaluation
The nurse continually evaluates the client's and family's responses to interventions in order to determine progress toward goal attainment and to revise the data base, nursing diagnoses, and plan of care.

Continued.

STANDARDS OF GERONTOLOGICAL NURSING PRACTICE[1] — cont'd

Standard VIII. Interdisciplinary collaboration
The nurse collaborates with other members of the health care team in the various settings in which care is given to the older person. The team meets regularly to evaluate the effectiveness of the care plan for the client and family and to adjust the plan of care to accommodate changing needs.

Standard IX. Research
The nurse participates in research designed to generate an organized body of gerontological nursing knowledge, disseminates research findings, and ues them in practice.

Standard X. Ethics
The nurse uses the code for nurses established by the American Nurses' Association as a guide for ethical decision making in practice.[2]

Standard XI. Professional Development
The nurse assumes responsibility for professional development and contributes to the professional growth of interdisciplinary team members. The nurse participates in peer review and other means of evaluation to ensure the quality of nursing practice.

Reprinted, with permission, from American Nurses' Association, *Standards and scope of geronotological nursing practice*, Kansas City, Mo, 1987, ANA.
[1]American Nurses' Association: *Standards and scope of gerontological nursing practice* (pp 1-27), Kansas City, Mo, 1987, ANA.
[2]American Nurses' Association: *Code for nurses with interpretive statements*, Kansas City, Mo, 1985, ANA.

Client Care Delivery Systems

Nursing is a service industry. We produce no products that can be sold or traded in the marketplace. Our product is the health care we provide for our clients.

Throughout nursing history, various approaches have been devised to deliver safe, effective, and efficient health and illness care (service) to patients (clients). Effective delivery of nursing and other client care requires adequate staff and an organized method or system for providing or delivering care. Four client care delivery systems are currently in use. The **delivery system used reflects the organization's philosophy, structure, staffing patterns, and patient population.** Refer to Figure 8-3 for a comparison of the organizational structure for each nursing care delivery system.

Case management method

The case management system (see Figure 8-3, *A*) is the oldest approach to client care. It first gained popularity during the Civil War and continued as the only nursing care delivery system until the early 1930s. With this method, **one nurse cared for one patient, meeting all nursing and non-nursing needs.** Early nurses (1880s to 1920s) graduated from nurse's training and found that the only option for employment was to become a private duty nurse, living with the patient (in the home or hospital) and providing 24-hour care. Today's private duty nursing specialty evolved from the case management system.

Characteristics. The case method is simply organized. A one-to-one ratio allows the nurse to coordinate and control all aspects of the client's care. In today's care facilities, one nurse is responsible for one client while on duty and reports to a charge nurse or unit manager. The case method emphasizes following physicians' orders and is used in emergency rooms, intensive care units, community health agencies, and by nursing students.

Advantages. The case method system has several advantages (Tappen, 1989):

- It is simple and direct.
- It has a clear line of responsibility.
- Care is comprehensive and continuous, and client needs are quickly met.
- It simplifies planning of assignments.

Disadvantages. Although considered the ideal management system by some, the case method also has disadvantages:

- It is expensive. Professionals do work that can be done by less skilled people.
- It cannot be used with ancillary (nonlicensed) staff.
- Confusion can result with different nurses independently interacting with various departments (dietary, laboratory, pharmacy, etc.).

Functional method

During the 1930s, nurses changed from private duty practitioners to hospital employees. Nursing developed to a point where nursing students could no longer provide all the patient care, which was a common practice prior to this time. Graduate nurses were now needed to cope with new technologies, medical advances, and more complex patient care.

Characteristics. Based on the 'assembly line' division of labor style, the **functional method** (see Figure 8-3, *B*) **divides nursing cares into specific tasks and assigns caregivers to different tasks.** The basis for making assign-

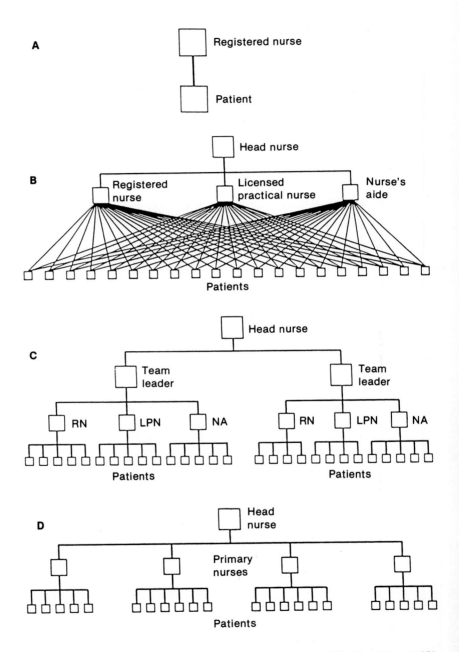

FIGURE 8-3 Organization of the **(A)** case method, **(B)** functional, **(C)** team, and **(D)** primary nursing care delivery systems. *(From Bernhard LA, Walsh M: Leadership: the key to professionalism of nursing, St Louis, 1990, Mosby.)*

ments is efficiency. A typical unit, for example, would be staffed with a charge nurse, a medication nurse, a treatment nurse, aides who take vital signs, and so on. The charge nurse supervises and coordinates all care. Each staff member is responsible only for assigned tasks. Functional nursing is bureaucratic, centralized, and hierarchical. It reflects the classical scientific management theory by focusing on tasks and efficiency.

Advantages. Functional nursing was further developed during World War II when the shortage of nurses was critical. Advantages of this method are as follows:

- Fewer professional nurses are required, for less skilled workers perform many tasks.
- Efficiency. Assignments are clearly defined and easy to monitor and coordinate.
- Workers become adept at tasks and can finish quickly.

Disadvantages. Some serious disadvantages exist with this system. The disadvantages are as follows:

- It may be efficient (tasks are performed) but not effective (client wonders who his nurse is).
- Fragmentation of care may result due to the emphasis on tasks instead of the person (patient).
- Work can become boring for the staff and lead to frustration.
- Communications may be minimal, and no one has the overall picture of patient care.
- Holistic nursing is not compatible with the functional method of nursing care delivery.

Team nursing

"Team nursing was introduced during the 1950s to improve nursing services by using the knowledge and skills of professional nurses and to supervise the increasing numbers of auxiliary nursing staff" (Marriner-Tomey, 1992).

Characteristics. Team nursing (see Figure 8-3, *C*) **is based on the philosophy of achieving goals through use of the talents and abilities of group (team) members.** It is a humanistic, decentralized system designed to motivate workers and satisfy patients. The team leader is an RN with the authority to make assignments by matching client needs with caregiver skills and abilities. Team members use a democratic interactional style, and the responsibility for the total care given to the assigned patients rests with the whole team. Communication is built into the system via written nursing care plans, assignments, and verbal conferences.

Advantages. Team nursing delivery systems are advantageous for both the client and the caregivers in the following ways:

- When done well, team nursing is satisfying for both clients and caregivers, for the client knows who his 'nurse' is, and caregivers feel they are giving good patient care.
- Team members' abilities are more likely to be utilized fully and recognized.
- The delivery of nursing cares becomes more comprehensive and holistic.
- Productivity improves through increased cooperation, communication, and morale.

Disadvantages. There exist some definite drawbacks to the team nursing care delivery system. The disadvantages are as follows:

- Poorly constructed teams are ineffective. Insufficient numbers of staff or nurses who refuse to delegate can disrupt the whole system.
- Much cooperation and communication among staff members is required.
- Some efficiency is lost because of the need for frequent interactions.
- Confusion can result if the composition of the team varies frequently.
- A large amount of patient care is given by non-nursing personnel.

Primary nursing

The **philosophy that patients, not tasks, should be the focus of nursing care delivery gave rise to the primary nursing method** (see Figure 8-3, *D*). It was developed by nurses during the early 1970s as an attempt to return to the 'my nurse, my patient' concept.

Characteristics. Each registered nurse is assigned as a primary nurse for four to six patients. The primary nurse is responsible for his/her client's care from admission to discharge, 24 hours a day throughout the client's stay. The nurse manager assigns the primary nurse, who then coordinates all aspects of the client's care after consulting the physician and other involved health care professionals. An ongoing nursing (patient) care plan is developed, and associate nurses provide the planned care when the primary nurse is not on duty. The primary nurse, however, retains the responsibility, authority, and autonomy for planning, implementing, and evaluating the care received by the client.

Advantages. Primary nursing has many benefits. The advantages of this system are as follows:

- An all-RN staff can provide more personalized and holistic care.
- Continuity and accountability of care is improved.
- Nurses have more autonomy and are challenged.
- Both patients and nurses are more satisfied due to the stability of the relationship.
- Research suggests that clients experience fewer complications and spend fewer days in the facility.

Disadvantages. Most drawbacks arise from problems with implementing the system. Drawbacks that may arise include the following:

- Costs may be increased with a larger number of professional nurses.
- Nurses may not be fully educated or trained to make extensive assessments and care plans.
- Role confusion can result when LPN/LVNs are used as associate nurses. CNAs may feel a sense of loss because direct patient care tasks are reduced.
- Communication problems may arise.

Nurse managers who are aware of the organization's care delivery methods are more able to recognize and use the system's advantages and compensate for its disadvantages.

◈ Key Concepts

- *Organization* refers to both a structure and a process.
- Classical organization theory occurs in a bureaucracy and is based on individual productivity.
- Humanistic organization theory is based on group productivity and workers' morale.
- Modern organizational theory uses a systems framework to focus on the interrelatedness of each part of the organization and emphasizes the process used to meet goals.
- Organizational structure provides the framework for the management process. It includes specific lines of authority, communication patterns, and delegation practices.
- Formal structures of an organization are illustrated in its organizational chart. Formal structures provide a matrix for functions, activities, and relationships.
- Formal structures define the organization's mission, philosophy, authority, levels of management, policies, and procedures.
- Types of formal organizational structures include the bureaucratic, functionalized, ad hoc, and matrix structures.
- Efficient organizational structures define goals, coordinate efforts, save labor, and identify chains-of-command.
- Informal organizational structures are characterized by lines of authority and communications, which are not seen in the organizational chart.
- Organizational culture is comprised of the assumptions, symbols, language, behaviors, and attitudes that reflect the company's values and norms.
- Authority is defined as the right to make decisions, take action, and direct others.
- Organizational authority can be centralized where all decisions are made by few persons at the top of the hierarchy or decentralized where managers function democratically and are involved in decision-making activities.
- Nurses and other managers exercise line, staff, and expert authority.
- Authority is granted, but respect must be earned.
- Levels of management are divided into top, middle, and first-line (supervisory) categories.
- A standard is an agreed-upon level of excellence.
- Standards for nurses define the scope and dimensions for professional nursing care.
- Nurses are held accountable for upholding the standards of the American Nurses' Association's Standards of Nursing Practice.

- Standards assist the nurse manager to plan, implement, and evaluate the quality of nursing care delivered.
- Client care delivery systems are methods for organizing and providing nursing care.
- The most commonly used client care delivery systems relate to case management, functional, team, and primary nursing.

ॐ Learning Activities

1. List the similarities and differences of the classical, humanistic, and modern organizational theories.
2. Draw a diagram of a hospital or long-term care facility with a bureaucratic structure.
3. Describe how you would use staff authority to improve a unit's bathing routine (procedures).
4. Divide the class into three groups. Group 1 is to write a structural standard. Group 2 is to write a process standard. Group 3 is to write an outcome standard relating to patient's personal hygiene (bathing).
5. Scenario: You are the charge nurse for a 20-bed skilled care unit in a long-term care facility. Your staff consists of two RNs, one LPN, and three CNAs.
   a. Plan care assignments using the case, functional, team, and primary care delivery systems.
   b. Which system works best (worst) in this situation?

References

Adair MN, Nygard NK: Theory Z management: can it work for nursing?, *Nursing and Health Care* 3(11):489, 1982.

Alidina S, Funke-Furber J: First-line nurse managers: optimizing the span of control, *Journal of Nursing Administration* 18(5):34, 1988.

Certo SC: *Principles of modern management: functions and systems*, ed 4, Needham Heights, Mass, 1989, Allyn & Bacon.

Davis K, Newstrom J: *Human behavior at work: organizational behavior*, ed 8, New York, 1989, McGraw-Hill.

del Bueno DJ: An organizational checklist, *Journal of Nursing Administration* 17(5):30, 1987.

del Bueno DJ, Vincent PM: Organizational culture: how important is it?, *Journal of Nursing Administration* 16(10):15, 1986.

Fayol H: *General and industrial management*, London, 1949, Pitman & Sons.

Gillies DA: *Nursing management: a systems approach*, ed 2, Philadelphia, 1989, Saunders.

Kimball DS: *Principles of industrial organization*, ed 3, New York, 1925, McGraw-Hill.

Likert R: *New patterns of management*, New York, 1967, McGraw-Hill.

Magula M, editor: *Understanding organizations: a guide for the nurse executive*, Wakefield, Mass, 1982, Nursing Resources.

Marriner-Tomey A: *Guide to nursing management*, ed 4, St Louis, 1992, Mosby.

McGregor D: *The human side of enterprise*, New York, 1960, McGraw-Hill.

Reinecke JA, Dessler G, Schoell W: *Introduction to business: a contemporary view*, ed 6, Needham Heights, Mass, 1989, Allyn & Bacon.

Roethlisberger FJ, Dickenson WJ: *Management and the worker*, Cambridge, Mass, 1939, Harvard University Press.

Rutkowski B: *Managing for productivity in nursing*, Rockville, Md, 1987, Aspen.

Straub JT, Attner RF: *Introduction to business*, ed 4, Boston, 1991, PWS-KENT.

Sullivan MP: *Nursing leadership and management: a study and learning tool*, Springhouse, Pa, 1990, Springhouse.

Tappen RM: *Nursing leadership and management: concepts and practice*, ed 2, Philadelphia, 1989, Davis.

Additional Readings

Adkins RD: Responsibility and authority must match in nursing management, *Hospitals* Feb 1:69, 1979. *When nurse manager's authority matches the level of responsibility, a highly responsive operational system results.*

Coeling H: Work culture is the key, *Nursing 92* 22(7):74, 1992. *Finding, enjoying, and keeping the right nursing position depends on how you fit in with the staff's style.*

Cohen MH, Ross ME: Team building: a strategy for unit cohesiveness, *Journal of Nursing Administration* 12(1):29, 1982. *The authors describe one hospital's efforts at improving intershift cooperation and communication via a team-building effort.*

Douglas LM: *The effective nurse leader and manager*, ed 4, St Louis, 1992, Mosby. *Chapter 3 presents an overview of organizational structure as well as a comparison of bureaucratic and humanistic approaches to management.*

Eliopoulos C: Nurse staffing in long-term care facilities: the case against a high ratio of RNs, *Journal of Nursing Administration* 13(10):29, 1983. *All RN staffs in long-term care facilities are unrealistic and may have significant negative impacts.*

Harragan BL: *Games mother never taught you*, New York, 1977, Rawson Associates. *The author offers many insights into the corporate gamesmanship skills necessary for women to climb the organizational ladder.*

Jernigan DK, Young AP: *Standards, job descriptions, and performance evaluations for nursing practice*, Norwalk, Conn, 1983, Appleton-Century-Crofts. *This book is an excellent reference text for nurses needing well-defined job descriptions and performance evaluation tools.*

Joel LA, Patterson JE: Nursing homes can't afford cheap care, *RN* 53(4):57, 1990. *The author suggests that hiring more RNs and giving them greater autonomy can improve resident's health.*

Monaco RJ, Smith TT: How supervisors can put systems to work in day to day management, *Hospital Topics* 55:34, 1977. *Managers of the future must learn to manage work rather than the worker.*

Schuldt S: Supervision and the informal organization, *Journal of Nursing Administration* 8(7):21, 1978. *Using a problem-solving approach, the relationship of the supervisor to the powerful informal structure is discussed.*

Shukla RK: Nursing care standards and productivity, *Hospital and Health Services Administration* 27:45, 1982. *The author describes a research study of three nursing care structures — team, modular, and primary — in relation to nurse productivity.*

Vestal KW: *Management concepts for the new nurse*, Philadelphia, 1987, Lippincott. *Chapter 2 discusses organizational theory and the roles of the nurse executive, middle manager, head nurse, and staff nurse.*

CREATIVE

9

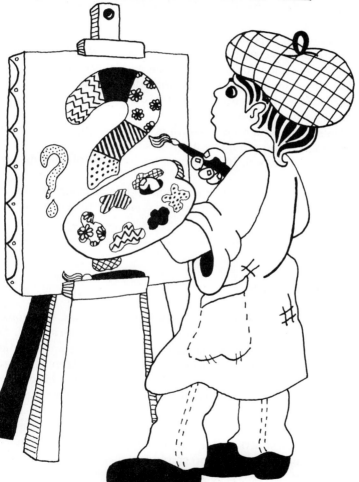

DECISION MAKING

Learning Objectives

Upon completion of this chapter, the reader will be able to:

1. State three ways to make any decision.
2. List three characteristics of good decisions.
3. Describe five causes of poor decision making.
4. Differentiate between job-oriented and people-oriented problems.
5. Identify five points to remember for making sound and timely decisions.
6. Explain four types of managerial decisions.
7. List two characteristics for each of the four decision-making styles.
8. Describe eight steps of the decision-making process.
9. List three steps for making 30-second (snap) decisions.
10. Explain the importance of objective and subjective evaluations in the decision-making process.
11. Identify four situations in which involving employees in the decision-making process would be appropriate.
12. List six characteristics of a mature (capable of making decisions) group.
13. Discuss four advantages and disadvantages of group decision making.
14. Describe five methods for adding creativity to the decision-making process.

General Considerations

Decisions are judgments. More specifically, decisions are choices made or courses of action selected from two or more alternatives. Decision making is a core element of management. In fact, it is an important component of all the basic management functions: planning, organizing, coordinating, directing, and evaluating. Nurses use decision making in every facet of practice. Decisions made by nurses may (and often do) have life or death significance.

Everyone makes numerous decisions daily. Some are made impulsively, emotionally, or superficially. Others require emotional stability, logic, and deep thinking. Many good employees make poor managers because of an inability to effectively make decisions.

Three approaches

Any decision may be approached in one of three ways. One may ignore, stall, or delay action; make no-thought decisions; or apply sound decision-making practices.

Ignore, stall, or delay action. Some personal decisions may be handled in this manner, but, as a manager, this wishy-washy approach is almost certain to guarantee failure. At risk is the loss of respect from your supervisors and productivity from your employees. Making decisions is an inescapable part of management. In most cases, stalling or delaying only compounds the original problem.

Make no-thought decisions. Quick decisions, made with no logic and little thinking, usually rely on hunches and create more problems than they solve. The no-thought method refuses to consider the side effects of the decision and applies the same off-the-cuff treatment to large, small, important, or routine problems.

Apply sound decision-making practices. Effective decisions follow a systematic, orderly process based on scientific principles. Decision making encompasses such topics as change, communication, conflict, and group dynamics. Managers with good decision-making skills improve productivity, build trust in employees, and engender respect from those in upper-management positions.

Good decisions, poor decisions

If decision making is the most important part of a manager's job, how do you know when a 'good' decision is made? Basically, **a good decision contributes to the organizational gain.** If the decision is poor, the organization or its members may suffer. Today's business environments increasingly demand that managers make good decisions as well as coach other staff members to do the same.

Characteristics of good decisions. According to Vestal (1988), "Good decisions are those that set the highest standards for action" (see box on p. 230). Decisions with these characteristics usually result in positive outcomes. The role of a nurse manager is to improve the odds for a favorable decision.

Causes of poor decisions. Many factors can contribute to poor decision making. Chief among these are factors relating to the following:

> *Incompetence of the manager.* If the supervisor is unable or unwilling to use each step of the decision-making process, the outcome of the decision will be ineffective.
> *Inadequate or too much data.* Prompt, timely, and accurate data are imperative for good decision making. If information is incomplete or inaccurate, decisions cannot be based on a full understanding of the facts. Conversely, if greater amounts of data than the manager

CHARACTERISTICS INHERENT IN A GOOD DECISION

- It is technically correct. Data have been researched or investigated. The decision is based on facts or technical competence. For example, nurses who make clinical decisions need extensive technical knowledge.
- It produces as few negative effects as possible. "Good deciding will anticipate potential downsides of the decision and weigh those against the expected positive outcomes" (Vestal, 1988).
- Action is taken. A good decision is of little value if it is not carried out. For example, if only a few staff members are following a new procedure, the odds are that it will not work. In order to be judged as positive, some action must be taken as a result of the decision.

can effectively process exist, decision making can become bogged down by too much information. Managers suffering from 'information overload' become incapable of making good decisions.

Confused responsibilities. Decisions that involve several people and departments can confuse the 'who is responsible for what?' question. Overlapping interests and areas of authority can split the power and responsibilities of the decision makers and drag out the process of making effective decisions.

Poor management atmosphere. "Few things are more detrimental to decision making than an atmosphere that breeds fear of making a wrong decision. One of the privileges a competent manager must enjoy is the right to be wrong. Although his overall performance will be measured on the number of correct decisions he makes, and their impact on progress, no successful manager can boast with justification that all his decisions have been 100 percent correct" (McConkey, 1974).

Failure to set time limits. Target dates or time limits by which an action must be taken are needed to prevent decisions from 'drifting' or becoming lost in other matters. When time limits are not applied, decisions fail.

Remembering the basic causes of poor decisions will help you to avoid them.

Types of problems

Managers (supervisors) are faced with making numerous decisions every day. According to Chapman (1975), most work-oriented problems will fall into one of two groups: job-oriented problems and people-oriented problems. As a manager, your task is to recognize and solve each type of problem.

Job-oriented problems. On any given day, many problems relate more to production than to the people who do the work. Two types of basic job-oriented problems exist:

Minor problems. These require decisions but have little influence on the organization's operations. Generally, small problems can be immediately solved then forgotten. Decisions are made in an orderly, efficient manner without consuming large amounts of time. The '30-second procedure' (discussed later in this chapter) provides an excellent tool for quick, frustration-free decisions for minor problems.

Major problems. Decisions that may have a permanent and lasting effect on the department's or organization's operations demand serious treatment and time. Because major job-related decisions may change policies or procedures, avoid the temptation to make a quick decision. Pay careful attention to all aspects of the problem and use your best logical thinking.

People-oriented problems. Problems that do not deal with things or procedures usually relate to people. These need special treatment. People problems exist inside the employee and fall into two basic categories:

Simple requests. Special requests involving such things as schedules, breaks, days off, and the like may be important to the worker but have an insignificant impact on the department's routine operation. Most of the time, after listening carefully, an on-the-spot answer may be given. However, three questions (criteria) should be answered when weighing each request. Is there a written policy relating to the request? Will relationships be damaged if the request is granted? Will the health or safety of others be compromised if the request is granted? When you are satisfied with the answers, graciously grant the request or explain your reasons for refusing.

Complex human problems. Problems involving one or more persons to the extent that they influence productivity are potentially serious. To reach a fair solution, listen carefully, gather information from all sides, weigh the facts carefully, and use good communication techniques to explain your decision to all involved employees. Encourage feedback but stand firm with your decision.

Points to remember
The process of making decisions effectively can be learned, practiced, and improved upon. As you grow in decision-making abilities, keep the following points about the 'real world' in mind.

Real-life decisions. "Real life decisions are usually called for in a pressure-packed environment of inadequate input, conflicting information, budget restraints, time squeezes, scarce resources, and many other elements that cloud the issues and threaten the quality of decisions [emphasis added]. Despite all this, poor decision making is not likely to be excused because of the complexities of the manager's workload. The manager needs a simple and logical framework for making decisions that stick" (Hersey, Blanchard, 1988).

A right to be wrong. As a manager, you have a right to be wrong. No one makes the 'right' choice 100 percent of the time. When decisions turn out poorly, examine the causes, learn, and move on. Every manager will occasionally make a 'wrong call.' The trick is to keep them at a minimum.

Unnecessary decisions. Do not make unnecessary decisions. Opportunities for making decisions will be thrust upon you from many sources. Prioritize and work with the more important ones first. A manager who makes unnecessary decisions is, at best, "viewed as a meddler rather than a manager. At worst you'll have ruptured the normal chains of command and confuse the organization" (Sloma, 1977).

Timing. Pay attention to timing. As Sloma (1977) so aptly states, "The right decision at the wrong time is always a bad decision." For example, do not present your director with a new and improved staffing plan the day after the quarterly budget figures were released showing the department was losing money. Appropriate timing can improve the effectiveness of the decision.

Decisiveness. The decisive person will prevail. Almost everyone is willing to share opinions, but few are willing to 'put their money where their mouth is,' or be decisive. Decisiveness is a willingness to assume the responsibility to act. To be an effective leader or manager, you must be decisive.

Remembering these five points will assist you to retain perspective during the many decision-packed days that lie ahead.

Decision Types and Styles

Decisions come in a variety of sizes, types, and styles. Management decisions are made throughout the day at various levels within the organization.

Levels of decisions

Decisions made by the management of an organization fall into three levels:

1. *Strategic decisions.* Decisions made by the company's top executives that are crucial to operations or long-range planning are strategic because they define and focus on major, long-term goals.
2. *Administrative decisions.* Middle managers make most administrative decisions. They resolve unusual problems and develop techniques to improve functioning.
3. *Operational decisions.* These are the routine decisions that relate to day-to-day events. Many are made in accordance with established policies, rules, regulations, and strategies. Middle and first-line managers make most of the operational decisions.

Types of decisions

A management decision may be classified as one of four basic types: programmed, nonprogrammed, optimizing, and satisfying.

Programmed decisions. These are the routine decisions that are faced over and over (repetitive). Most often the organization has developed methods for handling them. By following the preexisting policies, procedures, or guidelines, the manager ensures consistency and saves valuable time. Decisions relating to staffing are examples of a programmed decision.

Nonprogrammed decisions. No well-defined procedures or strategies exist for this type of decision. They are typically one-shot occurrences which call upon the manager for novel, creative decisions. An example might be the decision to admit clients with HIV/AIDS to the facility.

Optimizing decisions. The decision that results in **the ideal or very best outcome is optimizing.** It assumes that time was taken to explore all possible alternatives and, thus, the best decision was made. The luxury of time rarely exists in the high-pressure health care industry; therefore, optimizing decisions seldom are made.

Satisfying decisions. Most managers aim for solutions that are not ideal but meet minimal requirements. They realize that the perfect decision is not possible because of incomplete information, inadequate time, or conflicting goals and settle for a course of action that is tolerable. The manager who decides that two more CNAs are needed but settles for one is an example of a satisfying decision—the reality of give and take.

Decision styles

Decisions are made using one of four styles. **The most appropriate style for any given decision will depend upon the situation and the readiness of the followers.** Hersey and Blanchard (1988) suggest four basic styles: authoritative, consultative, facilitative, and delegative.

Authoritative style. The decision is made only by the manager when the authoritative style is employed. This style is very useful in two situations: those in which the manager is the only available resource, and those situations in which "the manager has the necessary experience and information to reach a conclusion and followers do not possess the ability, willingness, or confidence to help" (Hersey, Blanchard, 1988). Decisions related to scheduling, for example, involve an authoritarian style because the staff members are usually unfamiliar with scheduling procedures.

Consultative style. When the workers possess some degree of knowledge or expertise, the consultative style may be a valuable strategy. The manager obtains input from those people willing to help make a determination but remains the one who makes the final decision. To illustrate, asking workers for which days off they prefer and then developing the work schedule (i.e., their input, your decisions), illustrates the use of the consultative decision-making style.

Facilitative style. Employees who are willing and capable of sharing the authority and responsibility for decisions do well with facilitative style managers who are willing to work together in a cooperative effort to reach a decision. The decision-making process is shared, but you, as the manager, are responsible for the ultimate outcome. For example, when the manager and his/her staff members decide on the best method to feed Mrs. Jones, the staff's duty is to feed her, but the manager has the ultimate responsibility of preventing Mrs. Jones from losing weight.

Delegative style. The delegative style is most appropriate for followers with high degrees of readiness, experience, and information. With this style, the followers own the problem and will make the decision. Committees with committed members do well with a delegative style.

As a general rule, the most appropriate style for making decisions can be determined by looking at 'who owns the decision.' With the authoritative style, the manager owns the decision. The consultative style considers input, but the final decision rests with the manager. The facilitative style shares the decision-making ownership. With the delegative style, the followers own the decision.

The Process of Making Decisions

A successful decision maker possesses four important qualities: **courage, sensitivity, energy, and creativity** (Magula, 1982). Courage is needed for taking risks. Sensitivity to other people and the situation is necessary for a correct assessment. Energy is required to make things happen, and creativity helps to develop new ways to approach and solve problems.

These qualities may be innate or developed, but the process of effective decision making can be taught and learned. It requires practice and systematic thinking, but, once mastered, it can be quickly and effectively applied to any situation.

Problem solving or decision making

The ability to solve problems and make effective decisions are important tools for management. Both are processes that follow a logical sequence, but there are several important differences between problem solving and decision making.

Problem solving. The process of solving problems follows an orderly sequence of steps. The problem is first identified. Then solutions are considered, and one is chosen. The solution is implemented; the results then are evaluated. The goal of the process is to identify and solve the problem. Trial and error, as well as a number of other methods, are used to arrive at a solution.

Decision making. The decision-making process differs from the problem-solving process in two ways. First, although decision making may be triggered by a problem, it may be used in a manner that may not solve the actual problem. To illustrate, the nurse manager may deal with a conflict by separating the parties and sending them to different areas. A decision was made to quell the conflict, but the problem itself was not addressed.

Second, the decision-making process includes the important step of setting objectives (goals). "What do I want to accomplish by making this decision?" is an important question in the decision-making process.

How to make decisions

At least one dozen models for making decisions have been developed since the early 1960s. Some models list as few as six steps, while others describe as many as fifteen. Fortunately, all models follow the same basic procedures as the familiar nursing process: assess, plan, diagnosis (goals), implement, and evaluate.

Managerial decision making. Follow the important steps listed in the box on p. 236 for a method of learning how to **make quality decisions**. Practice until the process becomes second nature for you. This tool will serve you well, especially when others are indecisive or unable to make decisions.

Two types of evaluations are needed for making managerial decisions:

HOW TO MAKE QUALITY DECISIONS

1. **Observe the situation.** Gather accurate descriptions (what, when, how, who). Define the problem, if one exists, in clear and simple terms. Compare the present situation (what is) with the situation that could exist (what could be). Discard inaccurate, questionable, or irrelevant data. Clearly state your objectives (goals), then decide whether to take action.
2. **Search for alternatives.** Gather information to analyze the problem. Use as many resources as possible (e.g., people, records, computer data bases) but do not become bogged down in unneeded data.
3. **Develop alternatives.** List as many alternatives as possible. Identify any limiting factors such as time, resources, personnel, money, equipment, and facilities. Be creative. Elicit input from staff members. No alternative is perfect, but attempt to find the best choice.
4. **Evaluate alternatives.** Weigh the pros and cons of each potential solution by listing every possible advantage and disadvantage. Consider such constraints as cost, value, risk, feasibility, and acceptability of each alternative.
5. **Choose.** Select the best possible solution or decision by choosing the alternative that offers the fewest disadvantages and the most advantages within the limits defined. Be careful not to solve one problem and create another.
6. **Implement the alternative.** It is very important to communicate with everyone involved. The 'what, how, when, and why' of the alternative must be clearly shared if the process is to be successful. Prudent managers 'buy' the workers into the idea by 'selling' them on their roles and contributions needed for success. Plan to expect the unexpected.
7. **Monitor.** Check frequently to see if the alternative (solution) is working. Determine if responses are favorable or unfavorable.
8. **Evaluate.** This is a critical, but often forgotten, step (especially if the alternative is working well).

objective and subjective. To perform an objective evaluation, critically analyze all the data, responses, and reviews. Decide how well the alternative was implemented, then assess the results (both positive and negative). Decide what adjustments, if any, are needed.

To subjectively evaluate the alternative (and the decision-making process), determine if the 'human costs' were worth it. Consider the time, anxiety, or emotional discomforts inherent in the situation. Identify people's

---

✎ HOW TO MAKE QUICK DECISIONS

1. **Ascertain if this is the type of decision that can be resolved quickly and easily.** "When the consequences are major, careful deliberation is time well spent" (Calano, Salzman, 1988).
2. **If the decision meets the 'quick' criteria,** "take time to quietly restate the problem and review the facts in your mind (should take about ten seconds)" (Chapman, 1975).
3. **"Compare the first answer you think of with one or two possibilities** [emphasis added]. Weigh one against the other and try to come up with the best choice. If a decision is not obvious, make one anyway (about fifteen seconds)" (Chapman, 1975).
4. **"Have confidence that you have made the right decision** [emphasis added], announce it to those involved, and move on to something else (about five seconds)" (Chapman, 1975).

---

feelings of accomplishment, satisfaction, or insecurity associated with the decision.

Finally, and most important, do not hesitate to correct, change, or even discard the solution if your evaluation discloses that it was not the best alternative or did not meet the goal. A good decision maker knows when to stick by a decision as well as when to reverse a decision and try something new.

The 30-second snap decision. Did you know that "80 percent of the business decisions you're faced with should be made on the spot, 15 percent need to mature, and 5 percent need not be made at all" (Calano, Salzman, 1988)? Snap decisions can be perfectly adequate if made in a timely fashion. In fact, being decisive inspires support, intimidates any opposition, and often brings a new perspective to a situation. Follow the steps listed in the box above for making quick, frustration-free decisions. Solve minor decisions quickly. Move slowly and logically with decisions that may have a major impact or permanent influence.

Group Decision Making

With the introduction of modern organizational theory and its involvement of employees, managers are focusing on building a better working climate and increasing productivity by including their employees in the decision-making process. Groups can be highly effective in making decisions. Knowing when to involve the workers is a judgment that must be made by managers.

Criteria for group decision making

Employee or worker groups can (and should) be included in the decision-making process when

- the decision will have an influence on the employees,
- the decision is not urgently needed and time permits,
- company and departmental priorities permit, and
- the manager is willing to agree to and stand by the decision made by the group.

When the situation meets the above criteria, the group will benefit from involvement in the decision-making process. However, the nurse manager or supervisor must exercise judgment and assess the group for characteristics of maturity.

The mature group

Work groups, committees, task groups, and review panels are examples of groups who practice making decisions. Just as individuals grow and mature, so do groups. (See Chapter 3.) 'Mature' groups usually do well with decision making and possess the following features:

Awareness. Group members are aware of their own strengths and weaknesses as well as those of others. Each person is accepted as is.

Acceptance. "Individual differences are accepted without being labeled as good or bad" (Douglas, 1992). Group members realize the richness and diversity of individual differences.

Relationships. Interpersonal and authority relationships are developed, recognized, and accepted by the group. Each member is comfortable with the authority structure within the group.

Decisions. Rational discussion guides the group when they are working with the decision-making process. Individual opinions are considered and discussed. Dissent is welcomed, and members feel free to disagree. Eventually the group arrives at a decision that is acceptable to all members.

Conflict. Only the important issues, such as establishing goals or deciding upon methods to meet goals, generate conflict. Steps are taken to keep the conflict productive. Emotionally generated conflict issues are kept at a minimum, for the focus is on resolving any conflict that impedes decision making.

Process. Each member is aware of and cooperates with the group process. Roles within the group are known and accepted. Members are comfortable with the roles they fulfill. Again, the group process is focused on the steps needed to arrive at a decision.

Not all decision-making groups possess every characteristic. Mature groups, however, are able to move past individual idiosyncrasies and concentrate on the decisions at hand. Look for (assess) these characteristics when considering a group's involvement and contributions to decision making.

Emotional aspects of group decision making

Because problem-solving and decision-making procedures are a major concern to managers working with organizational groups, researchers began to study the emotional dimensions of group behaviors. Hill, Lippitt, and Serkownek (1979) studied the emotional dimensions of decision making and found that **predictable emotional responses were evoked during each phase of the group process.**

Needs assessment phase. The initial phase is begun when the group is convened with the focus of making decisions relating to problems or goals. Each group member has individual ideas, concerns, and levels of commitment. The emotional climate within the group tends to be hopeful and energetic. Members become acquainted, share personal information, and jockey for positions in terms of power and control. Group expectations are formed. A climate of team building and a sense of collective power emerges as individual concerns recede. The group and its leader often experience anticipation, hopefulness, and some anxiety about how well the group will function.

Creative intervention strategies for the leader include clarifying what needs to be done and establishing a nonjudgmental climate. Giving permission to dream by creating a 'nothing is impossible' atmosphere encourages creativity, divergent thinking, and many (rather than few) ideas. Instead of listing problems, have the group focus on what the organization would be like *after* goals are reached. In other words, focus the group's energies on what they want to happen rather than what they do not want to happen.

Goal-setting phase. The task shifts toward defining the dream (ideal goals) during this phase. Alternatives are developed, analyzed, and evaluated by sifting through data. Responses at this stage can be described as overwhelmed, confused, or dissatisfied. The enthusiasm felt earlier vanishes, and goals may now appear unattainable. Because this seems to be the most stressful phase, the group leader may respond to the confusion with doubt, anxiety, and fear of failure. He/she may try to 'save the group,' or the group may demand authoritarian leadership. This could be a critical mistake, however, because it short-circuits the group's development.

The most important strategy at this stage is to trust the group process. Attending to the emotional climate by keeping members in touch with feelings and goals helps to prevent the group from becoming overwhelmed. Patience is needed during this phase.

Action planning phase. With renewed energy the group begins to focus on turning goals into action plans. Trust and cooperation revitalize the group's interest and willingness to work. Some members may express concern about the group's ability to meet its goals or may feel cautious about making a commitment. The leader feels pride in the group's abilities but is concerned with their ability to design and implement the action plan.

The most important interventions at this stage are to provide the design help needed and encourage the group "to assume responsibility and ownership of the final design" (Hill, Lippitt, Serkownek, 1979). To assist with design planning, have the group develop a general outline (macro design). Then encourage them to plan the specifics (e.g., times, activities, resources) in a step-by-step manner (micro design). Last, be available for support and consultation.

Implementation. Teamwork pays off, for the group is now 'on stage' with its plan. Actually, this phase becomes a process of doing, evaluating, replanning, and doing again. Emotional responses vary from apprehension to realization of success. Leaders must resist the temptation to protect the group by covering or fixing mistakes. They share in the excitement but are concerned about a positive conclusion.

The leader's role now becomes one of active observer. Offer support. Participate but do not create dependency. Let the group do the implementing.

Evaluation. The final phase of the group process consists of review, closure, feedback, and celebration. The group reviews its development, evaluates how well the goals were met, summarizes its learning, and makes suggestions for improvement. Issues of closure and termination surface. Members may feel a sense of loss or sadness at termination, which may express itself as denial and resistance to closure activities. Others may experience a sense of relief, joy, and accomplishment. Ideally, group members share a sense of success and a willingness to apply their new-found knowledge to other situations.

The leader's responsibility at this phase is to ensure that the evaluation component takes place. Three areas of evaluation need to be addressed (see box on p. 241).

AREAS OF EVALUATION

1. Finishing and closure activities — directed at dealing with whatever interpersonal and task issues remain unfinished;
2. Feedback — directed at helping members learn from each other about their behavior and the program alternations that may be needed;
3. Celebration of the finished process. The evaluation phase can provide a wealth of learning for the group members and for the facilitator.

From Hill B, Lippitt L, Serkownek K: The emotional dimensions of the problem solving process, *Group and Organizational Studies* 4(1):93, 1979.

The emotional responses of any decision-making group are cyclic. Applying this knowledge helps the leader to understand and support the group during each phase of the decision-making process.

Pros and cons of group decision making

Although participatory (group) decision making is now encouraged by all but the most authoritarian organizations, you should be aware that disadvantages as well as advantages do exist. An awareness of the pros and cons can assist you in exercising your decision-making responsibilities in the most appropriate manner.

Advantages. Group participation in decision making offers several benefits to the organization:

- "Because of their broader experiences, groups have a wider range of knowledge to draw upon than the individual" (Marriner, 1977).
- Group members have opportunities to express and discuss their points of view, which encourages self-expression, innovation, and mutual problem solving.
- Members' acceptance of and commitments to the decision are fostered when they have had a say in the process.
- Problems with persuading the group to accept the decision are decreased because it is the group, not the management, who 'owns' the decision.
- Group decision making fosters respect and values each individual's contributions.

Disadvantages. The following are negatives of group decision making:

- It is a time-consuming process that may not be suitable for decisions that require immediate action.
- Social pressures may influence the group's decision. Members may be influenced by a need to be accepted or intimidated by hierarchical pressures (what the boss wants).
- The group may be dominated by one member or viewpoint.
- Competition (winning) may become more important than achieving the goal.
- The group may accept the first solution offered, thus ignoring other possible alternatives.

Weigh each of the above factors carefully. Be aware of the pros and cons of group involvement. Then, when you choose to involve others, the making of group decisions will become a highly efficient process.

Adding Creativity to Decision Making

The process of making decisions may be approached from different directions, "depending on the nature of the issue, the time and resources, and the needs of the organization" (Vestal, 1988).

The **logical, orderly approach** (discussed earlier) **involves a series of steps that lead to a sound conclusion.** Following these steps leads to a well-thought-out decision.

The **research or experimental model** follows the same logical steps but allows new solutions or experiments to be tried. This approach is often used in laboratory or computer studies and often leads to new knowledge.

Last is the **creative approach,** which calls for the addition of imagination to logic. It is particularly suitable for dilemmas in which a new solution may be the only answer. Although the situation usually dictates the approach, nurse managers need to "recognize opportunities to alternate approaches so that the best interests of the organization are met" (Vestal, 1988).

Creativity

Words synonymous to creativity include *originality, expression,* and *imagination.* Creativity is considered a 'right brain' function, independent of analytical 'left brain' thinking. The **creative process emphasizes the uniqueness of the solution.** It also serves the need for self-expression in all of us and can be a powerful tool for developing unique solutions to problems. The key to tapping the creative process involves "uninhibited creative thinking" (Marriner-Tomey, 1992). The right brain generates many ideas and solutions without regarding the realism or feasibility of

METHODS TO CREATIVITY

1. Brainstorming
2. Forecasting
3. Collective notebooks
5. Brainwriting
6. Lists
7. Flipping a coin
8. Drawing
9. Meditation
10. Developing open-minded thinking attitudes
11. Breaking down the seven blocks to creativity

the idea. The left brain then analyzes and evaluates each creative idea for workability. In today's complex world, managers and supervisors need to be able to exercise both sides of the brain. Fortunately, several methods have been devised to help us do just that.

Tools for creativity

The development of creativity can be fostered through practice. Most of us have been taught to be analytical, or 'left brained.' However, just as we have learned and practiced to think analytically, so can we learn to tap our creativity (see box above). Let us consider each technique a little more closely.

Brainstorming. To encourage a free flow of thoughts, the group leader calls for ideas. The object is to list as many ideas as possible. Any and all ideas are listed, no matter how silly, expensive, inane, or unrealistic they may seem. Later, each idea will receive the left brain treatment of analysis and evaluation, but for now, if it is an idea, it is worthy of consideration. Brainstorming often results in new combinations or improvements of old ideas and may even generate entirely unique, new thoughts (ideas, solutions). The technique works best for simple, specific problems in an atmosphere of permissiveness and encouragement.

Forecasting. By predicting future potential outcomes, choices are clarified. The process of forecasting involves placing each potential scenario into one of four categories: status quo, not likely, least preferred, and most preferred. Outcomes are analyzed for strengths and weaknesses. The present situation along with related factors within the environment is assessed. The 'preferred future' is identified, and a plan of action is devised for each potential outcome. The outcome with the best likelihood for success is then chosen and further developed. Forecasting is appropriate for situations in which time is not a factor.

Visualizing. The 'big dream' approach uses the technique of free association. The first thing that comes to mind is explored. In management, the desired outcome is first visualized and then 'run backwards' to the present situation. New ideas or approaches are generated in the process. Pretending you have what you want focuses energy in that direction and frees you to concentrate on how to get there (action plan).

Collective notebooks. After the goal or problem is identified, each group member records his/her ideas, observations, and thoughts in a notebook. After a specific time, the notebooks are exchanged and each is analyzed for patterns, content, ideas, and the like. The group meets to share the information and to generate possible solutions or action plans. Collective notebooks are a good technique for a mature group whose members work comfortably together.

Brainwriting. Each group member is given a blank piece of paper. The problem is identified. Without discussion, each member, using free association, writes at least three ideas, thoughts, and the like. Papers are then exchanged and read, and new ideas are added. When all ideas are listed, the group assesses the results.

Lists. Data are written, prioritized, and modified. Items are added and eliminated. Lists work best when the goal is well established. Action plans can be broken down into specific steps or tasks with the use of lists.

Flipping a coin. Michael Ray, an instructor of creativity at Stanford University, recommends that when making a yes–no decision, the flip of a coin is one way to coax your intuition. With heads for yes and tails for no, flip the coin and "watch your reaction to the result. If you feel good about the outcome, then your intuition is in agreement. If you want to go for the best two out of three flips, you'll know you weren't comfortable with your initial choice" (Lessnick, 1992).

Drawing. Sometimes symbols can express impressions better than words. Drawing everything that spontaneously comes to mind encourages creativity. Later, each drawing is analyzed for ideas, solutions, possible plans, or the like.

Meditation. In essence, meditation is the act of becoming quiet. When outside stimuli are shut out, a state of relaxed attention results. Creative ideas are stimulated both during and between meditative periods.

Attitude. The most important tool for making creative decisions is an open-minded attitude. Look at all the possibilities. Develop an inquiring mind. Many creative ideas such as the steam engine, x-rays, and airplanes were ridiculed before they were accepted. Practice seeing the world through the eyes of a child, discovering something new every day.

Breaking blocks to creativity. Because creativity is a right brain function, our stronger, more active analytical left brain can easily overpower it. There are seven basic blocks that tend to stifle the creative process (see box below). Conforming, or going along with the group, is appropriate in many instances, but be careful to maintain an open mind. New ideas cannot be found in old attitudes.

Because habits are unconscious acts, they can block creativity. "We have always done it this way" is a killer phrase that diverts the creative process every time.

Lack of confidence may not stifle creativity itself, but it sure impedes its expression. Expressing your ideas may be a little intimidating at first, but it becomes easier with practice. Everyone has worthy contributions to make.

Lack of effort may be due to apathy or too many other commitments. Creativity when making decisions requires effort. Without it, decisions and problems remain unresolved.

Negative attitudes wipe out the creative process. "It will never work" has stopped more good ideas dead in their tracks than any other phrase in the English language. "How can we make it work?" is a much better phrase for fostering creative decisions.

Relying on the authorities contributes to closed, dependent attitudes. Sometimes the most creative decisions are found outside the realm of the authority. Organizational climates of acceptance, trust, respect, and good humor foster creativity.

✎ CREATIVITY BLOCKS

1. Conformity
2. Habits
3. Lack of confidence
4. Lack of effort
5. Negative attitudes
6. Reliance on authority
7. Self-censorship

From Marriner-Tomey A: *Guide to nursing management*, ed 4, St Louis, 1992, Mosby.

Last, self-censorship not only can dampen creativity but also can erode one's confidence. Repeatedly telling yourself that you never were very good at something may prevent you from trying. Besides, most everything that you are not good at doing is a learned skill and an opportunity for growth. Encouraging the creative process in self and others optimizes the effectiveness of the nurse manager's decision-making abilities, encourages group participation, and improves organizational functioning.

ی‌ **Key Concepts**

- Decision making is the process of selecting or choosing from two or more alternatives.
- Decisions may be made without thinking, by ignoring or delaying action, or by applying sound decision-making practices.
- A good decision is one that is technically correct, produces few negative side effects, and is actually acted upon.
- Poor decisions arise from factors relating to managerial competency, confused responsibilities, a poor management atmosphere, and a failure to set time limits.
- Problems in the workplace are usually job-oriented or people-oriented. Both types of problems may be further categorized into major and minor problems.
- When making decisions, remember the real-life situation, your right to be wrong, the necessity of the decision, timing, and the decisiveness factor.
- Managers make strategic, administrative, and operational decisions.
- Four types of management decisions are programmed, nonprogrammed, optimizing, and satisfying. An optimizing strategy should be used whenever possible.
- Decision-making styles may be classified as authoritative, consultative, facilitative, and delegative.
- The process of making decisions is divided into orderly, sequential steps: identify objectives; search for, develop, and evaluate alternatives; choose and implement the alternative; monitor and evaluate the results.
- A snap decision can be perfectly adequate for situations that can be quickly and easily resolved.
- The evaluation process includes a consideration of both material and human factors.
- Employees should be involved in the decision-making process when time and departmental priorities permit, the decision's outcome will have an influence on the employees, and the manager is willing to abide by the decision.
- Characteristics of a mature group include awareness, acceptance, comfortable relationships, rational decision making, productive conflict, and an effective group process.
- Managers who are aware of the group's predictable emotional responses during each phase of the decision-making process are better able to therapeutically intervene and support the group.
- There are several pros and cons to group decision making. Advantages include a broader range of experiences from which to draw, opportunities for employees to contribute, and a stronger commitment to the

goal. Disadvantages relate to time, social pressures, domination, competition, and conformity.
- Creativity can be applied to the decision-making process by the use of such techniques as brainstorming, forecasting, visualizing, collective notebooks, brainwriting, lists, a coin toss, drawing, meditation, and changes in attitude.
- Blocks to creativity include conformity, habits, lack of confidence or effort, negative attitudes, reliance on authority, and self-censorship.

Learning Activities

1. Explain why you think use of the decision process is/is not important for effective management.
2. Discuss the meaning of this statement: "To do nothing is to do something." How does it apply to decision making?
3. Scenario: Top management has made a decision to cut the time allowed for lunch breaks by half. Your staff is very upset and asking, "What are you going to do?" Apply the eight steps of the decision-making process to this situation.
4. Do you think that involving employees to participate in decision making would be threatening to managers? Explain.
5. Try one of the techniques for developing creativity. See if it works for you.

References

Calano J, Salzman J: The careful manager's guide to snap decisions, *Working Woman* 13(5):86, 1988.

Chapman EN: *Supervisor's survival kit: a mid-management primer*, ed 2, Chicago, 1975, Science Research Associates.

Douglas LM: *The effective nurse leader and manager*, ed 4, St Louis, 1992, Mosby.

Hersey P, Blanchard KH: *Management of organizational behavior: utilizing human resources*, ed 5, Englewood Cliffs, NJ, 1988, Prentice-Hall.

Hill B, Lippitt L, Serkownek K: The emotional dimensions of the problem solving process, *Group and Organizational Studies* 4(1):93, 1979.

Lessnick N: Indecisive? Flip a coin, *Executive Female* 14:14, 1992.

Magula M, editor: *Understanding organizations: a guide for the nurse executive*, Wakefield, Mass, 1982, Nursing Resources.

Marriner A: Behavioral aspects of decision making, *Supervisor Nurse* 8(3):40, 1977.

Marriner-Tomey A: *Guide to nursing management*, ed 4, St Louis, 1992, Mosby.

McConkey D: *No-nonsense delegation*, New York, 1974, AMACOM.

Sloma RS: *No-nonsense management: a general manager's primer*, New York, 1977, Macmillan.

Vestal KW: Making good decisions: a key to managerial success, *Journal of Pediatric Nursing* 3(5):338, 1988.

Additional Readings

Caudhill M: Nursing assistant involvement in patient care planning, *Nursing Management* 20(5):112Y, 1989. *Increasing input from nursing assistants dramatically decreases staff turnover rate.*

Hendricks DE: Decisions made easy, *Nursing 90* 19(1):120, 1990. *As your responsibilities increase, so does your need to make decisions effectively and confidently. Suggestions to help are offered.*

Lachman VD: Nine ways to make better decisions, *Nursing 86* 15(6):73, 1986. *Ms. Lachman suggests nine techniques for making sound decisions.*

Ludeman K: *The worth ethic: how to profit from the changing values of the new work force,* New York, 1989, Dutton. *Chapter 4, "Personal Power," offers many suggestions for managing by sharing power which lets employees make a real difference in productivity.*

McKenzie ME: Decisions: how you reach them makes the difference, *Nursing Management* 16(6):48, 1985. *The author discusses logical methods for involving staff members in the decision-making process.*

Nierenberg J, Ross I: *Women and the art of negotiating,* New York, 1985, Simon & Schuster. *This book offers numerous techniques for achieving success in your business and personal relationships.*

Peterson ME: Motivating staff to participate in decision making, *Nursing Administration Quarterly* 7(2):63, 1983. *Nurse managers typically focus on motivating staff to participate in decision making, but the central issue may be the development of trust.*

Rowe AJ, Mason RO: What's your decision style?, *Working Woman* 13(12):28, 1988. *Because your decision style affects the way you visualize and think about situations, the authors have developed a set of 20 thought-provoking questions called the decision-style inventory.*

Schumer AA: Employee involvement: the quality circle process, *Vital Speeches* 54:563, 1988. *Mr. Schumer describes the benefits of involving employees in decision making and offers several suggestions for activities to promote participation.*

Strickland RS: Decisions: forging the missing link, *Nursing Management* 14(7):44, 1983. *Nurses cannot and should not wait for 'big brother' to hand over decision-making opportunities.*

Van Dersal WR: *The successful supervisor in business or government,* ed 4, New York, 1985, Harper & Row. *The author has developed seven principles for helping managers approach supervision on an intelligent, common-sense basis.*

Van Dersal WR: Building a power base to sway a decision your way, *Supervisory Management* 31(5):16, 1986. *This article defines the process of the "power persuasion analysis" and offers suggestions for its use.*

PLANNING

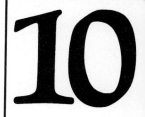

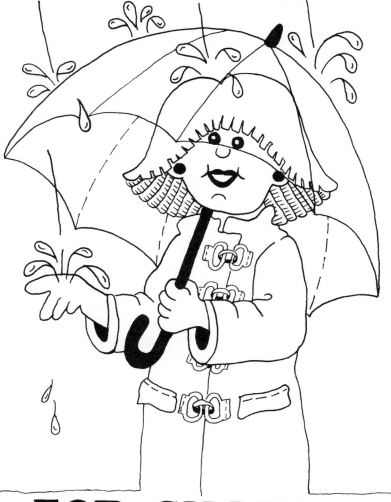

FOR CHANGE

Learning Objectives

Upon completion of this chapter, the reader will be able to:

1. Identify the fundamental purpose of planning.
2. List the six steps of the planning process.
3. Name three qualifications of an effective planner.
4. Compare the differences between driving forces and restoring forces.
5. Describe five factors to consider before planning a change.
6. Define three types of change.
7. Explain the role of a change agent.
8. Identify four reasons why people resist change.
9. List four techniques to help people cope with change.
10. Describe nine steps for planning change.
11. Examine five strategies for working with unplanned change.
12. State three basic characteristics of the management by objectives (MBO) system.
13. Name five steps of a successful MBO program.
14. Discuss four types of objectives within the MBO system.

Management Planning

Planning is the foundation of the management process. Without it, the organization will wander aimlessly and eventually perish. It is only through the process of planning that managers determine how the organization is to be structured, what its functions are, the use of resources, and the like. Because planning is the foundation step, it interrelates with and influences the outcome of all other management functions (i.e., organizing, coordinating, directing, and evaluating).

Planning defined

Very simply, "Planning is the process of determining how the organization can get where it wants to go" (Certo, 1989). Planning involves setting goals and devising the methods, action plans, and forecasts to achieve the goals. Unfortunately, planning is the easiest step to ignore. Most managers/supervisors spend their days being bombarded by interruptions, problems, and crises. The luxury of sitting quietly and planning eludes them. Despite the obstacles, planning must be done if the organization, company, or facility is to meet its goals.

Types of planning

The first and most fundamental purpose of planning is to help meet organizational goals. If the goals are clearly stated, understood, and accepted, all other plans are simply spin-offs of the 'master plan.'

Protective. C. W. Roney (1976), a management writer, states that the "**protective purpose of planning is to minimize risk** [emphasis added] by reducing the uncertainties surrounding business conditions and clarifying the consequences of related management action." If the planning process was successful, the organization is shielded from negative influences and still able to work toward achieving its goals.

Affirmative. This type of planning is done to **increase the degree of organizational success.** Affirmative planning involves the establishment of coordinated efforts, which leads to efficiency and goal achievement.

Strategic. Long-range plans which extend 3 to 5 years into the future are called strategic. "Strategic planning is the process of developing a broad plan for how a business is going to compete in its industry, what its goals should be, and what policies will be needed to achieve these goals" (Reinecke, Dessler, Schoell, 1989). Beliefs, values, and organizational direction are decided upon with strategic planning. It is important for nurse managers to be familiar with the facility's strategic plans. This knowledge helps the manager improve efficiency, eliminate duplication of efforts, concentrate resources, and coordinate activities that help meet organizational goals.

Operational. The process of **developing short-term plans for achieving the goals** of the facility's strategic plan is identified as operational planning. Day-to-day business is transacted and new programs are implemented through operational planning. For example, managers who prepare work schedules are using the operational planning process. Operational planning is sometimes referred to as 'tactical planning.'

Each type of planning is important to the success of the organization. Good planning also orients people to action instead of reaction, provides a framework for making decisions, and a basis for evaluating performance.

Pros and cons of planning

The necessity of planning is very clear when you consider how fast our society is changing. Planning has many advantages but also a few disadvantages. The astute manager is aware of both.

Advantages. Several benefits arise from a vigorous planning program:

- *It focuses managers on a 'future' orientation.* Managers are busy people. They tend to become so involved with everyday work problems that it becomes difficult to think about the future. Planning forces managers to consider the future.
- *Decisions are better coordinated.* Strategic plans provide the framework for decision making. When operational plans are coordinated, resources are used wisely, and duplication is avoided.
- *Organizational goals are emphasized.* Planning involves efforts to meet goals. When managers and employees are frequently reminded of these goals, resources and activities are focused in the direction of goal attainment.
- *Planning prevents the waste of duplicated or uncoordinated resources.* Time is an important resource, and it should not be wasted in unnecessary efforts. "I did all that work for nothing" is a frequently held thought when the planning process is poorly done.

Disadvantages. If planning is executed incorrectly or excessively within the organization, the results can be disadvantageous. Two basic drawbacks are:

- *Too much time.* An overemphasized planning program can involve time that could be better spent elsewhere. Managers and supervisors must strike a balance between time spent on planning and time spent on the other management activities.
- *Power plays.* The planning process, when used as a base for developing manipulative power, will function to fulfill individual goals at the cost of the organization's goals. Power can be a heady experience, but its use should be focused on and limited to meeting the needs and goals of the organization.

Overall, most managers agree that the benefits of planning far outweigh the disadvantages.

The process of planning

Work done inefficiently is work done haphazardly. Good planning is needed if both current and future work is to be effective.

Current work. When planning today's work (operational planning) several factors need to be considered. They include the following (Tappen, 1989):

1. *Priorities.* Something must be achieved today. Other work can wait until later. Learn to prioritize work in descending order, beginning with the most urgent and important items.

2. *Timing and sequence.* Learn which tasks must take place before others. For example, reports about the client's condition must take place before actual client care begins.
3. *Deadlines.* Time limits are frequently imposed on managers. These deadlines must be considered when prioritizing current work.
4. *Skill mix of staff.* Some nursing tasks are highly technical or require precise timing. Others require judgment and flexible timing. Staff members vary in education and experience, and this needs to be considered when planning current work.
5. *The work.* The amount, type, and special requirements of the work itself must be considered. Managers need to match the characteristics of the work with the abilities of the worker.

Future work. Strategic planning may be done on a large scale (throughout the entire facility) or on a small scale (your department, a procedure, yourself). Accurate planning for future work involves gathering information from several areas, including:

Major concerns. The health care industry is struggling with cost containment, economics, insurance, and infectious disease issues. How will each of these impact future work?

Major trends. As the delivery of health care services evolves, what role will nurses and other health care providers play? What plans have been made to relate to these trends?

Changes resulting from trends or concerns. Planning future work can be much easier if the nurse manager is aware of forces internal and external to the organization and the role they play in strategic planning.

Steps of the planning process. Six steps are involved in the process of planning. These steps are listed in the box on p. 256.

Effective planners are people who see the organization as a whole. They get along well with others, and they are able to detect and react to trends. By using the six-step process as a guideline, you will be able to provide a positive focus for the planning process.

Characteristics of Change

Change is a universal fact. Seasons change; plants change; people change; and organizations change. No one escapes it. A simple rule of thumb for change: "If you do not like the way things are now, wait a minute; they will change." The topic of change is important to managers who must keep pace with constant changes in the health care industry.

PLANNING PROCESS

1. **State the objectives (goal).** Simple, concise terms should be used. Everyone should understand, accept, and be willing to work with the objectives.
2. **List alternatives.** Consider as many ways as possible to meet the objectives.
3. **Develop premises.** Each alternative is based on assumptions. Based on these premises or assumptions, the planners forecast the possible outcome of an alternative. This helps to eliminate unreasonable alternatives.
4. **Choose an alternative.** The best alternative that meets the objectives should be selected.
5. **Develop plans.** Once an alternative has been chosen, both strategic (long-range) and operational (tactical, short-range) planning is begun. Action plans for implementing, monitoring, and evaluating the alternative are developed.
6. **Put plans into action.** Effective action plans provide both short-range and long-range directions for activity. This step includes the step of evaluating the alternative and planning for improvements.

From Certo SC: *Principles of modern management: functions and systems,* ed 4, Needham Heights, Mass, 1989, Allyn & Bacon.

The nature of change

Change is defined as the process of making or becoming different. Work change is any alteration that occurs in the organizational environment. Change is neither inherently good nor bad. It is the reactions of people involved in the process that tend to label change. Because **change is continually occurring, it is dynamic in nature and possesses several special characteristics.**

Change affects the organization. Change never occurs in a vacuum. When one part of the system changes, the whole organization is eventually affected. Organizations exist in a dynamic equilibrium (the status quo). Change disrupts this balance and triggers forces within the organization to work to restore equilibrium.

Opposing forces influence change. When the status quo is being maintained, all forces within the organization share equal amounts of power. When one of the opposing forces becomes unequal, change is triggered. Two kinds of opposing forces are:

- Driving forces — those people and energies moving toward change.
- Restoring forces — those people and energies working to restore the status quo or prevent the change.

Internal and external factors influence change. Widespread and varied changes in the health care system have occurred as a result of many technical, social, demographic, and economic forces. These forces are categorized as the following (Douglas, 1992):

> *Internal factors.* These are the influences that arise from within the organization. Changes within the work setting can be influenced by staffing patterns, the nurse/client ratio, the complexity of client care, and the quality of the working environment. Internal influences can serve as driving or restoring forces.
>
> *External factors.* Those forces existing outside the organization are external. Usually the organization exercises little, if any, control over these happenings. External forces effecting change include economic and legislative occurrences, the population explosion, as well as recent social and technological developments. Strategic planning is one way to cope with the changes brought about by external factors.

Change is a dynamic process. It is influenced by many variables, and its effects are widespread. Because organizations must change in order to survive, managers need to become astute users of the change process.

Factors to consider

Prior to planning for any organizational change, a manager must consider several major factors. How he/she deals with each factor will, to a large extent, determine how successful the change will be. Factors that determine the success or failure of a change process are the change agent, what is to be changed, the type of change, individuals affected by the change, and the evaluation of the change (Certo, 1989).

The change agent. One of the most important variables in the change process is the person responsible for the change. The change agent can originate from within the organization, such as an employee or manager, or be hired as a consultant from an outside source. Successful change agents possess several special skills. The ability to determine how a change should be made and how fast to proceed with the process is essential. Change agents also solve problems relating to the change in addition to using knowledge from the behavioral and social sciences to appropriately influence people during the change process.

What should be changed. In general, managers make changes in order to increase organizational effectiveness. To increase this effectiveness, people, structural, and technological factors must match and enhance each other.

People factors are the organization's human resources. They include the attitudes, communication, and leadership skills of the managers as well as the employees. When considering change, do not underestimate the impact of the people factor.

Structural factors are the organizational controls such as policies, procedures, and hierarchy. They, too, can strongly influence change.

Technological factors are the equipment and processes that assist employees to do their job. Changes involving complex equipment or procedures generate more anxiety than simple changes. **Matching the appropriate people with the appropriate structure and technologies is a major consideration in deciding what should be changed.**

The type of change. Organizations can be changed in various ways, but most changes fall into one of three categories: technological, structural, or people changes. Although the desired change may have elements of each type, it is categorized according to the area of emphasis.

Technological changes modify the level of skill within a system. When computers were first introduced into nursing, many nurses felt threatened and unable to cope. Once computer literacy skills were learned, the computer became indispensable, and skill levels increased.

Structural changes are aimed at increasing effectiveness by modifying the existing organizational structure. Changes can relate to clarifying job descriptions, modifying the chain-of-command to enhance communications and redefining the work environment.

People changes focus on "changing certain aspects of organization members" (Certo, 1989). A change in attitudes, skills, or behaviors can improve or dissolve organizational effectiveness. Industrial and organizational psychologists specialize in studying the process of people change.

The individuals affected. If organizational members do not support the change, it will be ineffective. Managers need to assess three areas when considering the impact of change. The usual level of employee resistance to change, methods or strategies to reduce the resistance, and the phases of change must all be thoroughly analyzed when looking at the impact of the change process on employees.

The evaluation. By spending time evaluating the change, managers can gain insight into the process, problems, and successes associated with the program. New ideas that may apply to future situations are generated, and the organizational benefits derived from the change increase due to the evaluation process.

Careful analysis of each of these five factors before deciding upon a change will increase the probability of successful implementation.

Resistance to Change

Change implies uncertainty, and uncertainty can bring about a disruption of the status quo. Because human beings exist in a state of dynamic equilibrium, we all resist change to some extent in order to 'rebalance the scales' and maintain equilibrium.

Reasons for resisting change

People resist change for many reasons. Although the status quo may have major deficiencies, it is known and comfortable. **Change disrupts the status quo and brings about discomfort.** Resistance to change can arise from several sources, which can be grouped into four categories: threatened self-interest, inaccurate perceptions, objective disagreement, and psychological resistance.

Threatened self-interest. When an employee feels or has reason to believe his/her job security, status, or paycheck is at risk, strong resistance can be expected. When organization members fear some type of personal loss, they will actively take measures to prevent the change from occurring. Union members striking when the management reduces wages or benefits is an example of resisting change due to threatened self-interests.

Inaccurate perceptions. When an individual does not understand the nature and implications of the change, he/she may believe that the change will not be beneficial. When these inaccurate perceptions are shared with others who hold inaccurate ideas, resistance to the change can grow. Ensuring that everyone has a clear understanding of the change helps to eliminate inaccurate understandings.

Objective disagreement. Some people will offer resistance to change because they truly believe the change will not benefit the organization.

> Objective disagreement often results when change agents and resisters have different information available to them. When the resister's judgment is based on more complete and accurate information, such resistance can be beneficial to the organization. This possibility is often overlooked by change agents (New, Couillard, 1981).

Psychological resistance. When individuals feel threatened they become motivationally aroused and begin to use psychological defense mechanisms in order to explain or defend their viewpoints. Frequently, when people are unable to explain the reasoning behind their viewpoints, they are psychologically resisting.

Psychological resistance also occurs when individuals have a low tolerance for change. Although they can intellectually understand the

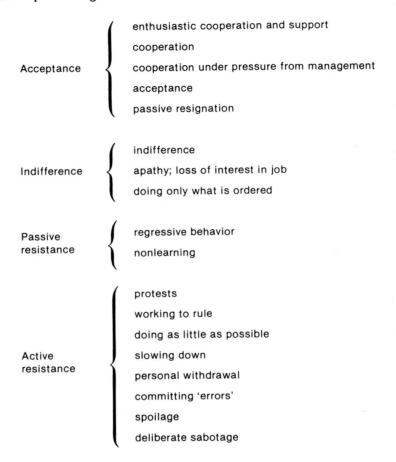

FIGURE 10-1 The spectrum of possible behavior toward a change. *(Reprinted, with permission, from Judson AJ: A manager's guide to making changes, New York, 1966, John Wiley & Sons.)*

change, they may be emotionally unable to make the transition. Some individuals have greater difficulty in coping emotionally with change. Problems due to low self-esteem, fear of risk or uncertainty, and failure can all manifest themselves as psychological resistance.

Resistance to change can arise from several sources. The astute nurse manager who can recognize these causes will be better able to soften the impact of change upon staff members.

Techniques to reduce resistance

Individual and group reactions to change range from enthusiastic support to deliberate sabotage. Figure 10-1 illustrates the spectrum of possible behaviors toward a change. One of the most fundamental techniques for the change agent is predicting the extent of the resistance to change.

Predicting resistance. "Management can attain their objective of minimizing resistance most effectively if they first focus their attention on trying to anticipate the reasons for and the intensity of resistant feelings and attitudes" (Judson, 1966). Assessing the following assists the manager to gain an understanding of the dynamics of the situation:

> *Potential gains and losses.* What are they? What is the extent, intensity, and importance of each gain or loss? Do the gains outweigh the losses? How?
> *Reasons for resistance and acceptance.* Who accepts the change and why? Who resists and why? What is the emotional level of intensity associated with each reason?

Answering each of these questions helps the manager to anticipate reactions and plan more persuasive strategies for reducing resistance to change.

Guidelines for the change agent. The manager who is acting as **a change agent must be prepared.** The following guidelines by Elizabeth Olson (1979) may be helpful:

> *Look at the organization as a system.* Know the goals, norms, and functions. Identify key people.
> *Enlarge the group favoring the change.* Cultivate allies inside and outside the organization.
> *Know your change.* Identify strengths, weaknesses, and outcomes of the change. Know what objections have been raised.
> *Analyze the other point of view.* Seeing the situation from the resister's view provides an increased perspective and aids in developing strategies for coping.
> *Use timing strategically.* Develop your sense of timing. Act when forces favor the change. Be aware of the staff's level of tolerance for change. Do not introduce too much change too quickly.

Techniques to help others. Once the change agent is prepared, attention shifts to assisting others in coping with change. The amount of assistance needed is determined by the individual and group reactions to the change. Because change affects each person differently, individual interventions will be needed. However, there are five basic techniques that apply to everyone (see box on p. 262).

In addition to the techniques listed in the box on p. 262, one more thing is needed to help others cope with change — a feedback system that moni-

✎ COPING WITH CHANGE

1. **Communicate.** Avoid surprises. People need time to digest and discuss the proposed change. Once they are comfortable with the idea, the actual change becomes less threatening.
2. **Participate.** When workers are included in the process, they have more invested in the outcome. Participation promotes a deeper understanding of the change and decreases resistance through a sharing of associated concerns and anxieties. Sell your ideas by investing time with staff members. Encourage them to share their feelings about the change. Ask for suggestions. Listen.
3. **Educate.** Promote understanding by supplying information about why the change is necessary and what is to be accomplished. Clearly explain the specific change and what its impact will be on individuals, departments, and the organization. If the change is technical, such as the operation of a new piece of equipment, provide for individual and group learning sessions.
4. **Support.** Changes generate stress. Stress influences worker performance. Be alert for clues that indicate unhealthy stress levels. Stress can be difficult to detect, but behaviors such as moodiness, increased fatigue, aggression, temper outbursts, and chronic anxiety need to be recognized as symptoms of stress. Measures can then be taken to provide support for the employee or group and reduce the source of the stress. Providing support for each individual involved in the change requires your best psychosocial skills. People are more willing to embrace change if they feel trust and support.
5. **Move slowly.** Gradually introduce the change. People have a built-in level of tolerance for change. When change occurs too quickly, they will entrench themselves and resist any attempts to change anything. Introduce a change on a trial basis. This allows the workers some control and reduces many of the fears associated with the change. Time must also be allowed for the change to become incorporated into daily functions and behaviors. A gradual introduction of changes reduces resistance and allows time for assimilation.

tors levels of resistance among staff members. Even something as casual as a "How's it going?" on a planned regular basis will provide information about how well or poorly the change is doing. A feedback system also allows the change agent to troubleshoot possible problems and intervene early with actual problems.

Resistance to change can be minimized through careful preparation, an understanding of the causes of resistance, and effective use of therapeutic psychosocial supportive techniques.

Planned Change

Most changes require the members of an organization to modify their behaviors. Managers who introduce change must be prepared to work with the related human behavior.

Process of change

Kurt Lewin (1947), a German social scientist, pioneered the study of field theory. He states that changes in behavior result from three distinct, but related, experiences.

Unfreezing. This is the state in which the employees have a need to learn new behaviors. They are ready to change. Disequilibrium occurs when people feel a need, unfreezing occurs, and the system becomes unbalanced.

Changing. Change occurs when people begin to examine, accept, and try out the change. Individuals *identify* with the change by modeling their behaviors after an expert. For example, after attending classes on computer operation, the employee tries out the new behaviors by operating the computer using the same steps as the class instructor.

After the change has been identified, the individual attempts to *internalize* the new behaviors by incorporating them into his/her normal behavior pattern. Change will be most effective after the individual or group has gone through the process of identification and internalization.

Refreezing. When the change has become an established part of the system, refreezing occurs. People now see their new behaviors and attitudes as part of themselves. Rewards play an important part, for they are usually received as a result of adapting and performing the new behaviors. Practicing the changed behaviors successfully helps to integrate the change.

When change has an impact on employees, all individuals must be allowed to progress through each of the three phases of the change process. Only then will the change become an integrated part of the organization.

Pace of change

Change comes in two basic varieties: planned and unplanned. Each has unique characteristics and requires special management techniques.

Planned change. "Planned change results because of an intended effort by one or more change agents to deliberately move the system" (Marquis, Huston, 1987). These changes are carefully planned and implemented slowly and deliberately. When done appropriately, planned change meets with minimal hostility and resistance.

Unplanned change. Also called accidental change or change by drift, unplanned change results from an imbalance in the system. Changes occur without personal involvement — no planning or preparation. Unplanned change is always met with more hostility and resistance because the involved individuals feel uninformed, surprised, and threatened. Too much unplanned change can erode an organization's ability to function.

Steps for planning change

"Planned change is a purposeful, designed effort to bring about improvement in a system, with the assistance of a change agent" (Spradley, 1980). A knowledge of the problem-solving process is an essential ingredient for planning change. **Planned change is always preferable to unplanned change.** To make change serve a specific purpose, the manager must plan and control the change process. Following the nine steps in the next section (Spradley, 1980) will help.

Recognize. Recognize the need for change. Be alert for evidence indicating that something needs to be changed. Patients, staff, administrators, or anyone else can supply valuable information. Monitor records and other paperwork. Discover ways to improve. Gather data.

Diagnose. Clearly define the change. When possible, use group interaction to identify the internal and external forces for change; to analyze the problem, its causes, and possible solutions; and to reach a conclusion about what needs to be changed.

Analyze. List all reasonable alternatives for courses of action. For each course of action, analyze its risks, obstacles, resources, consequences, time frame, and amount of expected resistance.

Select. Choose an action plan based on the nature and cause of the problem. Pick the easiest, most economical, and useful plan. Be prepared with other possible solutions (action plans) in case the primary alternative fails.

Plan. This is an important step. Time spent here enhances your chances for success. Develop a strategy to implement the desired change. Make sure the plan includes specific, measurable objectives with time frames; the activities and resources needed to meet each objective; a method to monitor and manage resistance; an evaluation method (tool); and a feed-back system for monitoring the change process. Include opportunities for communication in each step of the plan.

Implement. Put the change into action. Communicate. Let everyone in-volved with the change know what to expect. Introduce the change slowly, one step at a time. Be flexible and make adjustments or revise plans when necessary. Focus on the positive aspects of the change, but do not ignore the negative side.

Evaluate. Using the evaluation tool developed in the fifth step (plan), analyze each objective for evidence indicating that the objectives were met. When specific criteria are established in advance, evidence of success or failure is easily found.

Stabilize. Once the change has been made and all the 'bugs' are worked out, measures to maintain and reinforce the change are needed. Commu-nicate. Encourage use of new methods resulting from the change. Provide monitoring and follow-up until the change becomes well established in the organizational system.

Support. Stay upbeat and enthusiastic. Maintain a positive attitude toward the change. Use appropriate psychosocial techniques to provide support for others during each phase of the change process. Be an example. Lead and inspire your staff members.

Planned change is always preferable, but a poorly constructed and ex-ecuted planned change will do more harm than good. Practice working with each step of the change process. It will provide you with a basis for sound decisions and creative actions. As Barbra Spradley (1980) states, "Nursing leaders have no choice as to *whether* they will deal with change, only *how* they will deal with it."

Unplanned Change

"Expect the unexpected" is not a frivolous statement. Change happens whether it is planned or unexpected. In the health care setting, especially when caring directly for patients, unplanned changes are daily occur-rences. Health care providers and their managers need to be adept at cop-ing with unplanned changes.

Reactions to unplanned change

Change generates stress. When the change is unanticipated, it provokes more intense reactions in those people affected. Reactions range from simple acceptance to outright hostility, and they are highly individual. Basically, these emotional responses to unplanned changes can be categorized as anxiety, mistrust, or loss.

Anxiety. When the comfort of the daily routine is disrupted, workers become anxious. Planned change offers opportunities to reduce anxieties and provide emotional support, but unexpected change does not allow this luxury. People require extra emotional support during unplanned change.

Mistrust. When individuals and work groups are denied the opportunity to progress through each phase of the change experience (i.e., unfreezing, changing, refreezing), they feel threatened, and resistance develops. Mistrust with the change situation can evolve into 'us versus them' attitudes, and that can expand into a mistrust of the entire organization. Open communication lines help prevent mistrust from developing.

Loss. Change, planned or unplanned, involves loss and discomfort. Giving up old and comfortable behaviors, viewpoints, and attitudes in order to change generates feelings of loss. Phrases such as "in the old days" and "how we used to do it" are heard when people express feelings associated with loss. Focusing on the possible benefits of the change helps to replace loss with hope, especially with unexpected change.

Coping with the unexpected

Health care workers routinely deal with unplanned change. Managers are usually removed from the immediacy of life-or-death decisions associated with direct patient care. Therefore, they have the benefit of time, however brief, to plan a response appropriate to the situation. These five steps will enable you to respond constructively to unexpected changes.

1. Do not panic. Remain calm no matter what happens. Deal realistically with your own feelings and attitudes. Remember that decisions made during periods of high stress are more likely to be ineffective. Keep your reactions under control by staying in the 'thinking' arena.

2. Analyze the situation. Define the problems brought about by the change. Discover why the change is occurring. Assess the potential effects of the change. Consider the resources and restrictions and the driving and restoring forces, as well as the effects on employees. Work with the best information you have available at the time. Analysis can take place over a period of a few minutes or many hours.

3. Reprioritize. Determining what needs to be done will help you to cope with the unexpected change. Add these tasks to the 'priority list' and order it according to importance. Reassign and redistribute work loads if necessary. Share your plans or analysis of the situation with all staff members. Solicit feedback and do not be hesitant to pitch in and help when needed. Remember: you lead by example. When staff members see you coping with unexpected changes calmly and effectively, they will do the same.

4. Match resources with priorities. Line up your 'must be done' tasks and match them with the best available resource. For example, assigning the LPN to care for the critical patient is a better use of resources than assigning a CNA to the patient. The most important rule to remember here is "Do the best you can with what you've got." Resources, both human and material, are always limited. The successful supervisor meets as many priorities as possible with the resources available.

5. Evaluate continuously. The **evaluation step is even more important when the change is unplanned.** Evaluations at frequent intervals allow the manager to identify and support groups and individuals as they progress through the change process. Frequent evaluations also help the manager to monitor the situation's dynamics and anticipate other possible changes.

Coping with the unexpected will always be a part of every supervisor's day. Managing unexpected change calmly and competently increases worker, managerial, and organizational effectiveness.

Change and Management by Objectives

Change can be effectively managed through the use of a system known as management by objectives (MBO). The concepts behind MBO were developed in the early 1950s by Peter Drucker and have since been expanded upon by other management researchers.

Characteristics

Management by objectives is an attempt to integrate the goals and objectives of the individual with the organization. The system has several unique characteristics.

Definition. MBO is defined by Bell (1980) as a "system for setting organizational objectives for a given period, devising plans to implement the objectives, and providing periodic evaluation of progress." Simply stated, **MBO is a system for orderly change.**

Principles. Three basic principles guide the MBO system. First, the system is oriented toward results. Effective managers are those who can attain results. Second, MBO follows concepts of human motivation and behavior. By assigning responsibilities specifically, MBO offers opportunities for personal growth and commitment for all employees. Last, MBO provides orderly organizational growth through statements of objectives and measurements of actual achievements.

Theory bases. Peter Drucker, father of the MBO system, states that several concepts or theories of human behavior and motivation serve as a framework for MBO. Maslow's hierarchy of needs; Herzberg's two-factor theory; McGregor's X, Y, and Z theories; and the path–goal theory are all important concepts in the MBO system. MBO recognizes that most employees are willing to do their best, want to assume responsibility, and are motivated to satisfy their higher level needs.

The MBO process

When members of an organization jointly identify goals, plan, implement, and evaluate them, they are functioning with MBO. The process of management by objectives can be divided into five distinct, but interrelated, steps.

1. Goal setting. During the goal-setting phase, all the organization's goals are defined for the coming year. Goals and objectives should be clearly stated, concise, and attainable. They should be realistic, measurable, and include target dates for completion. Upon agreement by all supervisors and subordinates, the goals are adopted and used as a point of focus, or the decision-making framework, for the next full year.

2. Action planning. Once overall goals have been established, each manager devises objectives (see box below) and develops action plans to meet the goals. Routine objectives are concerned with everyday duties and activities. Most routine objectives can be found in the organization's job descriptions, policy and procedure manuals, and standards of per-

---

 TYPES OF OBJECTIVES

Routine
Problem-solving
Creative
Personal development

formance. It is important that each employee know his/her job description and performance standards (routine objectives).

Problem-solving objectives can be used to solve actual problems or prevent them from occurring. Use the problem-solving process to identify and effectively cope with problem objectives.

Creative objectives are the innovative contributions made to better the organization. New ideas may be integrated into old methods, but innovation and creativity are the result.

Personal development objectives are those associated with an individual's self-actualization. Although these objectives may not be job-related, the employee performs better when they are achieved. The total person is affected by his/her personal objectives.

Take into account each type of objective, then develop your plans for action (see the section on planning earlier in this chapter).

3. Clarify responsibilities. Once the action plan, including the methods and activities needed to accomplish the objective, is established, the manager assigns responsibilities and describes what is to be done, how, when, and by whom. Each action plan should include the specific activities that lead to the objective, the sequence (steps) for each activity, defined and assigned responsibilities, and an estimation of needed resources. Be specific. A well-developed action plan will aid in measuring and evaluating the objectives.

4. Develop control systems. Control systems consist of periodic reviews and annual performance appraisals. Frequent reviews enable managers to assess the progress being made toward each objective. Each employee and supervisor is evaluated in terms of goal achievement, and the action plan may then be modified. Objectives can also serve as guidelines for improving performance and assuming responsibilities. "The focus of this entire phase is upon solving problems and taking corrective action" (Cain, Luchsinger, 1978).

5. Performance appraisal. The annual performance appraisal is used to measure the results achieved by the individual and the organization. Both supervisor and worker prepare a report of the individual's achievements relating to the objectives. Accomplishments are recognized and praised, while poor performances are analyzed and plans developed for improvement.

Annual performance appraisals serve a second important function. They allow the organization to assess "where it stands now in order to begin planning for the next year" (Cain, Luchsinger, 1978). By reviewing where it has been, the organization will be better able to determine where it is going.

Management by objectives is becoming more widely accepted because of the societal shift from the authority to the individual. By providing opportunities for involvement, each person becomes directly responsible for decisions relating to job planning. Managers begin to assume a supportive rather than authoritative role, and this, in turn, fosters a greater commitment to meeting organizational goals.

☙ Key Concepts

- Planning is the process of determining how to get where you want to go.
- The most fundamental purpose of planning is to help meet organizational (or personal) goals.
- Planning can be protective (to reduce risk), affirmative (to ensure success), or operational (to meet short-term goals, the day-to-day business).
- The benefits of planning include better coordinated decisions; improved use of resources; and an emphasis on organizational goals, which provide a focus on the future as well as the present.
- When planning current work, consider the priorities, timing, sequence, deadlines, the skill mix of staff members, and the work itself.
- The six steps of the planning process are: state objectives, list alternatives, develop premises, choose an alternative, develop action plans, and implement plans.
- Effective planners are able to view the organization as a whole, get along well with people, and detect and react to trends.
- Change, the process of becoming different, is an inescapable fact.
- Change has several unique characteristics: it is a dynamic process that disrupts the organization's equilibrium, and it is affected by driving and restoring forces as well as internal and external factors.
- Factors to consider before planning a change relate to the change agent, what should be changed, the type of change, the individuals affected, and the evaluation process.
- Types of organizational changes include technological, structural, and people changes.
- People resist change because of threatened self-interests, inaccurate perceptions, objective disagreements, and psychological resistance.
- To understand the dynamics of resistance to change, the manager assesses the potential gains and losses of the change as well as the reasons for resistance or acceptance.
- Managers who act as change agents can be better prepared by knowing the organization's systems and dynamics, networking, having detailed knowledge of the change, analyzing resister's viewpoints, and using timing effectively.
- Techniques to overcome resistance to change are: communicate, participate, educate, support, move slowly, and monitor progress.
- Lewin's field theory model of the change process describes the phases of unfreezing, changing, and refreezing.
- Change may be planned or unplanned.
- The nine steps for planning change are: recognize, diagnose, analyze, select, plan, implement, evaluate, stabilize, and support.
- People react to unplanned changes with anxiety, mistrust, and feelings of loss.

- Five steps for responding constructively to unplanned changes are: do not panic, quickly analyze the situation, restructure priorities, match available resources with priorities, and continuously evaluate the process.
- Management by objectives is a system for defining, implementing, and evaluating change.
- MBO is a results-oriented system based on concepts of human behavior and motivation.
- The MBO process includes five interrelated steps: goal setting, action planning, clarification of responsibilities, developing control systems, and performance appraisals.
- MBO working objectives can be categorized as routine, problem solving, creative, and personal development.
- Both routine and annual performance appraisals are important for measuring the progress made toward goal achievement.

✑ Learning Activities

1. The situation: You are a wing supervisor at ABC long-term care facility with seven other supervisors. The administrator has just discovered that a new facility will be opening across the street. You and the other wing supervisors have been told to develop a plan for convincing the public that, although your facility may be older, it is better. Describe how you would meet the goal (develop the plan). Be specific. Use time frames. The new facility across the street is scheduled to open in 2 months.
2. Describe how a change agent can impact an organization.
3. A new checklist for documenting routine resident care was introduced 3 weeks ago. The checklist is not completed most of the time because the aides say they are "just too busy to sit around making checkmarks." Explain how you would cope with the staff's resistance and plan to meet the goal (checklists completed).
4. Suppose your instructor just changed your grade from an "A" to a "B." Describe your reaction. Would you resist this change? How? Now suppose you are old, arthritic, and poorly sighted. Your wing supervisor has just moved you away from your friend and into a new room. Describe your reaction. Would you resist this change? How?
5. Describe how the management by objectives system works.

References

Bell ML: Management by objectives, *Journal of Nursing Administration* 10(5):19, 1980.

Cain C, Luchsinger V: Management by objectives: applications to nursing, *Journal of Nursing Administration* 8(1):35, 1978.

Certo SC: *Principles of modern management: functions and systems*, ed 4, Needham Heights, Mass, 1989, Allyn & Bacon.

Douglas LM: *The effective nurse leader and manager*, ed 4, St Louis, 1992, Mosby.

Judson AJ: *A manager's guide to making changes*, New York, 1966, John Wiley & Sons.

Lewin K: Frontiers in group dynamics: concept, method, and reality of social sciences — social equilibria and social change, *Human Relations* 1(6):5, 1947.

Marquis BL, Huston CJ: *Management decision making for nurses*, Philadelphia, 1987, Lippincott.

New RJ, Couillard NA: Guidelines for introducing change, *Journal of Nursing Administration* 11(3):17, 1981.

Olson EM: Strategies and techniques for the nurse change agent, *Nursing Clinics of North America* 14(2):323, 1979.

Reinecke JA, Dessler G, Schoell WF: *Introduction to business: a contemporary view*, ed 6, Needham Heights, Mass, 1989, Allyn & Bacon.

Roney CW: The two purposes of business planning, *Managerial Planning* 25:1, 1976.

Spradley BW: Managing change creatively, *Journal of Nursing Administration* 10(5):32, 1980.

Tappen RM: *Nursing leadership and management: concepts and practice*, ed 2, Philadelphia, 1989, Davis.

Additional Readings

Beyers M: Getting on top of organizational change: process and development, *Journal of Nursing Administration* 14(10):32, 1984. *Ms. Beyers discusses the process of change, organizational development, and the critical management functions of nurse executives in dynamic organizations.*

Bowman RA, Culpepper RC: Power: RX for change, *American Journal of Nursing* 74(6):1053, 1974. *Nurse power is an idea whose time has come, say these authors, as they examine the concept and reality of power.*

Brooten DA, Hayman LL, Naylor MD: *Leadership for change: an action guide for nurses*, ed 2, Philadelphia, 1988, Lippincott. *The effective nurse leader is one who commands both a theoretical grasp of change methods and practical skills for planning and directing change.*

Curtin LL: Strategic planning: asking the right questions, *Nursing Management* 22(1):7, 1991. *To plan effectively with a sense of purpose, managers need to include key issues and trends in their information gathering.*

DeGeus AP: Planning as learning, *Harvard Business Review* 88:70, 1988. *The head of planning for the Royal Dutch/Shell Group of companies believes that planning means changing minds, not making plans.*

Dobyns L: Ed Deming wants big changes, and he wants them fast, *Smithsonian* 20(5):74, 1990. *The capitalist revolutionary who sold Japan on the notion that quality drives profits up is now trying to sell the same to American businesses.*

Gillen DJ: Harnessing the energy from change anxiety, *Supervisory Management* 31(3):40, 1986. *By using goal agendas, education, and sharing ownership, managers are better able to positively direct the employee's increased energies that result from change anxiety.*

Haffner A: Facilitating change: choosing the appropriate strategy, *Journal of Nursing Administration* 16(4):18, 1986. *This article describes a method for selecting an effective change strategy using a combination of three factors: change target, level of willingness to change, and ability.*

Hersey P, Blanchard KH: *Management of organizational behavior: utilizing human resources,* ed 5, Englewood Cliffs, NJ, 1988, Prentice-Hall. *Chapter 15, "Planning and Implementing Change," presents a general framework for understanding change and its impact on the total system.*

Sloma RS: *No-nonsense management: a general manager's primer,* New York, 1977, Macmillan. *Mr. Sloma clearly describes several principles for managers to follow when dealing with change.*

Sobkowski A: Damage control when a crisis hits, *Executive Female* 14:67, 1992. *Crisis consultants offer numerous tips and techniques for coping with unplanned changes.*

Ward MJ, Moran SG: Resistance to change: recognize, respond, overcome, *Nursing Management* 15(1):30, 1984. *Nurse supervisors who resolutely face challenges improve the shape, pace, and direction of change.*

Woodward WA, Miller P: Ten ways to make sure your project succeeds, *Working Woman* 13(12):92, 1988. *The authors offer advice on ensuring success of the changes brought about by your project.*

CREATING A POSITIVE

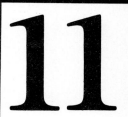

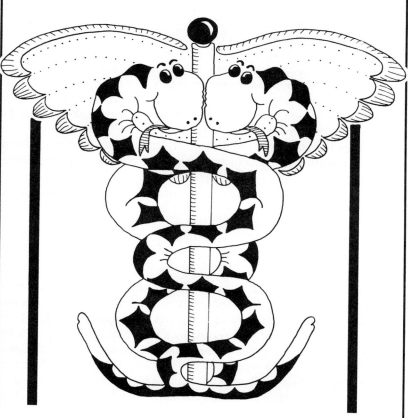

WORK ENVIRONMENT

✎ Learning Objectives

Upon completion of this chapter, the reader will be able to:

1. Discuss the concept of quality of work life (QWL) programs.
2. Describe how the worth ethic guides a manager's daily actions.
3. Examine how employees' attitudes influence the work environment.
4. List the five core dimensions of a job.
5. Discuss four personal traits to assess when analyzing your personal outlook.
6. Explain how the manager's attitudes and behaviors influence the working climate.
7. Discuss seven positive leadership traits.
8. Identify four steps to manage time wisely.
9. Describe six characteristics of a positive manager.
10. Explain the 10 commandments of negotiation.
11. Explain the importance of role models in the workplace.
12. Identify how each management function can be applied to creating a positive work environment.
13. Describe four steps for building an effective, motivated work team.
14. List two methods for decreasing physician–nurse and other interdepartmental conflicts.

New Work Designs

Traditional work designs (i.e., autocracy, bureaucracy) may have been productive, but they exacted high human costs. Productivity was emphasized; status symbols became measures of success; and front-line workers were driven, without regard to their needs, to produce in the name of profit. The paycheck was expected to purchase not only labor but loyalty as well. As a result, job satisfaction was low, and turnover rates were high. Organizations, realizing that there must be a better way, began to experiment with work designs that could provide high levels of productivity for the employer as well as a better quality of work life for employees.

Quality of work life

The **quality of work life** (QWL) refers to the impact of the work environment upon the individual. It is the favorableness or unfavorableness of the work climate. "Are the workers happy?" is a key consideration in the quest for profit. Programs for QWL were designed in order to "develop work environments that are excellent for people as well as for the economic health of the organization" (Davis, Newstrom, 1989).

Elements of QWL programs. Programs developed to improve the quality of work life focus on such topics as employee security, job design and improvement, open communication systems, and equitable reward systems. Many efforts relate to enriching workers' jobs through skill development, cooperative labor–management relationships, and techniques for reducing occupational stress.

Purposes. A more humanized work environment helps to meet workers' higher level needs. QWL programs are designed to emphasize the 'best fit' among the worker, the technology, the job, and the working environment. Organizations are redesigned in order to improve the environment, and jobs are redesigned to include the attributes desired by the workers. The results for workers are opportunities for growth and skill development, as well as chances to contribute individual ideas. Where traditional management systems *use* human resources, QWL programs *develop* them.

The worth ethic

The work force is changing. Workers want a sense of **identity, recognition, and worth** for the work they do. They are willing to commit their time, energy, and creativity only as long as they feel they are respected and a part of the team. As John Vasconcellos, Chairman of California State Legislative Ethics Committee, states, "Honoring and evoking the inherent worth of every employee is the surest way toward productivity, creativity, and the bottom line, profit making" (Ludeman, 1989).

Elements. Worth ethics (WE) programs begin with the managers. By developing commitments to building self-esteem (in themselves as well as their employees), all workers are provided with an environment that fosters growth, innovation, and risk taking.

Kate Ludeman, author of *The Worth Ethic: How to Profit from the Changing Values of the New Work Force* (1989), devised an eight-step process (changing) which empowers managers to build a belief system that fosters self-worth and respect in all employees.

Purposes. Because the work ethics system encourages personal contributions, broad organizational successes frequently result. Encouraging workers to do their best and test their limits satisfies needs for self-actualization and personal fulfillment. Workers become more cooperative, harder working, and committed. Loyalty to the company grows, and employees practice a high degree of integrity. Quality and profits improve, and worker satisfaction is enriched.

ATTITUDES OF CONCERN

1. **Job satisfaction.** The favorable or unfavorable feelings about the job determine the level of satisfaction. Like all attitudes, satisfaction with the job is developed over time and can improve or deteriorate. Job satisfaction is dynamic and reflects one component of the employee's broader satisfaction with life. Personal lives affect work lives, and attitudes about work have an impact in the personal arena. This 'spillover' effect is important for managers/supervisors to monitor. The employee's attitudes toward the job, the work environment, and his/her personal life all affect performance and satisfaction levels.

2. **Job involvement.** The degree to which employees dedicate themselves to the job determines the level of job involvement. Employees who are involved believe work is a central part of their lives. Doing a meaningful job well is important. Workers with high levels of job satisfaction are seldom late or absent, willing to work long hours, and try to perform at high levels.

3. **Organizational commitment.** Employees have various attitudes about their future with the company. People who identify strongly with the organization believe in its philosophy and goals. They are willing to work toward achieving the goals. They are loyal and committed to a long-term relationship with the company. "Organizationally committed employees will usually have good attendance records, willing adherence to company policies, and lower turnover rates."

From Davis K, Newstrom J: *Human behavior at work: organizational behavior,* ed 8, New York, 1989, McGraw-Hill.

Job enrichment

The term 'job enrichment' was coined by Fredrick Herzberg based on his research with worker motivators. The term was later expanded to include **anything (motivator) that made a job more rewarding.** An important component of job enrichment programs is the employee's attitude.

Employee attitudes. An attitude is a feeling, belief, or mental set that affects a person's perception or viewpoint. The attitudes of each employee affect the organization's productivity, performance, and costs. It is an important task of managers to understand, monitor, and influence employee attitudes (see box above).

Employees' attitudes are reflected in job performance, turnover rates, absences, tardiness, and theft. When attitudes are upbeat and positive, employees demonstrate high levels of performance and low levels of turnover, absenteeism, theft, and tardiness.

To apply job enrichment techniques, managers consider employee attitudes, gather information about what may enrich the job, and then collaborate with employees. The final judges of what enriches the job are the employees. Their attitudes define 'enrichment.' Managers assess the core dimensions of a job and apply the employee-defined enriching factors to each dimension.

The job's core dimensions. Although not all jobs contain each component, most employees view these components as basic for internal motivation. If one dimension is missing, motivation is decreased, and employees feel psychologically deprived. When the job contains each component and is enriched, motivation, job satisfaction, and quality of work are improved, while absenteeism and job turnover are greatly reduced.

According to management experts Davis and Newstrom (1989), there are five core dimensions of jobs:

1. *Task variety.* Jobs that involve different tasks and require various skills are more challenging. Repetitive work is boring, monotonous, and tiring. Employees who have variety in their jobs demonstrate higher levels of competency, enthusiasm, and involvement.
2. *Task identity.* Allowing employees to perform a complete piece of work identifies the worker with the task. This fosters a sense of responsibility, completion, and ownership in the employee. To illustrate, a CNA feels more identified with assigned clients than those he/she just feeds. When employees can identify with the task, they become more responsible and involved.
3. *Task significance.* People need to believe that the work they perform is important. Workers need to feel that their efforts will benefit the company, society, or the world. When staff members feel their work is making a contribution, the whole organization (and possibly society) benefits.
4. *Autonomy.* Workers with autonomy have some discretion and control over decisions relating to their jobs. Responsibility is encouraged when workers have a degree of freedom and can choose their own 'best way' of doing the job. Autonomy is necessary for self-actualization and a basic ingredient for job enrichment.
5. *Feedback.* The last core dimension is a simple, but often forgotten, item. Feedback is an exchange of information that tells the worker how well he/she is doing the job. These information exchanges can be formal and written, such as with progress reports, job evaluations,

and performance reviews, or informal and verbal. People invest much time in work, and knowing how well they are doing is important. Giving positive feedback frequently and negative feedback constructively is one way of enriching the job.

New ways of managing people in their work are evolving. Your company or facility may not have any of these innovative programs in place, but there are several things you can do to create your own positive work environment no matter where you work.

The Positive Personal Outlook

It is your first day on the job. You arrive at work a few minutes early to meet some of the staff members with whom you will be working. Everyone is welcoming and friendly. After a few minutes of casual conversation, you notice people glancing at the clock and the tension level rising. The nurse to whom you were speaking notices your puzzled expression and says, "The supervisor is due around this time. You never know what her mood is going to be. We all walk around on pins and needles until she decides whether to become civilized for the day. It's tough to work for a boss like that." Then she smiles and leaves the room. Little did she know that you were being oriented to the supervisor's position and would soon replace their retiring 'boss.' How will you establish your work environment?

Personal traits

To encourage a positive, nurturing work environment the manager must first develop a personal outlook. Leadership/supervision involves working with people, and, because each person is unique and may be very different, your personal outlook will be questioned and tested many times. One's personal viewpoints are dynamic and change with time and experience. It is important to consider the following areas when analyzing your personal outlook.

Philosophy. One's philosophy is composed of the **concepts and principles that motivate behavior.** Whether it is recognized or not, each individual possesses a system of fundamental values and beliefs by which he/she lives and governs behaviors. For example, if your philosophy values honesty, you would not steal, even when given an opportunity.

Your philosophy of life and work affects your staff members. Managers who adopt a philosophy of individual worth believe that every person is capable of making worthy contributions to the organization. This attitude affects every aspect of the work environment, for the manager will plan, organize, and so on from his/her own philosophical point of view.

Ethics. Ethics are principles or standards that govern 'right behavior.' Once a philosophy (of work in this case) has been adopted, individuals will base their behavior on what is viewed as right or wrong according to that philosophy. These views of what is right or wrong behavior provide the basis for a system of ethics. For example, a nurse who holds a philosophy of preserving life at all costs, would not apply for a job as a hospice nurse.

Integrity. Managers who practice integrity are honest, dependable, and fair. They make no promises that cannot be fulfilled. They do what they say they will do. During conflict situations they can be relied upon to listen to everyone's point of view. They apply sound decision making and conflict resolution skills to reach optimal solutions. Employees can consistently count on them.

Self-awareness. Self-aware managers practice looking at work situations from an outsider's viewpoint. They analyze their interactions and identify new, more positive responses. They focus on abilities but work for improvement, are willing to admit mistakes, take corrective action, and then move on. Managers with high levels of awareness respect themselves and look for ways to encourage respect in others.

Managers who function with a sound philosophical and ethical base create a stable working climate for staff members. By acting with integrity and practicing self-awareness, managers can set an example for employees to follow and foster a positive work environment. The personal traits of the supervisor have a strong impact on the working climate and resultant levels of productivity.

The working climate

Organizations, facilities, and companies all have individual and, sometimes, unique working climates. One of the most important factors in the work environment is the manager or supervisor. The atmosphere under which the employees work (working climate) is established by the manager. The best working climate generates the greatest productivity and encourages the growth of employees.

Working climates change according to the needs of the department; therefore, the manager must consider the working climate when planning for change. The addition or loss of staff members has a strong impact on climate, but the most influential factors are the attitudes and behavioral examples of the manager.

Attitudes. "All the employees in your department have a special kind of radar tuned to your mental attitude that permits them to read and evaluate your disposition each day" (Chapman, 1975). If you drag, grump, or grouch into work, your employees will receive your signals and back away from you. Opportunities for communication will be stifled. Staff members will go about their work with little enthusiasm and much negativity. Steps will be taken to actively avoid you.

Fortunately, the reverse is also true. When you arrive with an upbeat, 'can do' attitude and a smile, your employees pick up and reflect your outlook. They will show enthusiasm with their work and seek opportunities to communicate with you. Like it or not, **your attitude as a manager or supervisor sets the mood and climate for the entire unit.**

Examples. The behavioral examples set by the manager contribute more than anything else to the working climate. A manager sets the norms and standards of the department through personal behavior. The energy, enthusiasm, and creativity demonstrated by the manager are transmitted to the employees who act according to the messages received.

Because you are the 'boss,' you cannot afford to have a bad day. Your employees can be grouchy or undependable, but you cannot. You always strive to set the best example because you are the supervisor.

Emergencies. "The way you handle emergencies shows your real character more than normal circumstances do" (Chapman, 1975). Leaders who can 'keep their cool' during unexpected changes engender feelings of security in staff members. The security of employees becomes seriously damaged when they cannot trust their manager to remain calm enough to lead them through difficult situations.

When an employee's mistake creates an emergency, remember that your reactions will greatly influence the working climate you are establishing. Most of the time, the individual is aware of the error and feels remorseful and guilty. Acknowledge the error and take corrective action. Do not show anger, disgust, or impatience. These stand in the way of a healthy, productive working climate.

Pressures from above. Every supervisor will occasionally receive negative feedback or a 'chewing out' from someone higher up in the chain-of-command. When this occurs, a manager has two choices: pass the pressure down the chain-of-command to the workers, or absorb it without passing it along. Of course you must take steps to correct the cause of the complaint but use your leader's position to act as a buffer or shock absorber between upper management and workers. Your willingness to accept criticism on their behalf, without passing it on, will earn much respect and loyalty from your staff members.

The personal traits and outlook of the manager, coupled with the established working climate, determine the work environment. Creating a positive, healthy working environment is the responsibility of each health care supervisor.

The Positive Working Environment

Each department, unit, or work group's supervisor sets the tone, mood, and climate for the day; and each day the work climate differs. When productivity is up and employees are happy, the work environment is positive and enriching. Because managers play such an important role in establishing a positive work environment, applying upbeat leadership and management skills will assist you in creating and maintaining a superior work environment.

Positive leadership traits

Effective leaders project a charisma that attracts attention. For some reason, people are drawn to them. Their opinions are important; and their followers are eager, loyal, and productive. Chapter 4 discusses the traits of leadership in depth. Charismatic leaders in the work environment exhibit several characteristics that stand out.

Emotional maturity. The **emotionally mature individual is independent in thought and action.** He/she may thoughtfully consider differing opinions, attitudes, or stances before making a decision; but he/she will not be swayed by popular opinion or peer pressure. Managers with emotional maturity demonstrate self-confidence and operate with a strong sense of values. They assume responsibility and are accountable for their own actions as well as the actions of their workers. Above all, they are consistent and predictable. They can be depended upon to provide calm, stable leadership.

Assertiveness. Super managers are able to stand up for (defend) their rights without infringing on the rights of others. Aggressiveness is characterized by "stepping on people's toes" or getting your way regardless of the costs. On the other hand, assertiveness employs a win-win view. Assertive people reach their goals while considering and respecting the rights of others. Assertiveness is an important trait for effective managers, for it fosters the philosophy of respect for others during the process of attaining goals. Staff members appreciate a supervisor who is willing to take a stand without hurting others. Practice being assertive. It pays off in increased productivity levels as well as improved employee well-being.

Critical thinking. The ability to gather and sift through data in order to make an effective decision or solve a problem involves the ability to think. Critical thinking involves careful consideration of all the factors. The problem-solving process is used as a method for developing critical-thinking skills and arriving at sound judgments.

Critical-thinking skills can also be used by managers to examine their own employee-related behaviors. When supervising or providing guidance for staff members ask yourself if you (Smith, 1982):

1. clearly identified job performance expectations,
2. selected the best person for the job,
3. clearly communicated all expectations, and
4. provided necessary resources.

When things did not go as expected, ask yourself two additional questions:

1. *Why were expectations not met?* Gather as much information as possible and critically analyze it all with this question in mind. More often than not, important factors are revealed during this process.
2. *Was disciplinary action needed and used when appropriate?* When the source of the unmet expectations is directly related to inadequate employee performance, disciplinary action may be necessary. "It is important to take immediate action when work is below standards" (Smith, 1982). However, use your critical-thinking abilities to assist the errant staff member to improve job performance.

Using critical thinking to solve problems and arrive at decisions increases a supervisor's effectiveness. Applying these same skills to managing employees' work efforts improves both employee performance and manager effectiveness.

Time management. Richard Sloma, author of *No-Nonsense Management (1977)*, firmly believes that "your true adversary is time — not competition, not legislation, not the economy, but time." It takes time to plan, to implement, and to monitor activities, programs, and change. It takes time to consider modifications of plans and new ways of instituting them. Time is also required for people. Staff members need guidance, support, and training. All this takes time. The successful manager treats time as a precious resource. Both his/her time and the employees' time should be focused on achieving the best results for each minute spent.

There are three kinds of management time (Oncken, Wass, 1975):

1. *Boss-imposed time.* The activities imposed by your superiors cannot be disregarded without penalty. They fit into the 'must do' category.
2. *System-imposed time.* Requirements for your time are usually imposed by peers, policies, and procedures. Time is also required in order to move an item 'through the system.' Penalties exist when the manager

does not accommodate system-related time requirements.
3. *Self-imposed time.* Things that originate with or are agreed to by the manager take up self-imposed time. "Self-imposed time is not subject to penalty since neither the boss nor the system can discipline the manager for not doing what they did not know he/she had intended to do in the first place."

Managers have control over their self-imposed time but part of this time will be consumed by staff members (subordinate-imposed time). The remaining time belongs to the manager. It is referred to as discretionary time. It is this time that becomes a major area of focus for time-management techniques. Managers who forget about saving time and concentrate on spending it wisely are far more effective.

To manage time and make it work for you, follow the simple techniques listed in the box on pp. 286 and 287. You control your time resources. Be effective by managing your time productively.

Advocacy. When working with clients the nurse acts as an advocate by "informing and supporting a person so that he can make the best decision possible for himself" (Kohnke, 1980). As a leader or supervisor, the nurse broadens the sphere of advocacy to include two groups: the clients and the staff members for whom he/she is responsible. As a client advocate, the manager plans activities, tasks, and programs that encourage client participation in planning care. As a staff advocate, the manager informs and supports workers. He/she also represents, defends, and 'pleads the case' of the staff when interacting with other department or administrative managers. Advocacy also includes a consideration of the staff members when making decisions or planning for change. Employees who know that their manager is their advocate develop loyalty and trust in the organization. They reward their managers with high productivity levels (quality nursing care) and positive attitudes.

Caring. Managers who care for their employees are interested in each staff member. They believe in and respect the uniqueness and individuality of each person. The person is nonjudgmentally accepted and encouraged to grow. In short, they are nurtured—provided with opportunities to participate, to improve, to grow. Caring is not only the core of nursing, it is also the core of positive leadership and management.

An eye on the future. The rapid changes in the health care field demand that the manager plan and function with the future always in mind. New regulations, new equipment, new procedures, and new products all affect the health care organization. Become attuned to and monitor the current

✐| HOW TO MANAGE TIME

1. **Ask yourself, "What is the best use of my time at *this minute*?"**
The answer will help you to become aware of the alternatives, consciously make choices, and spend your time effectively.

2. **Take time to plan.** One hour spent in planning can eliminate several hours spent in reacting. Planning allows you to set goals and devise the many tasks that must be accomplished in order to meet the goals. Planning makes all management tasks easier.

3. **Use a list.** "Lists increase the certainty of achieving goals" (McCarthy, 1981). In order to do it, you must remember it. Upon arrival at work, make a list of tasks that need to be done for the day. Then divide them into "Urgent" and "Important" categories. Number each item under each heading in order of priority. Perform the urgent tasks first and then move to the important category. Be careful to keep the number of urgent tasks low (if possible) so that attention can be paid to the day's important tasks. Make a list every day and use it.

4. **Organize.** Organize your schedule, your physical workplace, and your energies. Plan on doing a task only once. Group tasks together. Look for and use shortcuts. Give your total attention to the task. Do it right the first time. Estimate the amount of time needed for each task and then remember that everything takes longer than you expect.

5. **Concentrate on the few things that get the most results.** Pare your activities down to the most important. Learn to selectively ignore those problems that are likely to resolve themselves. Concentrate on completing those tasks which clearly contribute to achieving the goal. Allocate time to tasks in order of priority and ruthlessly reject the lowest priority activities. Get the most impact for the time spent.

6. **Delegate appropriately.** Make the most of your time by involving others. Delegating relieves your time and fosters the professional development of your staff members (subordinates). Remember, though, that no matter what you delegate to whom, you (the manager) retain the ultimate responsibility for the task. Chapter 13 discusses the art of delegating in detail.

7. **Think before acting.** Is this activity the best use of your time? Do not let impulse or habit rule your use of time. Learn to say no when necessary. Expect interruptions. "The average manager is interrupted every eight minutes all day long" (Schwartz, Mackenzie, 1979). To minimize interruptions, group or consolidate phone calls

HOW TO MANAGE TIME — cont'd

and visitors. Return all your phone calls at a certain time every day. Schedule time for staff members rather than allowing them to interrupt you at whim. For urgent tasks that must be completed on time, close the door to the office or find a hideaway. Last, follow up on yourself. At the end of the day, analyze the tasks that were not completed. Find and weed out the time wasters. Think about tomorrow, then itemize and prioritize your task list. Thinking about the best use of your time before leaping into action allows you to determine how you will spend this important resource.

events or news. Learn to anticipate changes. Sharp managers keep one foot firmly anchored in the present and one foot cautiously floating in the future.

Practice developing positive leadership traits. Use your emotional maturity as the foundation for cultivating assertiveness, critical thinking, and time-management skills. Work your right brain to foster advocacy and caring abilities. These are the cornerstones of successful leaders.

Positive management traits

Managing means getting things done, usually through the efforts of other people. The most successful managers maintain an open, positive working environment by being very adept in six areas: communications, negotiation, building trust, group skills, conflict resolution, and motivation.

Communication. Probably the single most important factor for promoting effectiveness, a manager's ability to accomplish, depends on his/her ability to communicate. Because we do it every day, managers often fail to apply a conscious effort to improving their communication skills. See the box on p. 288 for suggestions.

Negotiation. Negotiation is the art of arriving at a mutually acceptable decision from different starting points. It is always a preferable method for dealing with conflict. It includes selling your ideas, give and take, and producing a win-win outcome. Aaron Levenstein (1984) has developed 10 commandments for negotiators (see box on p. 289). Review them when preparing for a situation which requires negotiations. Managers with developed negotiation skills understand "the mutual desire for satisfying needs" (Laser, 1981) while recognizing the inherent worth and uniqueness of each person.

✍ SUGGESTIONS FOR EFFECTIVE COMMUNICATION

- **Give instructions clearly and completely.** Share your expectations about the task.
- **Give credit where credit is due.** Support and reward unusual performance. Learn to observe behaviors that deserve recognition. Be sincere and generous with praise when it is due.
- **Involve others.** When possible, communicate with staff members when making decisions or solving problems. Listen to what they say and include them in the process of deciding about change. This helps reduce friction and misunderstandings.
- **Create daily two-way conversations.** Talk things over with the people you supervise. Personally communicate with at least one staff member every day and remember that it is sometimes more important to listen than to talk.
- **Provide feedback.** "To keep the supervisor-employee relationship in good repair, take time to let employees know how they are getting along" (Chapman, 1975). Staff members, especially new ones, need to know if their job performance meets your expectations and standards. Reinforce your staff for jobs well done and quietly work to correct or improve the negatives.

Trust. When trust exists in the work environment, workers feel free to try new methods or seek a better way of doing things. Trust evolves over time and requires consistent, caring behaviors. It is built on respect for each staff member and a belief that each person will do his/her best. Trust is an essential ingredient of any positive work environment.

Group skills. Because managers achieve results through other people, the ability to work effectively with good group skills helps create a more dynamic and creative working atmosphere. See Chapter 3 for an in-depth discussion of group dynamics.

Conflict resolution. The ability to solve the human problems (i.e., the conflicts) can greatly influence the quality of workers' lives. When staff members feel their conflicts are resolved fairly, they are willing to take new risks and work for improvement. Chapter 6 offers several techniques for resolving conflict successfully.

Motivation. Managers lead by example. Staff members are always observing and evaluating their supervisors. When they are met with enthusiasm and an eagerness to do the job, each worker becomes inspired to

10 COMMANDMENTS FOR NEGOTIATION

1. **Clarify the common purpose.** When each party is working to achieve a shared goal, concessions are easier to make.
2. **Keep the discussion focused on the topic.** To keep each side from 'talking past each other,' decide on what they are going to disagree about. With those points in mind, keep the discussion relevant but look for hidden motives.
3. **Agree about terminology.** "I'll look into it" can mean anything from a casual interest to a full investigation. Be clear with the words you choose. Clarify or define words that you think may have a different meaning to others.
4. **Avoid abstracts.** Concentrate on the facts. When both parties hold to 'the principle of the thing,' nothing is accomplished. Decide on the goal, then stick to the facts and focus on how you will reach it.
5. **Look for trade-offs.** Consider the goal, then decide what concessions each party is willing to make. Give a little and take a little.
6. **Listen.** Are you, the negotiator, hearing what is actually being said? Are either or both parties hearing each other? Paraphrase, restate, summarize. Use any communication technique necessary. Compel each party to pay attention.
7. **Avoid debate.** Do not argue. Confrontation widens the gap between each side. Use tactics of persuasion. Words such as "us" and "we" help convince each side that they really are in agreement.
8. **Remember the personal element.** Consider the background, goals, needs, interests, and feelings of each individual. Many times negotiations become easier when individuals get to know each other.
9. **Be logical.** Present a logical case that takes into account the needs of the patient, the department or unit, and the involved people.
10. **Search for integrated solutions.** Hopefully, arriving at the shared goal satisfies the real needs and interests of all parties. If the solution was devised and shared by both (all) sides, it stands a greater chance of succeeding.

From Levenstein A: Negotiation vs. confrontation, *Nursing Management* 15(1):52, 1984.

do his/her best. Chapters 5 and 12 discuss motivational techniques and their application in more detail.

Managing Positively

The five functions of the manager can be applied in a variety of ways. Some managers use the five functions to impose rigid controls upon employees. Others function so casually that no one knows where the limits lie. The key is to find the balance between these extremes.

Functions

Supervisors who apply each management function in a positive way create a working environment where employees can grow. To develop and nurture motivated workers who will achieve the organization's goals, practice applying the management process with the following points in mind.

Role model. The strongest messages are sent via behaviors. **To set the best example possible, rely upon your philosophy, your code of ethics, and the standards for nursing practice.** Use them as guidelines for planning, interacting, and all other activities. Incorporate the principles of worth and respect by recognizing each person as a unique individual who is capable of growth, initiative, and creativity. In short, practice the 'golden rule.'

Plan. Have a plan. The positive work climate is not created, developed, and monitored haphazardly. It is a planned event. Plan for today's work every morning but keep the larger future picture in mind. Work to plan for long-term goals that include rewards for performance and recognition for innovation, creativity, loyalty, and the like. Plan for workers to participate in setting goals. Establish priorities, identify resources and liabilities, and devise action plans for implementing. Do it all with one eye on the worker and one eye on the goal.

Organize. A well-organized workplace adds to a positive environment because work flows smoothly. An organized manager also helps work to flow smoothly by structuring work loads equally and appropriately, organizing staff members, and gathering resources necessary for doing the work. When work is organized, tasks can be performed efficiently, and goals become attainable.

Coordinate. Once the action plan is implemented, the manager's attention turns to ensuring that each work activity is providing the planned result. First-line health care managers monitor the clients, patients, or residents for the quality of care delivered; staff members who deliver the care; and the administration that provides the structure and policies for delivering the care.

The manager's **positive coordination activities also include staff development and retention strategies.** When steps for growth are planned and agreed to by both employees and supervisors, people become motivated to stretch their limits, become creative, and contribute to the organization.

Direct. Providing upbeat, positive direction is an important managerial function. Whether the goal is giving the best nursing care possible for that day or implementing a new client care documentation system, the supervisor must provide the motivation and leadership needed to accomplish the goals. Positive direction is provided when managers inspire staff members to do their best through guidance, training, and team building. When employees are involved in problem solving, provided with learning opportunities, and given recognition for work well done, they become active, productive citizens of the creative work environment.

Evaluate. Even when everything is flowing smoothly and all the staff members are happy, you still must evaluate the results of your efforts. **Measure the progress toward the goal and revise or adjust the plan,** if necessary. Evaluations allow us to find what was done right, where the plan went awry, and why the outcomes resulted in success or failure. More importantly, evaluations encourage us to grow, even when basking in the glories of success.

Inspire. Energize your staff to do their best. Encourage a can-do attitude and teamwork. Approach your position as a supervisor or manager with excitement, enthusiasm, energy, and a determination to be the best. Approach your staff members with respect, dignity, trust, and concern. Inspire by example. Your staff will grow in its trust and loyalty, and together you will accomplish great things.

Interdepartmental relationships

Because no unit, department, or section can function independently, managers must interact and establish satisfactory working relationships with people from other sections of the organization. Building good interdepartmental relationships requires good communication, team building, and conflict resolution abilities.

Team building. Most health care facilities employ people from diverse educational backgrounds. Because most, if not all, of the client's care is determined by several specialists, team-building skills are important for fostering an effective, upbeat work environment. "Team building develops a supportive group atmosphere in which members work together effectively toward specific goals" (Sullivan, 1990). Whether it is the daily work group or the interdisciplinary care committee, the principles remain the same.

To foster team building, concentrate on the following:

Cohesiveness. Using your knowledge of communications and group dynamics to develop a climate that fosters group togetherness and loyalty (cohesiveness).

Working together. Planning, setting mutual goals, and finding common ground all encourage team members to focus on the goals.

Conflict management. Assist team members to work through and resolve conflicts. Once the conflicts are resolved, relationships within the team tend to solidify and become more comfortable.

Effectiveness. Are the goals being met? Is work smoothly coordinated? Is the client receiving improved care? Monitor the effectiveness of the team, encourage suggestions, and revise or adapt plans as needed.

Respect people's differences. Listen to, acknowledge, and appreciate each individual. If you focus the combined energies of the team toward the goal, nothing becomes unachievable.

⤜ HOW TO STRENGTHEN PHYSICIAN–NURSE RELATIONSHIPS

- **Communicate.** Initiate communication. Find out what the doctor wants to know and provide that knowledge, but also politely insist that he/she listen to what you need to say.
- **Know your stuff.** Use data to communicate in an intelligent, meaningful way. The words *good, fair, well,* and *poor* only communicate value judgments.
- **Negotiate roles.** "The interdependent nature of medicine and nursing with the overlap of functions means that they must mutually work toward the sorting out of responsibility" (Kalish, Kalish, 1977).
- **Trust.** Communications are vital for establishing trust in the performance of others. Deal with conflict openly and directly. Remember that doctors are people, too, with varying abilities to resolve conflict. Use opportunities to teach physicians about what you do.
- **Respect.** Respect the physician, but, more importantly, respect your abilities as a nurse and a leader.

Physician–nurse relationships. Because of the special nature of the historic relationship between these two professions, building an effective team deserves a special look.

In a recent survey of over 1100 practicing nurses, the editors of *Nursing 91* (1991) found some interesting results: 68 percent of the respondents do not think doctors understand what they do as nurses, and 57 percent felt that nurses are subordinate to physicians.

In order to establish an equal relationship of colleagues working together as a team, we (the nurses and health care professionals) must concentrate on building more effective team relationships. Perhaps the suggestions in the box on p. 292 may be helpful.

Focus on building effective teams. A learning collegial working environment is as important (if not more important) than money. It can go a long way toward creating a positive atmosphere for clients, staff members, and other professionals.

Creating your own positive work environment requires patience and consistency. You, too, can become a positive and effective manager if you remember to always do the best you can with what you have.

✍ Key Concepts

- Three new work designs that focus on the work life of the employee as well as productivity are quality of work life (QWL) programs, the worth ethic (WE), and job enrichment strategies.
- QWL programs focus on creating work environments that are good for both people and profits.
- The worth ethic states that managers who are committed to building self-esteem and respect provide workers with an environment in which growth, innovation, and personal fulfillment are fostered.
- Job enrichment programs assess employee attitudes and the job's core dimensions in order to discover what motivators make the job more rewarding.
- Employees have three types of work attitudes: job satisfaction, job involvement, and organizational commitment.
- The five core dimensions of a job are task variety, task identity, task significance, autonomy, and feedback.
- When analyzing your personal outlook toward managing people, consider your philosophy, ethics, integrity, and level of self-awareness.
- The working climate is most strongly influenced by the attitudes and behaviors of the manager.
- Managers who project a charismatic leadership style are emotionally mature, assertive, critical thinkers, good time managers, future-oriented, and caring advocates.
- Management time can be divided into boss-imposed, system-imposed, and self-imposed time.
- To manage time wisely, find the best use of your time, plan, organize, write lists, delegate, concentrate on the few most important jobs, plan to be interrupted, and think before acting.
- Positive management characteristics include excellent communication, negotiation, and conflict resolution skills, in addition to an ability to engender trust in the work group.
- Negotiation is the ability to arrive at a mutually acceptable decision when each party holds a different view. By following the 10 commandments of negotiation, the manager can practice effective negotiation skills.
- Effective managers lead by example and act as role models for their staff members. They plan, organize, coordinate, direct, and evaluate by considering workers as well as productivity.
- Inspiring yourself and others contributes strongly to a positive working environment.
- To build effective interdepartmental relationships, managers need to practice good communication, team-building, and conflict resolution skills.

- Motivated, functional teams are built by focusing on communications, cohesiveness, conflict management, and effectiveness.
- To improve nurse–physician relationships, communicate, know your stuff, negotiate roles, and demonstrate as much respect for your profession, your job, and yourself as you do other professional people.

✒ Learning Activities

1. Describe what you feel would be the perfect working environment.
2. Divide the group into two sections. One section will argue the pro position; the other will take the con position. The objective is to convince the administrator to adopt or not adopt a QWL, WE, or job enrichment program.
3. Plan your own time-management program for one week. Use the suggestions in this chapter to establish goals and prioritize for best use of your time. At the end of the week, evaluate your effectiveness and plan revisions.
4. You are the manager of a 30-bed unit in a long-term care facility. The administrator wants to know if 8-hour or 12-hour shifts are preferred by the staff. Half the staff members want to work 8 hours, while the other half believes that 12-hour shifts are better. Apply the '10 commandments' to negotiate a solution.
5. Explain how you would go about building an effective, motivated work team.

References

Chapman EN: *Supervisor's survival kit: a mid-management primer*, ed 2, Chicago, 1975, Science Research Associates.

Davis K, Newstrom J: *Human behavior at work: organizational behavior*, ed 8, New York, 1989, McGraw-Hill.

Editors: The doctor–nurse game, *Nursing 91* 21(6):60, 1991.

Kalish BJ, Kalish PA: An analysis of the sources of physician–nurse conflict, *Journal of Nursing Administration* 7(1):51, 1977.

Kohnke MF: The nurse as advocate, *American Journal of Nursing* 80(11):2038, 1980.

Laser RJ: I win–you win negotiating, *Journal of Nursing Administration* 11(11):24, 1981.

Levenstein A: Negotiation vs. confrontation, *Nursing Management* 15(1):52, 1984.

Ludeman K: *The worth ethic: how to profit from the changing values of the new work force*, New York, 1989, EP Dutton.

McCarthy MJ: Managing your own time: the most important management task, *Journal of Nursing Administration* 11(12):61, 1981.

Oncken W, Wass DL: Management time: who's got the monkey, *Journal of Nursing Administration* 5(7):26, 1975.

Schwartz EB, Mackenzie RA: Time-management strategy for women, *Journal of Nursing Administration* 9(3):22, 1979.

Sloma RS: *No-nonsense management: a general manager's primer*, New York, 1977, Macmillan.

Smith J: Managing employee performance, *Nursing Management* 13(8):14, 1982.

Sullivan MP: *Nursing leadership and management: a study and learning tool*, Springhouse, Pa, 1990, Springhouse.

Additional Readings

Amedurl P: Making time work for you, *Nursing 90* 20(10):144, 1990. *Time can be used as a resource instead of a liability by following these four time-saving tips.*

Autry JA: *Love and profit: the art of caring leadership*, New York, 1991, William Morrow. *Written in poetry and prose, this book is a unique primer with an honest and humane approach to management.*

Coyne W: Nurses are the key to quality health care, *RN* 53(2):69, 1990. *Ms. Coyne offers several successful strategies, borrowed from one of the world's leading manufacturers, to build a commitment to quality.*

Dorney RC: Making time to manage, *Harvard Business Review* 88(1):38, 1988. *Time management is more about management than about time.*

Griffen M: Assumptions for success, *Nursing Management* 19(1)32u, 1988. *A manager's use of McGregor's Y-theory assumptions produces significant changes in staff attitudes and performance in this long-term care facility.*

Kane RA, Caplan AL, editors: *Everyday ethics: resolving dilemmas in nursing home life*, New York, 1990, Springer. *An excellent tool for analyzing the many ethical situations that arise when providing long-term health care.*

Lancaster J: Creating a climate for excellence, *Journal of Nursing Administration* 15(1):16, 1985. *The author discusses the steps for creating a climate for achievement based on trust and open communication.*

Leebov W: *Positive co-worker relationships in health care*, Chicago, 1990, American Hospital Publishing. *Taking an active role in promoting a productive work environment and understanding your co-worker will enhance growth and improve relationships.*

Lynch M: P-A-C-E yourself: tips on time management, *Nursing 91* 21(3):105, 1991. *The acronym PACE can be used to organize your time.*

Mitty EL: The nurse as advocate: issues in LTC, *Nursing and Health Care* 10(12):520, 1991. *The author explores the issues and barricades to good and equitable long-term care.*

Schneider P: Career charisma, *Working Woman* 13(5):79, 1988. *Follow these tips for developing optimism and the confidence to master change and empower others to face challenges.*

Smeltzer CH: The art of negotiation: an everyday experience, *Journal of Nursing Administration* 21(7/8):26, 1991. *Managers cannot communicate or make decisions without using the process of negotiation, an essential skill in today's rapidly changing health care environment.*

MOTIVATION

12

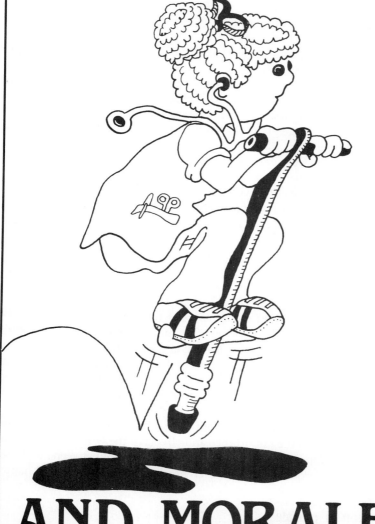

AND MORALE

✤ Learning Objectives

Upon completion of this chapter, the reader will be able to:

1. Describe the differences between motivation and morale.
2. List five principles of motivation.
3. Explain how each motivational principle can help managers provide high levels of morale.
4. Define organizational morale.
5. List five signs of low morale.
6. Discuss at least four important differences in motivating younger and older workers.
7. Explain the process for orienting a new employee.
8. Discuss the importance of a skills evaluation.
9. Explain why the first 100 days on a job are the most important.
10. Identify four stages that take place in the development of a nurse manager.
11. Identify four strategies for continuing your education and learning.
12. List six techniques for improving motivation and morale.
13. Describe four ways to avoid the 'Superperson syndrome.'
14. List four strategies for empowering yourself and others.

Principles of Motivation

One of the most important components of the work environment is the level of motivation and, consequently, morale of the workers. When employees are working only for the paycheck, morale and productivity are low. Things get done, but just barely. Staff members do their jobs at the minimum level of competency. They arrive as late as possible and leave as early as they can. Work is considered a way to 'bring home the bacon' and nothing more.

Fortunately, this is changing as both organizations and employees are beginning to realize the importance and effects of the workers' morale on productivity. Managers are recognizing the connection between employee satisfaction and productivity. In other words, we are learning that happy workers produce more.

Motivation or morale

Motivation and morale go hand in hand. Each is necessary and enhances the other, but there are differences.

Motivation. The internal drive that moves a person to act is a motivator. A motivator may be felt as an emotion, impulse, desire, or need, but each one provides impetus for action. The internal drive generated by these feelings can be satisfied only by the person experiencing them. Others may notice these needs and attempt to fulfill them, but unless the motivated person feels or believes that his/her needs are satisfied, they are not. We motivate ourselves by feeling needs and attempting to meet them. We motivate others by assessing their needs, offering appropriate support, and providing opportunities for them to meet their needs and, thus, grow.

Morale. When referring to the work organization, morale is defined as "the attitude workers have toward the quality of their total work life" (Straub, Attner, 1991). This attitude affects the quality as well as quantity of their work. When morale is high, so is productivity. Morale evolves from the employees' motivation level, the behaviors of the supervisors, and the philosophy of the organization. If employees are positively motivated to achieve, explore their creativity, and meet higher-level needs, morale will be high and the quality of work superior. If, however, employees are motivated by lower-level needs such as security or fear of reprisal, work output will be of poor quality and quantity. Motivation influences morale. Nurses who supervise should be aware of and learn to work with motivational principles. They are the keys to fostering high morale within your organization.

Five motivational precepts

Because motivation is an important concept, several theories have been developed to explain how motivation occurs. (Review the summary box on p. 120 for motivational theories.) Although each theory focuses on a different aspect of motivation, they all are based on five premises.

Unique individual. Each person is the combination of a particular past and the present. The influences of childhood, school, peers, and experiences mold each of us into a unique human being. We may look, talk, and behave alike, but each of us is one of a kind. Therefore, each individual has worth and is deserving of respect. Nurse managers who recognize the uniqueness of each staff member look for opportunities to support and promote each individual's growth.

Needs will be met. Every person has needs and strives to fulfill them. Whether the needs are for oxygen or self-actualization, the individual will do everything possible to fulfill his/her needs. Recall that lower-level needs will be met first. Accurately determining each staff member's needs will assist the supervisor in planning appropriate assignments and offering opportunities for growth and improvement.

You are not alone. The saying, "No man is an island," is a basic truth. Man is gregarious. Anthropologists even refer to man as a 'herd animal.' These all mean that people live, interact, and work within groups. People need each other and tend to form groups based on shared needs, ideas, or values. Within the work setting, various groups form, fill their function, and dissolve or change. Groups vary in importance for the employee. For example, changes in the group with whom the employee has lunch would probably have less of an impact than changes in the employee's work (task) group. Remember to consider the importance of the group to the individual when motivating others.

People are dynamic. Early theorists believed that people became static and unchanging as soon as they reached adulthood. They had learned everything they needed in childhood. Physical growth was completed, so, they reasoned, mental growth also was done. Adulthood was characterized by stability, routine, and uniformity. Fortunately, later theorists, such as Erickson, began to explore adulthood and found it to be a dynamic time characterized by the passage from one level of development to another. Therefore, people are always growing, changing, and developing. Offering staff members new opportunities and challenges is a good way to recognize the dynamic nature of individuals.

Pleasure–pain principle. All creatures, from the amoeba to man, move away from pain and toward pleasure. This is an important principle for supervisors to keep in mind. When employees are motivated *toward* achieving goals, morale is high, and work output is increased. The opposite is also true. Workers motivated by the desire to avoid punishment (pain) will demonstrate low levels of morale and productivity. Recall a basic guide from Chapter 1: Always work toward, not against. Do not fight against low motivation levels. Work toward improved morale by focusing energies in a positive, achievement-oriented direction.

Organizational Morale

The attitudes of workers toward the quality of their work lives make up the organizational morale. These attitudes are a direct reflection of the work environment. Astute team leaders, supervisors, and managers function with a strong consideration for the workers' morale.

Assessing workplace morale

Although each work environment (like its individuals) is unique, there are several factors that affect the quality of everyday work life.

Employee's perceptions. Each worker attempts to seek satisfaction and fill needs within the work environment. Therefore, each individual perceives or views the quality of the work environment uniquely and places importance on those factors that will help him/her receive satisfaction. The factors listed in the next section and their degree of importance should be examined when appraising the morale at your facility.

Factors affecting morale. According to business text authors, Joseph Straub and Raymond Attner (1991), the factors (determined by employees) that most affect the quality of work life and morale relate to:

1. Absence of apathy.
2. Absence of undue stress associated with the job.
3. Advancement based on merit.
4. Career goals progress.
5. Confidence in the management.
6. Development and utilization of skills, talents, and abilities.
7. Economic well-being (salary, benefits).
8. Employee commitment, involvement, and influence.
9. Employee state of mind.
10. Impact of job on personal life.
11. Physical working environment.
12. Relations with supervisor and work group.
13. Respect for the individual.
14. Union–management relations.

As you may have noticed, the above factors are listed alphabetically. During your analysis of the staff's morale, make sure you discover which factors are considered the most important by your employees. The list could be used by staff members to consider which factors are most important to them. Assessing the factors which affect the quality of work life allows the nurse manager to ascertain how each factor, individually and collectively, "aids in creating a work environment where workers receive satisfaction and are motivated in their jobs" (Straub, Attner, 1991).

Signs of low morale. By observing, listening, and asking, the supervisor can uncover the clues and causes of poor morale. Because both the employee and the work environment are dynamic and changing, supervisors must constantly monitor each for clues relating to the level of morale and motivation (see box on p. 302).

SIGNS OF LOW MORALE

- Increased lateness, absenteeism, and job turnover
- Decreased productivity and quality of work
- Disregard for rules
- Carelessness resulting in increased injury rates
- Heavy or extreme criticism of facility's policies, procedures, and rules
- Increased interpersonal conflicts

The more subtle indications of low morale can be uncovered by observing behaviors such as body language, group interactions, and informal communications (i.e., breaks, lunch, off-duty hours). These behaviors all give clues to employees' morale levels. If one behavior pattern is present, you (the supervisor) may have a personnel problem. If two or more behavior patterns exist, you may have a morale problem.

Health care worker burnout

The function of the health care industry is to provide direct and indirect health services to people. There are usually more people who need health or illness care than there are health care workers to provide the needed services. Because health care workers truly care about their clients, they respond by setting unrealistic goals, becoming unrealistically dedicated, and overworking. This eventually leads to the condition known as burnout.

Characteristics. *Burnout* is defined as a "syndrome of physical and emotional exhaustion, involving the development of a negative self-concept, negative job attitude, and loss of concern and feelings for clients" (Pines, Maslach, 1978). **The major cause of burnout is stress.** Nurses and other health care providers have a strong need or desire to alleviate suffering and improve the human condition. When this goal is unattainable, an intense stress is generated.

Over time, this stress begins to manifest itself on the physical level as feelings of fatigue and exhaustion, "frequent or prolonged colds, headaches, stomachaches, backaches, difficulty sleeping or getting up, depression, and a number of psychosomatic complaints" (Khalsa, 1978). To emotionally cope with this stress, nurses distance themselves from their clients. They intellectualize by treating cases, diagnoses, or room numbers instead of people. Some become very competent technically. Stress is reduced by using this method, but care becomes dehumanized. Many health care workers attempt to "reduce emotional stress by making sharp distinctions between their personal and professional lives" (Yee, 1981). This sounds like a workable idea, but, in reality, it is difficult to do. People in our society tend to define themselves and others by the work they do. It is difficult to separate the roles, for example, when everyone in the area where you live knows that you are a nurse.

All these signs and symptoms eventually affect the employee's morale and job performance, which now adds additional stress and more negative feelings. The final result is a loss of one more health care provider as the nurse transfers away from direct client care or leaves the profession altogether. To save ourselves and our co-workers from burning out, we must learn to recognize its signs and prevent its occurrence.

Coping techniques. The first and **most important technique for coping with burnout is prevention.** First, prevent an overwhelming situation from growing into a crisis by realizing that you (as a nurse or a supervisor) cannot be all things to all people (see box below). Realistically appraise what you will be able to accomplish, set priorities, and then focus on what needs to be done. This technique assists you to meet goals and decrease stress. If you are not lending energies to looking for stressors, then you are not interpreting the situation as stress-provoking. You are busy achieving goals, doing what you can, and feeling comfortable with your best. The secret lies in the amount of energy you choose to give to being stressed. The more situations that you choose to define as stressful, the more stressful each situation will become. Fortunately, the opposite is also true.

A holistic approach appears to help decrease the potential for burnout. On the personal level this involves "opening up communication with oneself" (Clark, 1980). Identify and work with any nonverbalized negative feelings. Other steps focus on good nutrition, physical exercise, relaxation techniques, and regular outlets for stress. See Chapter 1 for other suggestions about positively coping with stress and preventing burnout. Managers and supervisors can also take steps to approach burnout from a holistic point of view. Begin by identifying which staff members have unrealistic expectations or dedication. These individuals fall into the

---

COPING TECHNIQUES

- Create a pleasant and open working environment.
- Set reasonable and realistic demands on self and staff.
- Set shared, achievable goals.
- Prioritize.
- Identify and work on negative feelings.
- Rotate undesirable tasks with favored ones.
- Practice good nutrition, exercise, and various relaxation techniques.

high-risk category and need support to develop realistic goals. Rotating undesirable or frustration tasks is helpful. Schedule and insist that each staff member take breaks and lunches, preferably away from the unit or work area. When dealing with conflict, work for the win-win situation. Perhaps most important, establish a staff support system where each person has the opportunity to share experiences and receive supportive human contact. Other important prevention factors include a pleasant and open working environment; reasonable and realistic demands of staff members; and shared, achievable goals. Practice these techniques. They are the best hedges against burnout.

Morale and age differences

"The real strength of any organization comes from its people" (Chapman, 1975). Without enthusiastic and energetic employees, no organization will survive in the long run. Because workers are unique, changing, and growing people, leaders need to develop an awareness of what motivators are most effective for each individual. The prudent supervisor considers the impact of age on motivation levels when attempting to understand what stimulates each worker.

As a manager, you will be faced with one of two age-related situations: you are the older supervisor who must relate to and understand how to motivate younger workers, or you are the younger manager attempting to understand and relate to the mature worker. Understanding age-related differences is important for nurse managers who want to encourage a high level of moral in staff members.

Younger workers. To understand the younger worker, keep six factors in mind (see box on p. 305). The supervisor who accepts younger employees as they are, supports their career development, and provides guidance for their growth will motivate and retain high-caliber workers.

Older workers. The mature employee may have been with the organization for many years or could be a newcomer. In either case, the older worker needs understanding, especially by the young supervisor (see box on p. 306).

Strive to develop an awareness of the effects of age on motivation. Many motivational techniques work well with all age groups, but the sensitive and skillful manager can employ specific, age-related practices to encourage high levels of quality, productivity, and worker morale.

The new employee

New employees are in a special group. In the health care industry, they usually arrive with specialized training or education. Preparation (training, education) programs can take several weeks, as with a nursing assis-

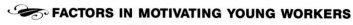 **FACTORS IN MOTIVATING YOUNG WORKERS**

1. **Younger people make commitments to the job more slowly.** In the past, people were happy just to work. Today, the job's probation period works both ways. Both the company and the employee decide if they will be happy with each other. It is more important for the younger worker to find the right job than to just work. Managers who understand this can help guide the employee toward making good career decisions while, at the same time, providing motivation for more immediate productivity.

2. **Young employees respond well to participative leadership styles.** Because they have been raised in a more permissive environment, young employees function better in a democratic, rather than autocratic, climate. They need to participate, feel that they are members of the group, and be stimulated. A participative leadership style helps meet these needs and benefits the organization as well.

3. **Money is not always the big incentive.** Although it is still important, it is usually outweighed by the opportunity to learn and grow. Challenge, excitement, and involvement are more important to the younger worker, at least in the beginning. Astute managers can recognize and support those needs that are more important than money.

4. **Attitudes toward physical work have changed.** Physical labor and endurance are no longer considered necessary for proving one's worth. Automation and affluence have eliminated the need for hard physical labor. Although younger workers want to be considered as members of the team, they are unwilling to use physical prowess as a method for gaining team membership.

5. **Loyalty to the job has changed.** Although young people today are more loyal to their professions, they do not demonstrate the company loyalty of the older generations. Managers who expect loyalty for the long term are frequently disappointed. Younger workers usually stay with an organization because they are motivated to do so, not out of loyalty.

6. **Time dimensions are different for younger employees.** They are not willing to wait 10 or 20 years to prove themselves, so they will push for opportunities. Many progressive companies recognize this and provide younger employees with graduated levels of responsibility and productivity.

From Chapman EN: *Supervisor's survival kit: a mid-management primer,* ed 2, Chicago, 1975, Science Research Associates.

FACTORS IN MOTIVATING MATURE WORKERS

1. **They need extra support and behavioral reinforcement during periods of change.** It is natural to refer and revert to 'the good old days,' especially during stressful situations. Frequent and consistent feedback helps the mature worker adjust to the change, evaluate how well he/she is doing, and gain positive reinforcement.

2. **Mature workers have survived many leadership styles.** People who have worked for 20 years or more have seen the rise and fall of autocratic, permissive, and democratic leadership theories. As a result, many have become suspicious of any new leadership technique. "The best method is to be very open and direct with them. If you wish their cooperation, ask for it; if you need their advice, ask for it" (Chapman, 1975).

3. **Performance and efficiency are very important to the older worker.** Most senior employees have worked for organizations with rigid rules and high productivity standards. Consequently, they expect and respect high standards in co-workers, especially supervisors. With this group, the manager who sets examples reflecting these high standards has a better chance of winning their respect.

4. **Mature workers need to be involved.** Because older workers carry a wealth of experience, they should always be included. Leaving them on the sidelines is a serious mistake. Older workers can act as consultants, problem solvers, and counselors. Responsibility can usually be safely delegated to a more mature employee. Involved older workers require no special treatment other than the recognition of making a contribution. Managers who provide this recognition foster a motivated employee to remain productive until retirement.

5. **Seniority counts.** Employees who have been with the facility for many years have developed certain patterns and characteristics. Work schedules, routines, and habits become deeply ingrained, and change may be more difficult for these people. Supervisors sensitive to this usually allow these behaviors to continue as long as they are not resented by others and do not adversely affect productivity.

tant program, or as long as 6 or 7 years (i.e., nurse practitioner, nurse administrator). No matter how great the education, all new employees share a common need — they must become familiar with the structure and function of the organization. This 'socialization' process begins with the preemployment interview and ends when the individual is a fully productive member of the work team.

The formal orientation. New employees are influenced by many different variables. Observations and impressions during the hiring process will be built upon during the orientation period. During this time, the supervisor has the opportunity to lay the groundwork for a productive, fulfilling relationship between the new employee and his/her company.

The **first step in orienting a new employee relates to personnel functions.** If not done earlier, describe the salary and benefits package. Then move to a discussion of the organizational structure which includes:

1. an overview of the company's philosophy, mission statement, goals, and plans for the future;
2. familiarization with policies and procedures;
3. an orientation to the organizational chart with an explanation of the management levels, lines of authority, and formal communication patterns.

Make sure the new employee knows where he/she 'fits' within the company's structure. Instilling organizational pride and personal commitment in the new worker begins here.

The next step in the orientation process is an introduction to the work setting. A tour of the unit or department and an explanation of how the job relates to other activities, persons, and departments takes place. This is followed by a discussion of the department's goals, standards of client care, the nursing care delivery system used at that facility, and the new employee's job description.

According to Vestal (1987), the job description offers "the fastest clues as to your employer's expectations." **The job description clarifies how the specific role contributes to the overall purpose and goals of the organization.** It contains the job title; a brief description of the job itself; specific qualifications, training, or skills needed; the job's functions, responsibilities, and essential tasks; and last, a description of the lines of authority to be followed. The new employee needs to be familiar and comfortable with his/her job description in order to become a fully functional member of the team.

Next, as part of each new employee's orientation, the manager arranges for a demonstration of the employee's skills. "Supervised practice with feedback will aid by developing agreement on job performance expectations" (George, 1986). The use of performance checklists, which list each step of a given skill, are very useful tools for the nurse manager. They allow for an accurate evaluation of the new employee's skills, assist in developing individualized training plans based on recognized needs, and encourage both manager and employee to work toward high standards of care. Evaluation of the new employee's skills is a critical element in the provision of quality client care.

The informal organization. Last, the employee needs some information about the organization's culture. Each facility has a unique combination of assumptions, attitudes, values, norms, behaviors, symbols, and language. During the orientation period, the new employee will be influenced by the behaviors of other employees as clues about the organizational culture are revealed. If the existing employees are committed to the facility's policies, procedures, and goals, it will be reflected in the culture and climate of the work environment. As the new employee adapts, he/she will slowly acquire the values and norms of the work group.

Instead of looking at the process of orienting new employees as something to be endured, consider it as an important investment that will yield high future dividends.

Manager Morale

Because you are the leader, supervisor, or manager, your attitudes set the tone for your entire staff. Being upbeat and knowledgeable is not always easy, but it is challenging. Managers who inspire others by their examples were not born with an ability to inspire. They began in ignorance, worked hard to learn, and practiced until they became effective leaders and managers. Like life, becoming an effective, motivated supervisor requires time and effort.

The new supervisor

Nurses and other health care professionals usually move into supervisory positions in one of two ways: they are promoted from a nonsupervisory position within the organization, or they are hired as a supervisor from outside the company. No matter how you arrived, you are now in a supervisory position, and the first few weeks are critical for establishing your credibility and effectiveness as a manager.

Making the transition. "The first hundred days on a job are the most important [emphasis added]. Not only will staffers and colleagues notice everything you do during your first days, but they will remember these things for a long time" (Austin, 1992). Once your employees form an opinion of you, changing it will not be easy. Use the suggestions listed in the box on p. 309 to survive the first weeks as a manager and encourage an effective transition.

Project confidence and enthusiasm. Begin to build relationships and a productive work climate. These guidelines will help your first few weeks become a strong foundation for future success.

⤳ TRANSITION TIPS

1. **Build good relationships.** If you are to lead people and manage their work, you need their cooperation. Ask their advice. Seek out different opinions. Involve staff members in making decisions. If you need help, ask for it. Do not become power-happy. Let your employees help you in the beginning. You usually need it anyway, and it is an effective way to begin building mutual trust and respect.

2. **Be patient with yourself.** Do not let the new job overwhelm you. The first days of any new job are hectic and frustrating. Do not set too many goals or try new innovations in the first weeks. Adopt a long-range viewpoint. Give yourself time to adjust and focus on building sound relationships with staff members.

3. **Do not neglect your staff members.** Resist the initial temptation of every new supervisor to impress management by increasing productivity. Make better use of these important first weeks by making personal, positive contact with every employee in your department. Begin to build sound working relationships by letting each worker know that he/she is respected as an individual and appreciated for his/her contributions to the organization. Devoting the first weeks to quietly getting to know your staff builds your credibility and encourages staff members to begin building trust in your abilities.

4. **Do not be influenced by previous relationships.** It is not uncommon for old work group members or friends to expect preferential treatment now that you are the boss. You cannot allow this. Your first responsibility is to treat each employee fairly and equally. The respect and confidence of every worker in the department depend on it.

5. **Act as a buffer.** Although you want to please your superiors and earn their support, be careful not to pass the pressures from above to your staff members. The job of a supervisor is to support the employee and make the work easier. Absorbing the 'flack' keeps your department operating smoothly and productively.

6. **Save some time for planning.** The first few days of any new job are hectic, but even new managers need a plan. Below are suggestions for the first week's goals:
   - Keep efficiency and productivity at established levels.
   - Discover the problems and potentials (strong points of the department).
   - Start building a relationship with each employee.

7. **Do not make changes too quickly.** The best supervisor can ruin the productivity and morale of staff members by introducing a series of rapid changes. People become anxious when there are changes. Let the staff adjust to *you* first, then involve people and slowly introduce innovations. See Chapter 10 for a detailed discussion of planned change.

From Chapman EN: *Supervisor's survival kit: a mid-management primer,* ed 2, Chicago, 1975, Science Research Associates.

Stages of growth. New nurse supervisors, like managers everywhere, pass through a series of stages when developing their management roles. As with other developmental stages, each phase of the nurse manager's growth has critical tasks which must be mastered in order to succeed. New supervisors who can identify these stages are able to cooperate with the process and facilitate their learning, adaptation, and growth. M. L. Etheredge (1985), a nursing educator at New England Medical Center, has referred to these stages as infancy, adolescence, adulthood, and the older years.

Infancy. This stage is ego-centered and characterized by dependency, passivity, and a low level of tolerance for frustration. The main developmental task at this level is to learn your job, the roles you play, and where you fit within the organization. New managers find it difficult to say no and may tend to personalize problems. It is easy to blame others during this phase. The new manager needs support, guidance, and understanding. At this stage, "A supportive boss is the best guarantee that a promising new manager will thrive" (Zetlin, 1992).

Adolescence. As the new nurse manager starts to trust in his/her judgment, he/she begins the struggle for a unique identity as a supervisor. Identifying and developing an individual leadership style is the critical task for the 'adolescent' manager. Like the teenager, the new supervisor's knowledge grows rapidly, and new information is integrated into the role. Conformity is important. The new supervisor may check with others before making decisions. Being accepted by other managers becomes important. Adolescent nurse managers also struggle for independence by rebelling against authority, being inconsistent, testing, and questioning almost everything. As the supervisor defines norms and sets limits, he/she begins to identify a management 'self' and "develop managerial judgement that's predictable, accurate, and reliable" (Etheredge, 1985).

Adulthood. The critical task here is to develop a fully integrated personality with an established philosophy, ethics, and convictions. He/she is comfortable with the role of leader and can now choose when to fight, flee, or do nothing. The ability to make objective assessments, formulate plans, and achieve goals is characteristic of the 'adult' manager. Supervisors at this level understand cause and effect and can tolerate mistakes without losing self-esteem. They are realistic and can approach situations with a sense of calm integrity.

The older years. If the manager has successfully mastered previous developmental tasks, he/she is able to integrate the knowledge and abilities of many years of experience into a mature wisdom. Characteristics of managers at this stage include tendencies to reminisce and make comparisons with the past. Forgetfulness may develop, and tolerance for frustration or conflict is low because the energy to deal with the issues is no longer there. The mature manager has been through it all before and now feels entitled to reap some peace and respect. Many managers at this stage live richly in the present by teaching, guiding, and sharing the wisdom of their experiences with newer, younger supervisors. Managers, supervisors, and team leaders — anyone who achieves through the efforts of others — will progress through each of these developmental stages. Cooperate with these dynamic growth processes and you will find the world of supervision challenging and exciting, both professionally and personally.

Professional development

Because of the rapid technological, social, and scientific advances, new knowledge is constantly influencing the health care industry. As a result, health care workers have an obligation to continue learning. Two methods for doing this are networking and continuing education.

Networking. Welsh (1980) defines networking as "the process of developing and using your contacts for information, advice, and moral support as you pursue your career." Meeting and sharing with other CNAs, LPNs, or RNs (or anyone else that does the same kind of work you do) offers many opportunities. New knowledge is shared. The latest technical advances are discussed. Teamworking skills are improved, and exposure to people with power, direction, and influence is gained. Networking also builds morale through the support of others who have had similar experiences. Start your own networking by volunteering to serve on committees at work. Join your nurses' association or specialty organization. Be a competent employee. Seek out and learn from the best in your field.

Continuing education. Your responsibility for learning does not end with graduation from school. On the contrary, your 'reality education' is a recurring, dynamic process that begins the day you leave school and continues throughout your career. Foster your own professional growth by consciously seeking out new opportunities for learning. Attend the educational programs offered by your work organization. Subscribe to and faithfully read professional journals. Attend association and networking meetings. Enroll in workshops or courses at the local community college and keep up with international, national, and local current events. Become an informed citizen, community member, leader, and health care provider.

Continuing education is so important to nurses that many states now require a minimum number of continuing education hours (units) (CEUs) for licensure renewal. **It is your responsibility to continue learning.** Do not avoid it. Both knowledge and morale levels improve when the manager is up-to-date and alert to the latest developments.

Building Morale

In today's world, the success or failure of managers will depend, to a large extent, on their ability to motivate other people. Employees who are highly motivated are more productive, stimulated, and creative. Morale levels are high, and attitudes are positive. To achieve this quality work climate, follow the guidelines in the next section when dealing with staff members.

What managers must know

A specific knowledge base is needed for building employee morale. Before you (the supervisor) actually do anything, be prepared with a knowledge of the business, the employees, and the goals.

The business. Know your job. "Develop yourself so that you will be technically and professionally qualified and proficient in your work" (Van Fleet, 1970). Your employees will respond by becoming confident in your abilities, developing loyalty, and respecting your knowledge. Understand the capabilities and limitations of the organization and realistically focus on what can be accomplished. Knowing the business gains the respect of others and increases your effectiveness.

The employees. Know your employees, their abilities, limitations, and attitudes. When your staff members believe you are looking out for their welfare, they will back and support you through the roughest of times. Be able to call each person by name. Discover each worker's individual characteristics, skills, and abilities. Treat each person equally. Recognize and praise good work and be willing to pass along the credit but absorb the blame. Your staff members are important. It is their efforts that determine your success.

The goals. Communicate goals and expectations clearly. Make sure the tasks are understood. People are more motivated to achieve when they know exactly what is expected of them. Emphasizing results instead of methods empowers employees to use their own ingenuity. When goals and tasks are clearly communicated and understood by everyone, confusion decreases, morale improves, and the staff functions more effectively.

What managers must do

Now armed with a knowledge of your business, employees, and goals, begin to build a high level of morale, just like the mason constructing a building — brick by brick. Numerous managerial behaviors help to motivate employees, but for simplicity, they can be grouped into three broad categories: practice, communicate, and empower.

Practice. First, be honest with yourself. Identifying your own strengths and limitations encourages you to responsibly focus your growth. Practice motivating yourself as well as others. Remember: success breeds success.

Practice delegation. Work to develop a sense of responsibility and confidence in your staff members. "Show faith in your subordinates and you'll motivate them to accept greater responsibilities for you" (Van Fleet, 1970). Techniques for delegating are explained in Chapter 13.

Also, do not forget to practice stress-reduction techniques and encourage or teach others to do the same. Avoid the 'Superperson syndrome,' where you try to be all things to all people. To be the perfect mate, parent, family member, and employee is not only unrealistic, but it is also exhausting. It also is an express ticket to burnout.

Practice these steps to avoid the Superperson syndrome (LaBella, Leach, 1985):

Recognize, establish, and respect your limits. Be willing to make choices. Let some activities go before taking on others. Find the balance in life.

Clarify your values and priorities. Energy is drained by nondirected behavior. Decide on your long-range and short-range goals. Arrange them in order of importance, then decide how much time and energy should be devoted to each goal.

Gain the cooperation of others. "The cooperation of those people you live and work with can make all the difference in your ability to balance home, family, and career" (LaBella, Leach, 1985). Learn to motivate, delegate, and reward people for their efforts.

Commit to replenishing your energy. Give yourself permission to pay attention to yourself. Replenish physical energy by eating, exercising, and resting wisely. During stressful situations, take a minute to breathe slowly and deeply. It has a calming effect that decreases muscle and emotional tension. Last, practice relaxation techniques faithfully. The technique you choose is not as important as practicing it daily.

Practice is the tool for becoming effective, competent, and confident. Do not hesitate to try it. As your staff sees you develop through practice, they will become motivated to improve themselves.

Communicate. Perhaps one of the greatest morale builders is the ability to communicate clearly. **Always keep your staff informed,** especially if the subject will have an effect on them. Praise quality work. Encourage participation in solving problems. Keep communication channels open. Establish a feedback system. Give each employee feedback about performance and ask for the same. Praise the whole person but be careful to criticize only the behaviors. A well-informed staff is cooperative, effective, and loyal.

Empower. Supervisors who empower their workers encourage each person to control and direct his/her resources in order to succeed in the workplace. Empowering others is based on the values of individual worth and respect as well as the belief that everyone wants to be successful. A **win-win strategy is a core element of empowerment.** Managers who empower their staff provide them with information about what is to be done and how; resources needed to meet the goal; alternatives that can remove barriers or assist in reaching the goal; and opportunities for skill improvement through training, decision making, and participation. Empowerment also means respecting and encouraging employees, building an effective work team, and providing opportunities for success.

Building morale is not always an easy task, but try to stay positive and upbeat. With practice and experience, you will continue to grow, develop new abilities, and provide inspiration for others.

✑ Key Concepts

- Workers' morale level directly influences productivity.
- Motivation is an internal drive that stimulates a person to act.
- Organizational morale is the attitude employees have toward the quality of their total work life.
- Five general principles of motivation relate to the uniqueness of the individual, his/her needs, the group, the dynamism of people, and the pleasure–pain principle.
- To assess the level of morale, consider the employee's perceptions, what factors affect morale, and which signs of low morale and burnout are present in the work setting.
- Burnout is a state of exhaustion resulting from prolonged stress and unrealistic expectations.
- Age affects morale. There are several differences to consider when motivating the younger or older worker.
- The orientation process for the new employee establishes the foundation for his/her relationship with the organization.
- New employees should be introduced to the company's structure, philosophy, work settings, and job descriptions.
- A skills demonstration allows the supervisor to accurately evaluate the new employee's abilities and develop appropriate, individualized training plans.
- To make the transition to manager, get to know your staff, build good working relationships, treat everyone fairly, make changes very slowly, and be patient.
- Managers and supervisors adapt to management roles by mastering critical tasks during each stage of role development.
- Professional development is an obligation to continue learning. Networking and continuing education activities are two methods for fostering professional growth.
- Before beginning to build morale, the supervisor must have a thorough knowledge of the business, the employees, and the goals.
- Motivating others requires the manager to practice, communicate, and empower staff members.
- To avoid the Superperson syndrome, the supervisor must learn to define values, goals, priorities, and limits; gain cooperation; and commit to replenishing his/her energies regularly.
- Managers who empower staff members provide them with information, resources, alternatives, and opportunities.

✑ Learning Activities

1. Discuss your reasons for agreeing or disagreeing with the following statement: Without motivation there would be no morale.

2. Explain how each of the five principles of motivation would apply to your job (as a health care worker or student).
3. Develop a checklist for assessing morale at home, work, or school.
4. Devise a plan for orienting a new student or worker to your environment.
5. Attend one professional meeting (ANA, NLN, state nurses' association) or continuing education class, program, or workshop. Discuss your experiences and impressions.

References

Austin NK: When you're the new boss, *Working Woman* 17(3):42, 1992.

Chapman EN: *Supervisor's survival kit: a mid-management primer,* ed 2, Chicago, 1975, Science Research Associates.

Clark CC: Burnout: assessment and intervention, *Journal of Nursing Administration* 10(9):39, 1980.

Etheredge ML: Nurse–manager . . . try that title on for size, *Nursing 85* 15(8):26, 1985.

George RT: First impressions: how they affect long-term performance, *Supervisory Management* 31(3):2, 1986.

Khalsa RK: *Healing the healer: a holistic/transpersonal perspective,* Los Angeles, 1978, Center for Health and Healing.

LaBella A, Leach D: *Personal power: the guide to power for today's working woman,* Boulder, Colo, 1985, Career Track.

Pines A, Maslach C: Characteristics of staff burnout in mental health settings, *Hospital and Community Psychiatry* 29(3):233, 1978.

Straub JT, Attner RF: *Introduction to business,* ed 4, Boston, 1991, PWS-Kent.

Van Fleet JK: *How to use the dynamics of motivation,* West Nyack, NY, 1970, Parker.

Vestal KW: *Management concepts for the new nurse,* Philadelphia, 1987, Lippincott.

Welsh MS: *Networking,* New York, 1980, Harcourt Brace Jovanovich.

Yee BH: The dynamics and management of burnout, *Nursing Administration* 12(11):14, 1981.

Zetlin M: How to help new managers succeed, *Executive Female* 10:9, 1992.

Additional Readings

Bauman A: Good beginnings, *Entrepreneur* 19(10):149, 1991. *A well-thought-out orientation gets employees off to a great start and paves the way for a good working relationship.*

Block P: *The empowered manager,* San Francisco, 1987, Jossey-Bass. *"This book presents a path to the empowerment of each employee."*

Heine CA: Burnout among nursing home personnel, *Journal of Gerontological Nursing* 12(3):14, 1986. *Ms. Heine discusses strategies to treat and prevent burnout for caregivers who work with dependent, confused elderly.*

Hoerr J: The payoff from teamwork, *Business Week* July 10:56, 1989. *When jobs are challenging, workers are committed and perform superbly. The quality gains from teamwork are substantial.*

Jernigan DK, Young AP: *Standards, job descriptions, and performance evaluations for nursing practice,* Norwalk, Conn, 1983, Appleton-Century-Crofts. *The authors thoroughly describe the purpose, structure, and function of job descriptions, performance evaluations, and standards of care. Excellent examples and usable tools are also provided.*

Leebov W: *Positive co-worker relationships in health care,* Chicago, 1990, American Hospital Publishing. *Taking an active role in promoting a productive working environment will enhance personal growth and help you better understand your place in a smooth-running organization.*

Ludeman K: *The worth ethic: how to profit from the changing values of the new work force,* New York, 1989, EP Dutton. *Inspiring high integrity and sharing power with employees gets the job done better.*

Manthey M: Committing to your co-workers, *Nursing 91* 21(7):85, 1991. *To build strong, supportive work relationships, review this list of commitments.*

McCaffrey C: Performance checklists: an effective method of teaching, learning, and evaluating, *Nurse Educator* 3:11, 1978. *The performance check list is a tool, based on accepted standard procedures, that lists each behavior required to successfully perform a given skill.*

Porter-O'Grady T: What motivation isn't, *Nursing Management* 13(12):27, 1982. *The author offers a convincing argument for changing organizations to provide an environment for truly professional, humane practice.*

Silber MB: The motivation pyramid in nurse retention, *Journal of Nursing Leadership and Management* 12(4):45, 1981. *The costly incidence of "on-the-job retirement" in health care facilities can be alleviated in part by an understanding of the motivation that comes from within the facility's employee.*

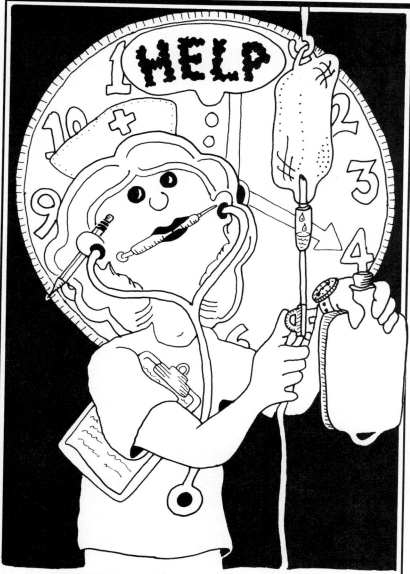

Upon completion of this chapter, the reader will be able to:

1. Describe the management process of directing.
2. List the basic reason for maintaining discipline.
3. Identify four responsibilities of managers when delegating.
4. Describe three principles of delegation relating to employees.
5. Explain the importance of job descriptions, policies, and procedures in planning for delegation.
6. Discuss four organizational barriers to effective delegation.
7. Describe three personal barriers to effective delegation.
8. Explain how group dynamics can influence the delegation process.
9. Relate how a supervisor's management style can affect the process of delegation.
10. List the six steps of the delegation process.
11. Explain the necessity of planning prior to delegating.
12. Identify four steps for assigning a delegated task.
13. Describe three minimum requirements for accepting a delegated responsibility.
14. State three characteristics of an effective delegatee.

Management Functions

The ability to competently delegate is an integral component of management and supervision. Delegation, however, is only one component of the broader management function known as controlling or directing.

Directing

Providing direction that efficiently moves the group toward goal attainment is a basic responsibility of the supervisor. Douglas (1992) describes direction as "the connecting link between organizing for work and getting the job done." Without direction, staff members tend to scatter their energies with each person, focusing on what they feel is most important. Team leaders, supervisors, managers, administrators, and even the owners must provide direction and focus for the organization.

Purpose. Providing effective direction results in goal attainment, efficient use of human and material resources, and the opportunity for staff members to contribute to the organization. Managers with competent directing skills inspire confidence and loyalty in their staff, as everyone knows where to focus their work energies. Morale levels improve when employees are efficiently directed and creativity is encouraged when supervisors and employees combine forces to solve problems that relate to goal attainment. **The art of directing individuals and focusing them on a common course of action is an essential ingredient** of effective management and supervision.

Process. Tasks associated with the directing process include:

- assigning, ordering, and instructing employees;
- solving problems, making decisions;
- productively managing conflict;
- planning delegated tasks, projects, etc.;
- teaching, counseling;
- monitoring progress; and
- evaluating performance and progress.

The manager's or supervisor's responsibility is to direct the resources and energies of the department toward meeting goals. Without this direction, the staff wanders though the work day, and the leader (no matter how hard he/she works) remains ineffective.

Work to develop and improve your directing skills. Remember your goals and focus staff energies to meet them. The goal, for example, may be to provide physical and psychological care for a certain group of clients. Ascertain what tasks must be done in order to provide the care (according to standards of nursing practice), then gather together the human and material resources available and focus or direct them to meeting the goal (good nursing care for a certain number of clients).

Discipline

Although *discipline* has become synonymous with *punishment*, the two are separate and disparate concepts. The concept of punishment is "based on the assumption that if the person who makes a mistake is made to feel enough pain, they will not make another" (Manthey, 1989). Unfortunately, our nursing heritage is rich in the tradition of punishment, and with the advent of the scientific method management theories, a 'zero tolerance' standard for mistakes developed. Today, we are beginning to recognize this as unrealistic because human beings are incapable of perfection. They will make mistakes, and no amount of intentionally caused pain (punishment) can prevent this from occurring.

Purpose. Discipline is the process of maintaining "a state of order based on submission to rules and authority" (Morris, 1976). The basic purpose of discipline is to maintain order within an organization. When work progresses in a smooth, orderly manner, employees perform more effectively, and morale is high. When a staff member becomes disruptive or impedes work progress, it is the supervisor's responsibility to take corrective action. These corrective actions are referred to as discipline.

Process. To use discipline effectively, the manager attempts to "reduce undesirable behavior by controlling the consequences of that behavior" (Matejka, Ashworth, Dodd-McCue, 1986). Two basic approaches can be adopted. First, the supervisor can impose the more traditional punitive method where the consequence of the employee's undesirable behavior is perceived as unpleasant. For example, Sally's paycheck is reduced by one hour's pay for every time she arrives late for work. Because Sally needs the money, she perceives the consequence of her tardiness as uncomfortable and begins to arrive on time. Punishing Sally changed her behavior and solved your problem, but it did absolutely nothing to solve Sally's problem (the reason for her chronic lateness). Also, Sally is now a less-than-happy employee because she is motivated by the desire to avoid discomfort (hygiene factors) rather than to achieve. The punitive approach may be effective in the short run, but it seldom has lasting effects.

The second approach attempts to "replace destructive behavior with productive, cooperative behavior" (Steines, 1982). In essence, the supervisor 'coaches' the staff member into recognizing the negative consequences of his/her current behaviors and then taking the responsibility for replacing them with more desirable, productive conduct.

Supervisors should respond to each situation early and thoroughly. This way, small discipline problems are prevented from enlarging (see box on p. 323).

As a last resort, the employee is terminated — not as a punishment, but because after all the corrective efforts, it becomes obvious that the employee and the organization do not mesh.

Discipline is a necessary component of the directing process; punishment is not. When *consistently* and fairly applied, discipline becomes a useful tool for ensuring order and productivity.

Delegating

Delegation is the process of "assigning job activities and corresponding authority to specific individuals within the organization" (Certo, 1989). It is a method for channeling work activities toward goals. As a tool, delegation proves itself to be very useful. As a process, delegation helps to develop both manager and employee abilities.

Purpose. If managers or supervisors are to effectively function, they must delegate. The purpose of a manager is to achieve results through the efforts of others. Delegation is one of the tools that helps to achieve those results. Managers plan, organize, coordinate, and direct through the use

---

❧ HOW TO DISCIPLINE EFFECTIVELY

1. Define the undesirable behavior and list its effects on the working environment.
2. Define the more appropriate, corrective behavior.
3. Determine the consequences of both the corrective and undesired behavior.
4. Confer with the employee. Define the problem (the undesirable behavior) and attempt to determine its cause. Mutually solve the problem with the employee if at all possible. Discuss your expectations and ways to eliminate the problem. Develop an action plan with each person's responsibilities clearly stated and write it down.
5. If no improvement is noticed, progress to the oral warning. Remind the employee of the action plan and document the discussion. "The key question that the employee must answer is whether or not he is prepared and able to abide by the rules in the future" (Steines, 1982).
6. The next step is the written warning. The problem is again discussed with the employee, only this time a description of the situation is placed in the employee's personnel file. Many managers then send the employee home to consider the situation. Sending the employee home enforces the seriousness of the situation and prevents an angry, hostile worker from disrupting the work environment. In any case, "The employee is apprised of the fact that another incident will require termination of the employee–employer relationship" (Steines, 1982).

---

of delegation. They also evaluate team members' abilities and performance by delegating both tasks and authority. Delegating well-defined tasks or projects also allows the supervisor more time for other management activities.

Process. For the most part, delegation involves three main steps: assign duties, grant authority, and create an obligation (Newman, Warren, 1977). The process is simple, but the dynamics can become perplexing.

Principles of Delegation

Delegation is essentially a contract between the delegator (the manager, supervisor, or team leader) and the delegatee (employee, team member, or worker). Upon entering into this contract, each person assumes certain responsibilities and roles. The concepts of authority, responsibility, and accountability must be mutually defined and agreed upon. Role requirements and tasks must be clearly communicated, understood, and accepted. Fortunately, several principles can serve as guidelines for practicing effective delegation.

The delegator

Supervisors must delegate if they are to accomplish goals. Many, however, overdelegate and cannot control the results, or underdelegate and lapse into exhaustion from trying to do it all themselves. The balance must be found if the supervisor is to be effective. Examining the responsibilities and tasks of the delegators and applying these principles is one way of finding the balance between too much and not enough.

Responsibilities. To delegate well, managers must remember a few basic principles:

Delegate the activities you know best. If you know how it should be done, then you are in a better position to assign, monitor, and evaluate the activity.

Clearly assign duties. Once the duty, activity, or project has been assigned and accepted, the manager must be willing to trust in the worker's abilities and commitment. Along with each duty comes the responsibility to carry it out. A watchful eye from the manager (monitoring) should be carried out, but interference with the worker's area of responsibility needs to be avoided.

Delegate the authority; retain the responsibility. The nurse manager retains the overall responsibility for the final outcome of the delegated activity. The employee to whom the activity was delegated assumes the authority for completing the assigned duties.

Managers who delegate frequently challenge their staff members, encourage creativity, and provide opportunities for growth.

Delegate when you need time for work only you can do; want to involve employees; and are willing to spend the time and effort to skillfully plan, monitor, and evaluate the delegation process.

The organization's policies, procedures, and job descriptions provide the manager with guidelines for delegating.

Always match the assignment with the employee's abilities. Know your staff members' abilities, skill levels, and needs for improvement. Writing client care plans, for example, is never delegated to a nursing assistant because the assignment is out of the realm of the assistant's abilities. Be careful here. Follow legal and ethical standards. Use job descriptions as guidelines when determining what to delegate. Also, remember to delegate those assignments that result in success, for every employee needs to feel capable.

Tasks. When acting as a delegator, the supervisor must be willing to do the following (McConkey, 1974):

> Exercise control broadly. This means maintaining control without stifling the employee. Trust becomes an issue here, and many problems often originate with the manager's reluctance to supervise only the big picture and trust those people to whom the assignments were delegated. Avoid overcontrol. It stifles initiative, creativity, and morale.
>
> "Let others make the mistakes. Continual checking to eliminate all mistakes will make true delegation impossible." Besides, employees need the opportunity to grow by learning from their errors. Make sure to intercede before critical mistakes are made but, otherwise, monitor the situation quietly from the sidelines.
>
> Allow the delegate to exercise the authority to accomplish the task. Concentrate on the crucial tasks that you, as supervisor, must do. Delegate the other tasks (even if you can accomplish them better) and allow the delegatee to achieve the goals as he/she determines.
>
> Establish and agree upon the results and the standards of performance for the delegated duties. You cannot arrive at the same place if you do not know where you are going or how you are going to get there.
>
> Encourage ideas. Give staff members the opportunity to share and discuss their ideas.

These five basic tasks serve as guidelines for effective delegating. Remember them when planning delegated activities, and they will serve you well.

The delegatee

The contract between manager and employee for delegated responsibilities does not stop with the manager's role. If the delegation process is to be successful, the delegatee must play an active part in fulfilling the delegation contract. There must be a meeting of the minds as well as a mutual understanding and agreement relating to goals, tasks, and performance standards. Each person must play an active role in this dynamic process.

Responsibilities. In order to ensure the success of the delegated activity, the staff member to whom the responsibility was delegated (in short, the delegatee) must be willing to follow the duties outlined in the box on p. 326. During the delegative process, responsibilities become an important component of each person's role.

Tasks. The role of the delegatee carries with it several basic tasks. Effec-

---

✒ DELEGATEE'S DUTIES

1. **Accept the responsibility for the delegated activity.** When the delegatee agrees with the goals and accepts the responsibility, he/she must take the initiative to execute the assigned duties.
2. **Operate within the limits of authority granted.** Authority must be exercised to accomplish the goal, but the use of inappropriate or excessive authority stifles progress and embitters co-workers.
3. **Put forth a best effort.** If the delegatee reacts to the tasks in a halfhearted, unenthusiastic manner, it may be better to consider someone else. Success is much more likely when the delegatee is a willing and eager participant.
4. **Be accountable for the results.** Whether the outcome is negative or positive, the delegatee must be willing to share ownership for the delegated activity.

---

tive delegatees make sure each step is taken during the process of achieving results. According to McConkey (1974), the following steps should be taken:

Take the initiative. Assuming an active rather than passive role allows the delegatee to plan, organize, and coordinate the delegated activities. Rather than waiting for the supervisor to do it, the delegatee establishes his/her methods for meeting the goals.

Relate to the manager. Plans, problems, and progress must be shared with the delegator. Disagreements can be healthy and lead to better performance, but they must remain private. Loyalty to the boss must be demonstrated throughout the process, even when discord exists.

Accept delegation realistically. Many problems during the delegative process stem from overly optimistic delegatees who accept unrealistic delegations. Knowing one's capabilities helps here.

Set up a feedback system. Managers have a critical stake in feedback. They rely on accurate, succinct data in order to monitor, troubleshoot, and evaluate the process. They must be kept informed.

Carry out the task. Delegatees who develop and follow concrete, realistic plans successfully achieve their objectives. Devoting time and energy to performing the duties well results in success for the delegatee, manager, and the organization.

When both the supervisor and the delegatee understand and assume their roles and responsibilities, the delegative process becomes highly effective and enhances opportunities for development.

Barriers to Effective Delegation

The process of delegating is simple, but the dynamics that surround the delegation process are not. Although delegation is a major managerial function, many supervisors fail to do it skillfully. "The problem with delegating is that most supervisors know they *should* do it and most *think* they do it, but few really *do* it and those who do often go about it awkwardly" (Chapman, 1975). Managers, leaders, and supervisors, in order to become effective delegators, need to be aware of the obstacles to the delegation process and be able to function around them.

Barriers to delegation can be broadly categorized as organizational, employee-, and supervisor-related. Let us look at each in more detail.

Organizational obstacles

Certain characteristics of the organization itself may present difficulties relating to delegation. Barriers may be structural obstacles — that is, they are there because of the way the facility's organizational structure is arranged — or functional obstacles rooted in the methods used by the organization to carry out its business.

Structural barriers. Delegation obstacles are structural in nature when they are related to the organization itself. McConkey (1974) lists these hindrances as

> *A slippery organizational chart.* Organizational charts may reflect job titles and reporting channels, but they do not reflect the degree of delegation. Many managers feel that, by giving the delegatee an organizational chart and a lengthy job description, their job of delegation was complete. The delegatee knew what to do and to whom to report. These attitudes led to the belief that the more levels and spans of control, the greater the degree of delegation. This is not usually the case. Organizational charts describe what a company says it is. How it *really* functions is not seen in the chart.
>
> *A nondescript job description.* Job descriptions may be lengthy or short, broadly stated or highly detailed, but whatever the case, they serve as a main vehicle of delegation. A typical job description contains four sections. The first section describes the basic functions of the job. The second section explains the job's nature and scope. The third and fourth sections relate to responsibilities and the dimensions of the job. Study your staff's job descriptions. Analyze them in detail. Too often, vague or ambiguous job descriptions hinder effective delegations.

Functional barriers. The way or manner in which a company operates may pose obstacles to delegation. Some of the more common functional barriers are

> *Its history.* If the organization has historically delegated few activities and responsibilities, an attempt at delegation may make employees apprehensive and reluctant to cooperate, especially if earlier attempts resulted in failure.
>
> *Lack of authority.* Authority is the power to act. When delegates are given responsibility (to meet the goals) without the authority (to do the job), failure is eminent.
>
> *Job confusion.* If the delegatee or the supervisor has any question about the content of the delegated activity or area of responsibility, the outcome is likely to result in similar confusion.

Organizational barriers may be subtle and difficult to define, but a watchful eye and an awareness of how the organization actually functions can improve the odds for effective delegation.

Employee-related obstacles

Some barriers to the delegation process arise from the delegatee, especially those employees who are inexperienced or unsure of themselves. The most common problems with staff members relate to fear, uncertainty, and a hesitancy to take risks.

Fear. Staff members "may be reluctant to accept delegated authority for fear of failure or because of a lack of self-confidence" (Certo, 1989). Individuals may lack confidence in their leader and, as a result, be unwilling to risk the possibility of failure. When one is unwilling to accept delegation, he/she is safe and risks little.

Lack of guidance. When employees feel the delegated activity is 'dumped in their laps,' they are resistant because of lack of guidance. Part of the delegation contract includes the supervisor's responsibility to be supportive and available for guidance during the entire process. Managers who do not monitor progress and provide guidance have few eager delegatees.

Responsibility. Some employees avoid accepting any more responsibility than necessary. Much of the time, this is due to a lack of self-confidence or poor communication skills. Other causes can include a fear of complicating comfortable working relationships with co-workers, inadequate organizational skills, and a lack of interest in the job. These employees require special attention if they are to be included in the delegation process.

Supervisor-related obstacles

Although the ability to delegate remains one of the most important tools for the supervisor, many fail to delegate skillfully or frequently. Delegating seems to be difficult to put into practice for several reasons. For the sake of discussion, obstacles to the delegation process that relate to managers are categorized as self-, activity-, or group-related. Recognizing and correcting these problems goes a long way toward becoming an effective delegator.

Relating to self. Several roadblocks to delegation arise from within the supervisor. Manager-related obstacles can arise from the following:

Lack of knowledge. Managers who know little about the process of delegation cannot work effectively. An inadequate knowledge of the "staff capabilities and talents results in ineffective delegation" (Brown, 1986).

Inadequate organizational skills. Planning delegation takes time. Supervisors need the organizing abilities to balance work loads with the uncertainty associated with delegated tasks in order to meet goals. Refusing to delegate a responsibility today does not save time for tomorrow. Time expenditures can be more wisely spent when the supervisor is organized and prepared for delegating duties.

Insecurity. Some supervisors resist delegating because they enjoy their authority and feel insecure when they relinquish even a small amount. Others feel insecure about the members of the work team, which leads to a lack of faith in the employees. Insecurities also stem from anxieties related to loss of control, apprehension about how well or poorly the job will be done, and a reluctance to take risks.

Fear. Anxieties about delegation can stem from many sources, the chief one being a fear of failure. Fear of criticism from superiors or peers can impede delegation. Managers and supervisors also "recognize that they are ultimately responsible for the activities of their subordinates and are often unwilling to allow others to make mistakes. They feel the risk factors outweigh the rewards" (Brown, 1986).

Desire for personal recognition. When a supervisor's ego needs overshadow departmental productivity, little control is relinquished. Doing (and receiving credit for) the most important work becomes more important than motivating employees through the use of delegation.

Inadequate or insufficient role models. If no one in the company practices delegating, it will be difficult for a single supervisor to do so. When the role models who do practice delegation lack the knowledge or skill to be effective, poor examples are set. Managers observing the process may become hesitant to try themselves when the outcomes are less than positive.

✍️ TASK OBSTACLES

1. A belief that the task, activity, or project may be too difficult to delegate.
2. A belief that the performance of the activity requires a specific person if it is to be successful.
3. A belief that too much time is required to plan, delegate, and monitor.
4. A belief that the possibility of legal ramifications exists.

From Bernhard LA, Walsh M: *Leadership: the key to professionalization of nursing,* ed 2, St Louis, 1990, Mosby.

Relating to the activity. How the manager views an activity or task affects the decision to delegate. See the box above for a list of obstacles relating to the task. The manager's particular like or distaste of the activity can influence the delegation process.

Relating to the group. Feelings and attitudes that the leader may have about delegation and the work group relate to:

- A lack of trust in group's experience, willingness to communicate, and ability to do the job.
- A hesitancy in adding another task to an already overworked staff.
- An insecurity that the group may become too good and demand more money or (worse yet) want to compete for the supervisor's job.

Managers may also find the cause of failed delegations within the work group's dynamics. The two primary reasons that groups resist delegative authority are a lack of confidence and a fear of failure.

Learning to recognize the barriers, obstacles, and hindrances to effective delegation is the first step for empowering employees toward higher levels of productivity and morale.

To Delegate Effectively

The ability to effectively delegate is an acquired skill. As a result of numerous management studies, steps for understanding and using the process of delegation have been developed. However, **the first focus of a good delegator is to build a strong foundation with employees.** The success of all future delegating activities rests upon the strength of this foundation.

Build a foundation

Delegation does not take place in a vacuum. The environment within which delegation takes place is as important as the actual delegation. The effectiveness of any delegated activity is strongly affected by the company's atmosphere and management style. These two factors comprise the foundation for the delegating process.

Management style. Each particular management style rests upon a specific foundation. Autocratic management styles, for example, have a foundation or support system that differs greatly from more participatory styles. Organizational charts, policies, procedures, and the degree of decentralization all support the company's style of management (see Chapter 8).

Differences in management styles can also be seen in supervisors. The autocratic type emphasizes control while the more participatory manager focuses on the importance of motivating workers. As you may imagine, autocratic managers tend to delegate less and concentrate more on actual performance than the level of contributions made to the organization. Participatory supervisors delegate easily because they view control as secondary to employee development. Their staff members enjoy greater job satisfaction and perform more competently than autocratically managed employees.

Management atmosphere. A certain atmosphere, or management environment, is necessary for a solid delegation foundation. Managers and supervisors themselves must be motivated to share in the delegative process. How the upper-level management views change, attacking sacred cows (unrealistic practices, policies, customs, and mandates), making mistakes, recognition, rewards, and work performance affects the success of the delegation process. Achievement-oriented management atmospheres encourage cooperative goal setting, self-improvement, and recognition of achievements. Discussing ideas, emphasizing task completion instead of fear of failure, and believing in the worth of each employee all create a higher probability of success for the supervisor, the employee, and the organization.

Observe and assess your facility's management style and atmosphere. Then use that knowledge as your framework for mastering the skill of delegation.

How to delegate

Delegation is a contract that involves an agreement, transfer of power, accountability, and an obligation. Supervisors who delegate well have a knowledge of the process, the activity, and the employees. They communicate clearly, play a supportive role, appreciate differences, and focus on success. Delegating skillfully is a learned process that requires **prepa-**

ration, practice, and patience; but by following the six-step process in the next section, you will greatly improve your skills.

1. Prepare. Understand the delegation process. If you know *how*, then doing becomes easier. Assess your strengths, limitations, and feelings about power, leadership, authority, and delegating; then do the same for each staff member. Work to understand the work group's readiness or willingness to assume responsibility for the delegated task. Read, understand, and consult the job descriptions and standards of performance before delegating. You must be aware of each team member's practice limitations (e.g., CNAs do not give IM medications) and job requirements in order to delegate appropriate activities. Last, plan the delegated task or activity, the standards for its achievement, required monitoring activities, and resources needed. Planning and preparing for delegation is a very important, but often ignored, first step.

2. Select the task. Choose delegated activities carefully. "Analyze *your* [emphasis added] job and identify tasks that you can delegate" (Brown, 1986). Activities that can be delegated should meet these criteria:

They take too much of the supervisor's time.
They are low in responsibility when compared with other duties.
They should provide some feelings of satisfaction or success for the delegatee.

For each activity or task to be delegated, clearly define its elements. "Without a clear understanding of what you want done and why, you cannot possibly communicate effectively with someone else" (Volante, 1974). Know the delegated activity. Write down the key factors describing the task. A clearly defined activity (task, project) stands a much greater chance for success.

3. Select the person. One of the keys to competent delegating is the selection of the right person for the job. To figure out who is best suited for the task, consider the employee's current work load, need for challenge, enthusiasm, skills, abilities, and willingness to assume more responsibility. How the delegated activity fits with the staff member's job description, as well as the facility's policies and procedures, is important in defining limits and responsibilities. Staff members to whom tasks are delegated "should be selected carefully, given accountability and authority, and then provided with the opportunity to develop to carry out his [her] delegation" (McConkey, 1974).

4. Communicate. Prepare your staff for a change. Sudden, unannounced changes disturb both people and productivity. Protect the delegatee and his/her co-workers by ensuring that everyone is informed of the decision, misunderstandings are cleared up, and opportunities for questions are provided.

When actually assigning a delegated task to an individual staff member, keep these points in mind:

Arrange for sufficient time and privacy.

Communicate the task (job, activity, etc.) *step by step.* Communicate clearly, completely, and competently by sharing exactly what is to be done, the reasons for doing the task, its purpose, and expected performance standards and outcomes.

Elicit feedback. Ask for and take time to answer any questions. Explore for any misunderstandings. Determine if specific instructions on how to do the task are necessary. Then have the employee paraphrase or repeat the basic points.

Establish the contract. Spell out the goal, resources available, evaluation criteria, and areas of responsibility. Each person then obligates himself/herself to fulfill the terms of the agreement. Delegation contracts are seldom written. Their real purpose lies in defining and clarifying the terms (parameters) of the delegated activity and responsibility.

Once the agreement is in place, be available for support and guidance. This becomes especially important with inexperienced delegatees.

5. Assign and monitor. This step involves making assignments that relate to the delegatee's area of authority and monitoring tools. First, each staff member who has been delegated a responsibility must be assigned authority that is appropriate to the activity. Without this authority, the staff member will be unable to meet the goal of the delegated activity.

Second, assigning 'checkpoints' during the process allows progress to be judged and provides both parties with feedback. **Periodically monitoring what is happening demonstrates interest** and allows the supervisor to remain responsible for the delegated work.

6. Evaluate. The last, but an important, step to effective delegation is to **evaluate the results.** Evaluation becomes a simple step if the progress monitoring was done. To use the evaluation process as a learning experience, follow the steps in the box on p. 334.

When all these steps have been done, celebrate. Reward the delegatee or group for successfully assuming the responsibility. Celebrate the accomplishments. Even a simple thanks can provide the motivation to accept future delegations.

Delegating is a critical skill for leaders and supervisors everywhere. It is a skill that you cannot afford to be without. Practice each step of the

---

EVALUATION PROCESS

1. Compare actual outcomes with the goal. Did we meet the goal?
2. Analyze areas of failure and success. Identify potential problems for future delegations. Remember to keep your expectations consistent with the goal.
3. Review the process (what happened) with the delegatee and then with the work group.
4. Give praise and recognition for accomplishments.
5. Provide opportunities for instruction or problem solving for failures.

---

delegating process. "If you learn to delegate frequently and skillfully, you'll eventually worry less, feel less pressured, have more time to plan and organize, build better relationships with your employees, and motivate greater productivity in your department" (Chapman, 1975).

To Accept Delegation

It is just as important to the overall success of the organization to be an effective delegatee. Many times supervisors and managers are the recipients of delegated activities. Before accepting a delegated responsibility, however, **each must agree upon the parameters and limitations of the process.**

Information requirements

To competently fill the role of delegatee, certain information is needed. The agreement or 'contract' between the delegator (e.g., your manager) and the delegatee (in this case, you) must address three basic issues: the responsibility (task, activity, project), the time frame, and the outcome. Without this essential information, the delegation process is apt to be ineffective from the start.

The responsibility. In order to execute the duties assigned and define the scope of authority for the delegation, **the delegatee must have a clear definition of the task.** First, thoroughly understand the goal from the delegator's point of view. Paraphrase or repeat your understanding of the goal. Next, focus on the tasks necessary to achieve the goal. Agree upon their order of priority. Actively listen and communicate. Be sure you clearly understand the goal, the tasks, and the priorities.

Last, discuss the type and amount of authority that is being granted. For example, do you have the authority to order supplies or materials; to schedule, assign, or discipline staff members? Take time to clarify the limits of the delegated authority. Take notes if necessary, but clearly understand the authority associated with the responsibility.

The parameters. The goals, tasks, priorities, and amount of authority have all been determined. Now pay attention to the setting (context) in which the delegated activity will take place. Consider such factors as available resources (human and material), impact on staff members or clients, time frames for completion or progress checks, possible problems, and what coordination efforts with other departments may be needed.

The outcome. The feedback system for communications and monitoring progress must be clearly established prior to beginning the process. Because the delegator retains the ultimate responsibility, he/she must be kept informed of the progress, actual or potential problems, and how the delegation may be affecting staff members. Communicating frequently encourages early problem resolution, and monitoring progress allows both parties to measure each step toward goal achievement.

The effective delegatee

Once a meeting of the minds has taken place, the employee to whom the task was delegated now becomes responsible for competently executing the assigned duties. To do a first-rate job, keep in mind the following three simple, but succinct, points.

Take the initiative. If your manager trusts your judgment and abilities enough to delegate a responsibility to you, trust yourself enough to be proactive rather than passive. Determine what you are accountable for, then seize the opportunity to make things happen. Use your management skills to plan, organize, and create a successful outcome.

Communicate. Relate to the boss and your co-workers. Share your plans. Ask for ideas. Elicit cooperation and motivate others to meet the goals. Keep people informed of the progress. Good communications foster success and prevent misunderstandings.

Develop. The delegative process is an opportunity to learn and improve. Most of the best delegators started as delegatees who were willing to accept the "responsibility for developing [themselves] in whatever manner the delegation requires or provides" (McConkey, 1974). Your supervisor may provide the opportunity, but you must do the work of developing. Encourage yourself and provide opportunities for others. Recognize and praise the efforts of staff members to improve their skills and abilities.

Develop, foster, and nurture attitudes that breed success. Use the delegative process to grow.

The art of giving and receiving delegated responsibilities is an essential component of the management process. Effective use of delegation can foster teamwork, trust, and confidence and go a long way toward meeting the recognition and self-actualization needs that are present in all of us.

☙ Key Concepts

- Delegation is one component of the broader management function known as directing.
- Managers provide direction in order to achieve goals, use resources efficiently, and provide employees with opportunities for growth.
- Discipline is the process of maintaining order based on compliance with the organization's rules and authority.
- The positive approach to discipline involves working with the staff member to replace undesirable behaviors with more productive ones.
- Delegation is the process of assigning specific responsibilities, activities, and authority to a certain individual within the facility.
- If they are to function effectively, supervisors (leaders) must learn to delegate skillfully.
- The process of delegation consists of assigning responsibilities, granting authority, and creating an obligation.
- Delegation is a contract or agreement between supervisor and employee. Both must understand their roles and responsibilities.
- Supervisors must be willing to give up authority and let others make the mistakes while still retaining the ultimate responsibility for the delegation.
- Delegatees must be willing to assume responsibility, exercise limited authority, be accountable, and put forth a best effort.
- Organizational obstacles to quality delegation include inadequate organizational charts and job descriptions, job confusion, lack of authority, and the historical behavior of the management.
- Employee-related barriers to delegation stem from fear, lack of guidance, or an unwillingness to assume new responsibilities.
- Delegation obstacles relating to supervisors may arise from a lack of knowledge, organizational skills, insecurity, fear or anxiety, a desire for personal recognition, opinions about the activity or task, or attitudes relating to the work group.
- Effective delegation requires a solid foundation built on the company's atmosphere and management style.
- The process of delegation consists of six steps: preparation, task selection, delegatee selection, communication, assignments and monitoring tools, and evaluation.
- The planning step is critical for success of the delegation.
- Delegated tasks should meet specific criteria and be commensurate with the delegatee's abilities.
- Communications need to be clear and understood when determining activities, responsibilities, and other parameters of the delegation agreement.
- Monitoring activities show progress toward goal attainment, provide feedback, and allow for ease of evaluation.

- Evaluating the delegating process exposes its successes and allows the supervisor to engage in corrective planning for its failures.
- To accept delegation effectively certain information relating to the responsibility (delegated activity), the parameters, and the outcome (goals) of the delegation is necessary.
- Once the delegation contract is agreed upon, the effective delegatee takes the initiative for bringing about a successful outcome, communicates frequently to all involved staff, and works to develop himself/ herself as well as others.

✍ Learning Activities

1. You are the team leader for Wing A at XYZ long-term care facility. For several weeks, Mary Smith, a nursing assistant on your staff, has returned from lunch 10 minutes late. Several other nursing assistants are beginning to complain, and yesterday you overheard a CNA wondering how she could get away with it. Describe how you would handle this situation and what (if anything) could be delegated.

2. Locate job descriptions for a Certified Nursing Assistant and a Licensed Practical Nurse. Using the job descriptions as a guide, make a list of the tasks that could appropriately be delegated to each job level. What activities could be delegated to the LPN that could not be delegated to the CNA?

3. Compare the organizational obstacles to effective delegation. Describe how the authoritarian and participatory approaches to management would attempt to overcome these obstacles.

4. You are the supervisor of a 25-patient, long-term care unit. The director of nurses and the quality assurance committee has decided to assess each client's intake and output for 24 hours. You have been assigned the task of measuring I&O for each client on your unit. Fortunately, your senior aide is intelligent and cooperative. Since you are already incredibly busy and this must be accomplished within the next 30 days, you decide to delegate the task to your senior aide. Using the guidelines given in this chapter, develop a detailed plan for effectively delegating this task. Include monitoring and evaluating activities.

5. You are now the senior aide to whom the task described in activity #4 is being delegated. What information must you have before accepting the delegated task? Devise a plan to meet the goal (accurate I&O measurements for a 24-hour period for 25 clients within a 30-day time frame).

References

Bernhard LA, Walsh M: *Leadership: the key to professionalization of nursing*, ed 2, St Louis, 1990, Mosby.

Brown ST: Don't hesitate to delegate, *Nursing Success Today* 2(12):27, 1986.

Certo SC: *Principles of modern management: functions and systems*, ed 4, Needham Heights, Mass, 1989, Allyn & Bacon.

Chapman EN: *Supervisor's survival kit: a mid-management primer*, ed 2, Chicago, 1975, Science Research Associates.

Douglas LM: *The effective nurse leader and manager*, ed 4, St Louis, 1992, Mosby.

McConkey D: *No-nonsense delegation*, New York, 1974, AMACOM.

Manthey M: Discipline without punishment, *Nursing Management* 20(10);19, 1989.

Matejka JK, Ashworth DN, Dodd-McCue D: Discipline with guilt, *Supervisory Management* 31(5):34, 1986.

Morris W, editor: *The American heritage dictionary*, Boston, 1976, Houghton Mifflin.

Newman WH, Warren EK: *The process of management: concepts, behavior, and practice*, ed 4, Englewood Cliffs, NJ, 1977, Prentice-Hall.

Steines PA: Employee discipline: be positive not punitive, *Nursing Management* 13(3):29, 1982.

Volante EM: Mastering the managerial skill of delegation, *Journal of Nursing Administration* 4(1):20, 1974.

Additional Readings

Hansten RI: Delegation: learning when and how to let go, *Nursing 91* 21(4):126, 1991. *Whether you are a manager or not, you will be a more effective nurse if you learn to delegate.*

Hansten R, Washburn M: Delegation: how to deliver care through others, *American Journal of Nursing* 92(3):37, 1992. *Many nurses are reluctant to let go of traditional tasks and delegate to others. Are you one of those?*

Hansten R, Washburn M: How to plan what to delegate, *American Journal of Nursing* 92(4):71, 1992. *The "Four Rights" of delegation (the right task, person, communication, and feedback) are used to simplify the complex task of delegation.*

Hansten R, Washburn M: What do you say when you delegate work to others, *American Journal of Nursing* 92(7):48, 1992. *The 'right communication' when delegating involves the skill of effectively giving and receiving directions.*

Hansten R, Washburn M: What's your feedback style?, *American Journal of Nursing* 92(8):56, 1992. *The 'right feedback,' which involves evaluation and sharing, completes the loop of the delegation process.*

Jernigan DK, Young AP: *Standards, job descriptions, and performance evaluations for nursing practice*, Norwalk, Conn, 1983, Appleton-Century-Crofts. *An excellent source of information for generic job descriptions, performance standards, and evaluation tools for all levels of nursing from CNA to shift supervisor. (This is a great resource for Learning Activity #2).*

Jung FD: Teaching registered nurses how to supervise nursing assistants, *Journal of Nursing Administration* 21(4):32, 1991. *The author describes a program to improve nursing assistant supervision and discusses how the program has led to improved distribution of work loads and increased nursing assistant productivity.*

McConnell EA: What kind of a delegator are you? *Nursing 78* 8(10):105, 1978. *The author offers a humorous look at several types of delegators, from Autocratic Annie to Vague Vera.*

Manthey M: Trust: essential for delegation, *Nursing Management* 21(11):28, 1990. *The trust upon which the partnership system is based, is a necessary prerequisite to delegation.*

Mason JG: *How to build your management skills*, New York, 1965, McGraw-Hill. *Chapter 11, "Build Your Delegating Skills," suggests several ways to become adept at the art of delegation.*

Wilmoth EE: The art of delegation, *Nursing Management* 22(9):67, 1991. *Practicing four easy steps (communicate, appreciate, advocate, and participate) can introduce the art of delegation into any nursing unit's management.*

TECHNIQUES FOR 14

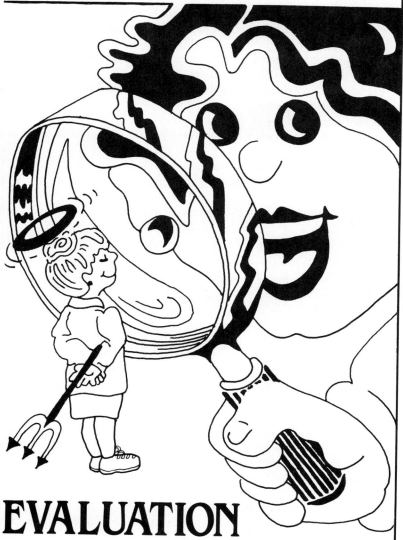

EVALUATION

Upon completion of this chapter, the reader will be able to:

1. Define *evaluation*.
2. Describe two types of evaluations.
3. Explain three applications of the evaluation process in health care settings.
4. List five reasons for using the evaluation process.
5. Discuss how the 'halo effect' or 'horns effect' could influence the evaluation process.
6. Differentiate between contrast errors and conflict errors.
7. Identify four data-collection tools.
8. Explain the importance of establishing criteria during the first step of the evaluation process.
9. Describe three types of criteria.
10. List three possible judgments or outcomes that result from the evaluation process.
11. Explain the purpose for performance evaluations.
12. List six topics to be addressed during the supervisor–employee conference.
13. Discuss how a supervisor's objectivity may influence the evaluation process.
14. Identify three guidelines for giving feedback effectively.

Management Functions

The management process is incomplete without the last step—**evaluation.** In fact, the last step of the scientific process, the nursing process, and the developmental process all include the step of evaluation. Even the child learning new skills unconsciously evaluates the outcome of his/her actions. Every parent knows that when a behavior is rewarded the child is likely to repeat it. The child has discovered that a certain behavior is effective in getting what he/she wants. In essence, the child has made an evaluation that "this behavior works or does not work." The evaluation then becomes a part of the child's knowledge base for use in coping with future situations.

Evaluations are an important part of everyday life. In business, health care, and most work environments, the process of evaluation is an integral component of the organization.

Evaluation

Supervisors use evaluation daily. If a staff member calls in sick, for example, the supervisor must evaluate the work situation and make decisions based on the results of that evaluation. Caregivers continuously evaluate their patients and their work surroundings. A manager, supervisor, or team leader with good evaluation skills also is better able to effectively carry out the other four management functions (plan, organize, coordinate, and direct).

Definition. *Evaluation* is derived from the Latin term that means "to value." **Evaluation involves a judgment or placing a value on something.** It is, then, a process for judging the value of an action. Managers need to know if the actions of their staff members resulted in success. To do this, they must evaluate and make judgments.

Types. Basically, the evaluation process is one of two types—informal or formal. The **informal evaluation** process is also called the formative evaluation. These are the types of evaluations done continuously throughout the day. They are the ongoing evaluations that help guide the leader to modify, refine, or improve the current situation. Informal evaluations focus on the "What needs to be done now?" question. They become very useful for guiding the manager effectively through the day.

The **formal evaluation** is also referred to as the summative evaluation process. As the name implies, these evaluations are more structured and formalized. They usually consist of a written summary covering a specific time interval, or they may occur at the end of a project. Their purpose is to summarize events and provide a method for determining the effectiveness of each action taken.

Both formal and informal evaluations are important tools for the nurse supervisor if he/she is to keep a 'finger on the department's pulse.'

Applications

Within the health care environment, formal evaluations are applied in many areas. Because our 'product' or 'commodity' relates to the well-being of people, it is extremely important for health care workers to use the evaluation process. Formal evaluations are tools that can be employed in many settings. Four of these applications are of prime importance for the nurse supervisor/manager—performance appraisals, quality assurance, utilization review, and risk management.

Performance appraisals. Formal evaluations of an employee's behaviors are often the responsibility of the immediate supervisor. Also known as work or performance evaluations, these reviews allow both the staff member and the supervisor an opportunity to discuss behaviors and set goals. The process of how to do a performance appraisal is detailed later in this chapter.

Quality assurance. In recent years, programs have been designed with the specific goal of monitoring and evaluating the level or quality of care provided to clients. Hospitals, extended care facilities, and numerous other health care agencies are required to "demonstrate a consistent endeavor to deliver patient care that is optimal within available resources and consistent with achievable goals" (Joint Commission on Accreditation of Healthcare Organizations [JCAHO], 1983). To simplify, health care organizations are now accountable for delivering the best care possible. Quality assurance (QA) programs for nursing were developed to monitor and evaluate "the quality and appropriateness of patient care provided by the nursing service" (JCAHO, 1983).

The goal of any QA program is to evaluate. These evaluation processes are ongoing, systematic, and comprehensive. QA committees are usually permanent (standing) committees involved in the long-term process of improving patient care. Their task is to compare specific aspects of patient care to established standards and introduce changes that result in improvement.

QA programs make use of several tools and monitoring activities in order to gather data. See the box below for a list of data-collection techniques.

The process of ensuring quality consists of eight steps. With each aspect of client care the quality assurance committee follows each step of the

---

⤞ METHODS OF DATA COLLECTION

- Incident reports
- Nursing audits
- Peer reviews
- Client satisfaction surveys and questionnaires
- Infection control reports
- Organizational statistics
- Utilization review reports
- 'Quality indicators' (measurements) devised by the QA committee itself

From Long BC, Phipps WJ: *Medical–surgical nursing: a nursing process approach*, ed 2, St Louis, 1989, Mosby.

QUALITY ASSURANCE PROCESS

Step One is to identify the values that are important to the organization.

Step Two defines the structure (environment, setting), the process (how to), the outcome (results), standards, and criteria (measurements) of the activity or subject. Levels of performance, which are specific, observable behaviors, are established for each measurement. "The CNA will be able to obtain a blood pressure reading within 5 mmHg of the nurse's reading 95% of the time" is an example of an objectively stated level of performance.

Step Three involves collecting data and measuring the degree of goal attainment (if the goal was met).

Step Four evaluates and interprets the strengths and weaknesses of the nursing care actions.

Step Five is to correct the weaknesses and reinforce the strengths by identifying possible courses of action. As with Step Four, the assets and liabilities of each possible solution must be evaluated.

Step Six selects a course of action. Decisions are made about implementing the plan. Resources are gathered. The plan is communicated to all concerned personnel, and all preparations are made.

Step Seven is to take action. The plan is implemented as soon as the details of time frames, responsibilities, and monitoring dates are developed.

Step Eight, evaluate, brings the process full circle. Once an action has been taken, it must be monitored and evaluated for effectiveness, and that begins the quality assurance cycle over again.

QA process. These steps are based on the American Nurses' Association's (1976) model of quality assurance review (see box above).

The quality assurance process is important because it serves as a vehicle for staff members to monitor and evaluate their nursing care quality. By taking action to monitor, evaluate, and improve our own patient care, we are assuming the accountability and responsibility necessary to determine our own professional destiny in addition to ensuring the highest quality client care.

Utilization review. The goal of the utilization review committee is to evaluate the use of the organization's resources. Quality assurance programs evaluate the nursing services provided to *people,* while utilization review programs focus on how well each *resource* is used. Although utilization review committees expand their scope to include the entire facility, the use of many resources relates to and requires nursing involvement.

Risk management. Quality assurance programs work hand-in-hand with risk-management programs to ensure that standards of care are efficiently, competently, and safely provided. Risk management's unique job is to decrease the organization's risk for mishaps, incidents, and accidents. Committee members analyze incident, unusual occurrence, and other reports for patterns suggesting a trend. They then evaluate the data and develop corrective action plans, anticipate new learning needs, and recommend actions to decrease any risk to the organization.

The common thread that runs through each program is the formal evaluation process. By using the evaluation process as tools, these programs contribute to a "better preparation for meeting the challenges of change by providing a sound base for decision making and problem solving" (Maciorowski, Larson, Keane, 1985).

Purposes

The act of evaluating is done by all of us daily. Such simple tasks as shopping, driving, and managing time all require evaluations. The ability to evaluate allows us to improve ourselves and move toward achieving our goals.

Organizational. Institutions employ the evaluation process for two basic reasons — to provide feedback and to improve work performance. Data derived from the evaluation process are used to develop new action plans which, when implemented, should lead to a higher level of performance as well as increased productivity. In other words, evaluations help organizations to get the biggest 'bang for their buck.'

Personal. Although many employees dread the annual formal work appraisal, evaluations can also prove to be very useful for staff members as well as supervisors.

According to Tappen (1989), evaluations serve three purposes. Evaluations:

> *Clarify performance expectations.* When the details of the task are in question, a review and evaluation of the activity can point out any areas needing special attention.
> *Modify behavior.* Evaluations foster rewards and recognition for desirable work behaviors. They reinforce positive conduct and allow for opportunities to recognize and correct unsatisfactory work behaviors.
> *Promote change.* The opportunity for learning is present in each evaluation process. Seeing where we have been encourages us to look to

where we are going. It is this self-awareness, derived through evaluation, that **fosters our growth.**

Common Evaluation Errors

Evaluating involves making a judgment. Becoming an objective, accurate evaluator is difficult because of our 'humanness.' As human beings, we are subject to the influences of pride, bias, and other subjective factors; but an awareness of this subjectivity helps prevent the supervisor from making many common errors in evaluation.

Influences

The manager/evaluator is affected by some strong influences. Chief among these are the 'halo' and 'horns' effects (Marriner-Tomey, 1992).

Halo effect. When evaluators generalize one trait and allow it to color their whole impression, they are guilty of 'haloing.' Supervisors tend to evaluate an employee with one outstanding characteristic higher in related areas. Also, employees who are more compatible with the supervisor tend to receive better evaluations. Employees who do not complain receive more favorable evaluations.

To help minimize the halo effect, use the job description and its performance standards as the basis for comparison (see Appendixes A and B for an example of each). This reduces subjectivity and allows for a more accurate evaluation.

Horns effect. With the horns effect, the cause of the misperception is rooted in a hypercritical evaluator. If the manager is a perfectionist, staff members will tend to be evaluated at lower levels than their performance deserves. When the supervisor compares the job with the way he/she did it, ratings will be lower. When effective workers are part of a weak work team or the nonconformists speak out, they are likely to receive less favorable evaluations. Personality differences may also influence the evaluation process. Again, use of the job description will help minimize the horns effect.

Differences

Evaluators are also subjected to the influences relating to genuine differences. Errors of contrast and conflict serve as good examples of evaluation errors based on differences.

Contrast error. Supervisors who tend to evaluate their employees opposite of the way they see themselves produce the contrast error. For example, if the manager has a high level of motivation, he/she may rate the employee's motivational level as low.

Conflict error. When individual differences exist between a supervisor and a staff member, the evaluation process is influenced. Many leaders have difficulty in 'agreeing to disagree,' and this can color the outcome of the evaluation process. If conflict exists, the staff member is surely to receive a lower evaluation, for most supervisors are unable to treat the conflict situation as a single event. The tendency to judge the whole based on a single factor is difficult to overcome, especially if the issue is emotionally charged.

Every supervisor who evaluates comes equipped with his/her "own built-in set of standards or frames of reference" (Marriner-Tomey, 1992). It is the manager's individual viewpoint which serves as the basis for evaluating. This explains why some supervisors are lenient and others are severe with their evaluations.

Methods

Subjectivity in the evaluation process cannot be eliminated, but it can be controlled. Use the following data-collection methods (tools) to minimize judgment errors.

Anecdotal records. These are descriptions of the actual behaviors observed during a specific time period. The record includes a description of the setting, the behaviors observed, and staff members involved. Observations are objective. Value-laden words (e.g., good, bad, fair, excellent, etc.) are strictly avoided. These observations allow both the supervisor and staff member to evaluate the effectiveness of an action, although they can be time-consuming.

Lists. Checklists can help the evaluator to assess for the presence or absence of a certain behavior. Skill checklists identify the behaviors essential for successful performance of the task. The employee's performance of the specific task is then compared to the established criteria, and recommendations are made.

Scales and ranks. Rating scales note the presence or absence of a behavior and then locate that behavior at a point on a scale. How well or poorly the task was performed determines placement on the scale.

Ranking is similar to rating except it requires the supervisor to make comparisons among staff members. Both scales and ranks evaluate the quality as well as the presence or absence of a given behavior.

Peer review. Peer review is the process of evaluating each other's work performance. Several people who do the same type of job appraise the employees' abilities using available evaluation tools. The results are then shared, and recognitions and recommendations are made. The peer review process may be intimidating at first, but within a supportive environment, the process provides a feedback mechanism for sharing, comparing, and recognizing performance.

The methods and techniques listed above are designed to document work performances with an objective eye. Evaluations which are based on objective data can be shared. This sharing of objective data allows the employee to take responsibility for improving his/her work performance by cooperating with the evaluation process.

The Evaluation Process

Because the purpose of an evaluation is to obtain feedback (information), the process can be applied to any situation. The three basic steps of **establishing criteria, collecting data, and making a judgment** appear simple, but the actual procedure involves the consideration of several necessary factors. By practicing the process and applying it to both formal and informal evaluations, the manager becomes more effective with both staff members and administrators. To be a capable evaluator, follow the steps discussed in the next section.

Establish criteria

"Criteria are statements of expected performance and must therefore relate to the thing or person being evaluated" (Bernhard, Walsh, 1990). This is where the planning function of management really pays off. If the performance standards (statements) were developed during the planning stage, it is now a simple matter of applying them to the evaluation process. If no performance statements were developed earlier, they must be established now.

The criteria must also fit the task or the person being evaluated. For example, evaluating a licensed practical nurse's performance by comparing it to a registered nurse's job description would be an inappropriate fit of criteria to person. This evaluation would be invalid due to unsuitable criteria.

The foundation. Criteria answer the question, "How do I know when I have arrived?" Establishing good criteria is of prime importance because the criteria serve as the foundation for making judgments. Although the evaluator may be able to control his/her personal biases, if the criteria are not appropriate, the evaluation process will be inaccurate.

Criteria (statements of performance) can be one of three types. Each type relates to a different aspect of evaluation.

Structural criteria refer to the organization's performance. They include the evaluation of the facility's physical layout, safety features, its mission, financial base, management practices, accreditation status, and nursing care delivery systems. First-line supervisors/managers are seldom required to help develop broader organizational criteria, but they are often called upon to participate in composing departmental or unit criteria relating to structure.

Process criteria refer to "what is actually done by the provider of care on behalf of a client" (Douglas, Bevis, 1983). This type of criteria measures nurses' performance—the therapeutic interventions and the decision-making process. Douglas and Bevis (1983) state that process criteria allow the evaluator to review

- the steps taken in the care of a patient,
- the rationale (reason) for taking the steps, and
- how well these measures helped the patient meet the specified goals.

The nursing process not only serves as a tool for systematically providing client care, it also provides excellent process criteria. Other appropriate sources of process criteria are job descriptions and their performance standards (see Appendixes A and B for an example), the American Nurses' Association's standards of nursing practices, and the facility's policy and procedure manual.

Outcome criteria relate to the end results, expected outcomes, or goal attainment. If structural and process criteria were met, then the outcome criteria will also yield success. "Outcomes are the products of actions, and without measuring outcomes, it cannot be determined whether . . . goals were achieved" (Brett, 1989).

The criteria. No matter what type of criterion is established, each measure must meet the requirements listed in the box on p. 351 in order to be effective. Criteria are the underpinnings of the evaluation process. Establishing usable criteria provides us with a sound foundation for conducting accurate, effective evaluations.

Collect data

Once the criteria have been developed, the collection of information relating to each criterion is begun. The evaluator may use one of several data-collection tools available. Generally, the simpler the criterion, the easier

CRITERIA REQUIREMENTS

1. **Simplicity.** Complex performance statements are difficult to remember and even more difficult to do. Simple criteria, written in understandable terms, stand a greater chance of being met.
2. **Attainable.** Resources, both human and material, must be considered when developing criteria. You would not expect four CNAs to finish blood pressures on 30 patients in 10 minutes if only three blood pressure cuffs are available, for example.
3. **Acceptable and positive.** At the very least, each criterion must be acceptable to staff members. Those employees involved must believe the measures are 'doable.' When people feel the criteria are a measurement of how well (not how poorly) they are performing, they are more motivated to work toward achieving them.
4. **Communicated.** Whether supervisor write their own criteria or adapt existing criteria, they must be communicated. Just as with delegation, all parties affected by the evaluation process must have the same understanding of the criteria. Unless shared, criteria remain only as statements written on a piece of paper.
5. **Accurate.** "An acceptable criterion is one that is a valid indicator of the expected performance" (Bernhard, Walsh, 1990). Accurate criteria actually measure what they are supposed to measure. Most of the time, they are written in observable, objective, assessable terms. For example, "Mr. Z. will remain hydrated" is too vague. How can you tell (measure) that he is hydrated? "Mr. Z. will drink 2000 ml of fluid every 24 hours," or "Mr. Z. will maintain a urinary output of 1000 ml/24 hours" gives objective, measurable criteria for judgment.

the data collection. Whether lists, scales, notes, or recordings are used to gather data, the accuracy of the data collected depends primarily on the evaluator's objectivity. If the evaluator has bias, so will the data.

Type of data. Subjective data are very difficult to measure. With such topics as pain or how one feels about something, measurements usually are objectified through the use of rating scales or ranking exercises. The nurse manager, supervisor, or team leader will want to choose the data-collection tool that collects the most objective (sharable, measurable) data.

Data-collection tools. Tools for collecting information may be as simple as using a checklist or as complex as the peer review process. Checklists, rating scales, and ranking scales can be used by the evaluator alone, while tools such as anecdotal notes, performance appraisals, an peer reviews all require the interaction and cooperation of other people.

Evaluate

The last step of the process includes compiling the collected data into an organized, usable form. Data may be ordered chronologically, by significance, by rank or score, or by the number of positive or negative incidents. Whatever the format, the data should be well organized to facilitate comparison with its predetermined criteria.

Compare data. Once the data are arranged in an orderly format, the evaluator compares them to each established criterion. When making each comparison, it is important to consider the source of the data. "Direct data are collected by observing the actual performance or event being evaluated. Indirect data are collected by assessing the product or outcome of the event, or from written records that document the event" (Bernhard, Walsh, 1990). Data derived from direct sources usually have a higher degree of accuracy. To illustrate, the supervisor may evaluate a CNA's ability to feed helpless clients by observing her/him feed a client (direct source) or by reading the client records and discussing the CNA's performance with the nurse (indirect source).

During the comparison process, it is important to be alert for any biases, opinions, or attitudes that may affect the outcome of the evaluation. The objectivity employed during the criteria-development and data-collection phases will directly influence the comparison process.

Make a judgment. After comparing data with criteria, the evaluator will arrive at one of three conclusions:

1. *The data have surpassed the established criteria.* The goal has been achieved above and beyond expectations, and special recognition is warranted. This is the best possible outcome of the evaluation process, and it needs to be recognized and rewarded if future performances at this level are to be encouraged.
2. *The data have met the criteria.* Objectives have been achieved, so praise and recognition should be given. Attention is paid to any difficulties or factors that slowed progress, and plans for improvement are carried forward for use in similar situations.
3. *The data did not meet the criteria.* This judgment calls for use of the problem-solving process in order to ascertain why the criteria were not met, what went awry, and how improvements can be made.

Rather than disciplining staff members for not meeting the criteria, provide the support, assistance, or direction necessary for achieving the desired aims.

Once the judgment has been made, documented, and shared, the evaluation process is complete. Next, we will look at guidelines for conducting a formal evaluation using the performance (work) evaluation as an example and techniques for providing effective feedback, the most important component of informal evaluations.

Conducting a Work Evaluation

Performance evaluations are only one example of the many applications for the formal evaluation process. It is, however, one of the most important tools for the first-line supervisor/manager.

The employee

The evaluation of staff members' performance may be done by the peer review process, but, more commonly, it is conducted by the immediate supervisor or unit manager. Work evaluations are also called performance appraisals or performance evaluations. They can be rewarding and offer opportunities for positive change, or they can be viewed with dread and discomfort. *How* the supervisor conducts the evaluation has a strong impact on the staff member's performance and morale.

Purpose. Theoretically, the performance evaluation was designed to be a positive experience (see box below). The ultimate goal of the evaluation process is to improve work performance through constructive recogni-

 FUNCTIONS OF PERFORMANCE EVALUATIONS

- Provide an opportunity to set goals
- Reinforce positive behavior
- Correct unacceptable behavior
- Provide the basis for advancement, reward, and recognition

From del Bueno DJ: Performance evaluation: when all is said and done, more is said than done, *Journal of Nursing Administration* 7(12):23, 1977.

tion, feedback, and guidance, "not to anger employees or to create a negative milieu characterized by disrespect and antagonism" (Loraine, 1982). Remember the purpose of the work evaluation. It will help to keep the process upbeat and positive.

Process. The most inappropriate and ineffective way to conduct a performance evaluation is to check the boxes on the form and hand it to the employee who reviews the form, becomes intimidated by any adverse comments on this official document, and immediately assumes a self-protective, defensive stance. This is no way to evaluate the work of others. Not only does it stifle opportunities for growth and improvement, but it also removes the respect for the dignity and worth of the staff member as a fellow human being. If work evaluations are to be at all effective, they must be done within an employee–supervisor conference setting that fosters an honest exchange of ideas, opinions, and information.

The conference

The goal of the employee–supervisor conference is to provide a positive, growth-promoting analysis of the work performed by the staff member. Supervisors must do their homework prior to the conference date. Most often, the facility's job description and its performance standards serve as criteria for making judgments. (See Appendix A for a sample job description and Appendix B for its performance standards.) Data about the employee's performance are collected and compared to the criteria. Strengths, as well as areas needing improvement, are identified; and notes for the conference are made. Although the completion of an official form may be required, this can be intimidating. If possible, use a plain writing tablet during the conference and complete the official record later.

Setting. The success of the evaluation can be influenced by the environment and atmosphere of the conference. To promote trust and facilitate open communication lines, the conference must be conducted in private and without interruption. The staff member needs your full attention. Also, remove the physical barriers that separate you. Come out from behind the desk and sit next to (not facing) the staff member at eye level. Use your best listening skills to discover the employee's thoughts or opinions, and the setting will foster, not inhibit, success.

Process. Begin the conference by focusing on positive aspects. "Tell me about all the good things you are doing" opens the discussion with the employee identifying with the positive aspects of the job. Listen and encourage new ideas but never downgrade a comment. Then acknowledge the employee's strong points and recognize any improvements made in weak areas. Next, direct the discussion to include these categories (Loraine, 1982):

- Quality and quantity of work.
- Job performance as compared to preestablished standards of performance.
- Attitudes. Be careful here. The tendency to be subjective is very strong.
- Learning needs. Any learning needs that are identified by the staff member must be addressed. If the employee was motivated enough to express the need, it is important to him/her, and the wise supervisor will take steps to provide the appropriate learning opportunities.

If negative comments must be made, focus them on the behavior (not the personality) and include options, techniques, or suggestions for replacing the undesired behaviors with more effective actions. If you cannot suggest improvements, do not mention the behaviors. "Some employees have many faults, but if you believe that they are working at their capacity it may be wise to overlook them" (Loraine, 1982).

Goals. The final step of the work performance evaluation is to establish goals for the next 6 months or until the next evaluation. The staff member should develop and write his/her goals, but they should be centered around improving areas that need strengthening. Each goal should be specific and attainable. "To improve my IV skills" is not specific. "To attend one workshop on IV techniques and perform three successful IV starts" establishes more objective criteria.

Keep the work evaluation process positive and you will soon see loyal, productive staff members who are motivated to do their best.

Guidelines for Effective Feedback

Most informal evaluations occur spontaneously and without specific preparations. Most often, the evaluation is unwritten and given in the form of verbal feedback. Techniques for sending and receiving verbal messages are discussed in Chapter 2. By applying those techniques as well as the guidelines discussed in this section, the nurse supervisor will be able to give effective evaluative feedback. There are three simple, but important, guidelines for giving evaluations informally: be objective, be positive, and plan for growth.

Be objective

Objectivity is just as important during the informal evaluation process as it is during formal appraisals. Emotions can distort perceptions and effect the validity of the evaluation. During informal, dynamic situations the

---

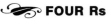 **FOUR Rs OF FEEDBACK**

1. **Right purpose.** Feedback that maintains or builds effective working relationships, improves performance or efficiency, or motivates employees is constructive and purposeful. Feedback that finds fault, criticizes, or belittles staff members serves no positive purpose and eventually becomes detrimental to the entire organization.
2. **Right time.** When evaluations are appropriately timed, the results can be very effective. As a general rule, give positive feedback immediately and save negative comments until you can communicate privately.
3. **Right place.** An informal evaluation (feedback) is more effective when the successes are publicly shared, but the criticisms are not.
4. **Right approach.** The manager's tone sets the stage for the acceptance of the feedback. If the focus is on what is wrong, the employee will accept the feedback differently than when emphasizing what to do in order to improve.

---

supervisor or leader is allowed little or no time to sift through emotional biases or opinions. The evaluator must approach the situation with extra objectivity and a knowledge of his/her own preconceptions.

Techniques. Several methods for maintaining objectivity and effectiveness have been developed. The first and most fundamental guideline is to base the evaluation on *observable* behaviors. Data derived from direct sources help reduce subjectivity and eliminate personal feelings. Then, take advantage of the four Rs of feedback (see box above).

Be positive

There are two basic ways to give feedback—positively or negatively. Any given work situation or employee behavior is neither good nor bad. It just *is*. It is only through interpretation that behaviors or situations receive value. During the evaluation or feedback process, the supervisor has the choice of which viewpoint to adopt. He/she can choose to focus on and emphasize correcting 'wrongs' or on motivating employees toward higher performance levels (and correct the wrongs in the process).

Respect. New management systems such as total quality management or participatory management encourage goal achievement through staff member participation. Inherent in these upbeat systems is the concept of individual worth, where each employee is considered unique and capable of making contributions to the organization. Because of this conceptual framework, employees are treated with respect. This, in turn, fosters a more accepting attitude with feedback and a willingness to make changes. Giving feedback with respect enhances the message and encourages a more positive response.

Plan for growth

If the overall goal of any evaluation process is to improve performance, then the informal evaluation (feedback) should include at least one suggestion to **encourage growth**. Recalling Maslow's hierarchy of needs reminds us of the human needs for learning, improving, and growing toward self-actualization. As managers, supervisors, team leaders, or bosses, we can take advantage of every feedback situation to encourage employees to grow.

Communicate. The growth of the employee, the supervisor, and the organization is enhanced when a 'communicating spirit' is established. People become willing to share, evaluate, disregard, or adopt new ideas. Staff members and managers establish goals and develop performance/evaluation criteria together. These mutual efforts enhance the group's abilities and improve its effectiveness while also promoting growth in each individual.

The evaluation process is truly "a cooperative between managers and employees" (Council, Plachy, 1980). It works best in an environment where supervisors and staff members have a "healthy respect for one another, a genuine concern for each other's success, and cooperation for mutual benefit" (Council, Plachy, 1980).

✍ Key Concepts

- Evaluation is the last step of the management process.
- Evaluation is a process for judging the value or effectiveness of an action.
- Two types of evaluations are the informal (formative) and the formal (summative) evaluation.
- Formal evaluations are used in performance appraisals, quality assurance programs, utilization reviews, and risk management programs.
- Purposes for evaluations are to provide feedback, clarify performance expectations, modify behaviors, promote change, and improve work performance.
- When working with the evaluation process, supervisors must guard against such subjective influences as the 'halo' or 'horns' effect, as well as contrast and conflict errors.
- Tools for collecting evaluation data include anecdotal records, lists, scales, ranks, audits, and peer reviews.
- There are three steps of the evaluation process: establish criteria, collect data, and make a judgment.
- Criteria are statements of expected performance that serve as the foundation or framework for making judgments.
- Three types of criteria are structural, process, and outcome criteria.
- Each criterion should be simple, attainable, acceptable, positive, accurate, and communicated.
- Objective data provide a more accurate basis for making judgments.
- The evaluation process results in one of three judgments: the data has surpassed, met, or did not meet the criteria.
- Performance (work) evaluations are done to reinforce positive behaviors, correct undesirable behaviors, set goals, and provide a basis for recognition and reward.
- The employee–supervisor conference is an effective method for conducting a work evaluation.
- Discussion during the work evaluation conference should focus on the quality and quantity of work, job performance, time management, attitudes, learning needs, and specific goals for improvement.
- Informal evaluations rely on feedback for effectiveness.
- To give informative, effective feedback, be objective and positive and plan for growth.
- Techniques for giving effective feedback include the four Rs: the right purpose, the right time, the right place, and the right approach.
- Respect for staff members, as well as a positive approach, enhances the effectiveness of the evaluation process.
- The evaluation process, when carefully planned and conducted, results in growth and improved performance.

✌ Learning Activities

1. Describe how a supervisor's 'gut reactions' may affect the evaluation process.
2. Keep a diary of your activities for one day. Then analyze the activities and list the number of times a judgment or evaluation was made.
3. Scenario: You are the day-shift team leader for a 28-client long-term care unit. You supervise four CNAs. The director of nurses has assigned you the responsibility for ensuring that each client receives nail care at least twice a month. She expects an evaluation of the nail care program at the end of one month. For this situation:
   a. State the goal of the project.
   b. Refer to Appendix B and establish the criteria for performance of nail care.
   c. Devise a plan for meeting the goal. Include data-collection tools and time frames for monitoring and evaluating.
   d. Describe how you would evaluate the effectiveness of the nail care program.

References

American Nurses' Association: *Quality assurance for nursing care,* Kansas City, Mo, 1976, The Association.

Bernhard LA, Walsh M: *Leadership: the key to professionalism of nursing,* ed 2, St Louis, 1990, Mosby.

Brett JL: *Outcome indicators of quality care.* In Henry B, Arndt C, DiVincent M, Marriner-Tomey A, editors: *Dimensions of nursing administration: theory, research, education, practice,* Boston, 1989, Blackwell.

Council JD, Plachy RJ: Performance appraisal is not enough, *Journal of Nursing Administration* 10(10):20, 1980.

del Bueno DJ: Performance evaluation: when all is said and done, more is said than done, *Journal of Nursing Administration* 7(12):23, 1977.

Douglas LM, Bevis EO: *Nursing management and leadership in action,* ed 4, St Louis, 1983, Mosby.

Joint Commission on Accreditation of Healthcare Organizations: *Manual for hospitals,* Chicago, 1983, JCAHO.

Long BC, Phipps WJ: *Medical–surgical nursing: a nursing process approach,* ed 2, St Louis, 1989, Mosby.

Loraine K: Work evaluations: are they effective?, *Nursing Management* 13(4):44, 1982.

Maciorowski LF, Larson E, Keane A: Quality assurance evaluate thyself, *Journal of Nursing Administration* 15(6):38, 1985.

Marriner-Tomey A: *Guide to nursing management,* ed 4, St Louis, 1992, Mosby.

Tappen RM: *Nursing leadership and management: concepts and practice,* ed 2, Philadelphia, 1989, Davis.

Additional Readings

Ammentorp W, Gossett KD, Poe NE: *Quality assurance for long-term care providers*, Newbury Park, Calif, 1991, Sage. *This manual, written for those managing nursing home care in the 1990s, describes quality management systems for providing better care and living environments for the elderly of our society.*

Anderson PA, Davis SE: Nursing peer review: a developmental process, *Nursing Management* 18(1):46, 1987. *A new approach to nursing peer review, based on staff involvement, yields substantive results.*

Bell DF, Bell DL: Effective evaluations, *Nurse Educator* 4(6):6, 1979. *The authors discuss the process of applying both formative and summative evaluations to a variety of situations.*

Coyne W: Nurses are the key to quality health care, *RN*, 53(2):69, 1990. *A commitment to quality is a must in today's environment. Mr. Coyne, vice president of 3M, offers several strategies for committing to quality and, thus, success.*

Curtis BJ, Simpson LJ: Auditing: a method for evaluating quality of care, *Journal of Nursing Administration* 15(10):14, 1985. *The authors have developed an audit tool that provides an organized approach for evaluating independent nursing actions based on the nursing process.*

Davis K, Newstrom JW: *Human behavior at work: organizational behavior*, ed 8, New York, 1989, McGraw-Hill. *Chapter 7, "Appraising and Rewarding Performance," describes performance appraisals and their relationships to several economic incentive systems.*

Hatton J: Performance evaluation in relation to psychosocial needs, *Supervisor Nurse* 8(7):30, 1977. *Ms. Hatton offers a data-collection tool for evaluating the level of therapeutic psychosocial responses to patients.*

Heinter WL: Relieving the pain of performance evaluations, *Management World* 17(3):7, 1988. *This article focuses on building a manageable long-term system for tracking your employees' progress.*

Huntsman AJ: A model for employee development, *Nursing Management* 18(2):51, 1987. *Learner-centered programs, clearly geared to the work setting, promote the best use of our most important resource — people.*

James J: Dealing with criticism during an evaluation, *Nursing 91* 21(9):103, 1991. *Ms. James suggests eight techniques for making negative feedback work for you.*

Vestal K: *Management concepts for the new nurse*, Philadelphia, 1987, Lippincott. *Chapter 9 offers a thorough discussion of risk-management and quality assurance evaluations.*

Washing HA, Boveington KW: Keeping account of employees' skills, *Supervisory Management* 31(5):20, 1986. *The authors discuss the use of the skills–functions model as a method for tracking employees' skills and strengthening the human resource functions within an organization.*

LEGAL IMPLICATIONS 15

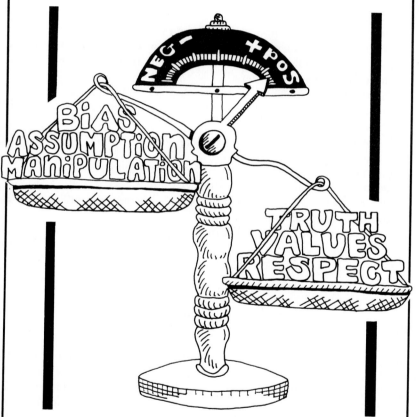

FOR SUPERVISION

Upon completion of this chapter, the reader will be able to:

1. Differentiate among licensure, registration, and certification.
2. Describe how standards of practice, policies, procedures, and job descriptions affect the practice of nursing.
3. Identify four legal roles of the nurse.
4. Explain the difference between a crime and a tort.
5. Define six torts that relate to nursing practice and give an example of each.
6. Describe five legal implications of the nursing process.
7. List at least two guidelines for the supervisor to follow when working with informed consents, incident or accident reports, patients' rights, and code or no-code orders.
8. Discuss three guidelines for receiving physician's orders.
9. Explain two legal duties that relate to teaching clients and staff members.
10. Name at least two legal implications of teaching specifically about medications.
11. Interpret the 'reasonable and prudent nurse' theory.
12. Describe six legal duties of a supervisor/manager.
13. Demonstrate how quality assurance and risk-management programs monitor the quality of client care.
14. Discuss how one's personal commitments affect the quality of client care delivery.

Legal Dimensions

During the past 30 years, nursing has evolved from a vocation to a profession. Along with this evolution came legal and ethical responsibilities, but exactly what is the difference now? What does being a professional mean?

Professions are distinguished from vocations by the presence of five characteristics (see box on p. 363). Nurses have worked hard to establish themselves as professionals and are still struggling with such issues as autonomy, scope of practice, and reimbursement. With this professionalism comes a greater responsibility, accountability, and a need for knowledge of the legal parameters that govern nursing.

Relating to nursing practice

All nurses are ethically and legally accountable for actions taken in the course of nursing practice as well as for actions delegated by the nurse to others assisting in the delivery of nursing care. Such accountability may be accomplished through the regulatory mechanism of licensure, through criminal and civil laws, through the code of ethics of the profession, and through peer evaluation (American Nurses' Association, 1985).

In order to be legally and ethically accountable, nurses and (especially) their supervisors must have a working knowledge of the legal dimensions that effect their practice.

Licensure, registration. In order to practice nursing, a person must be licensed. "Licenses are legal permits granted by a government agency to individuals to engage in the practice of a profession and to use a particular title" (Kozier, Erb, 1987). Licensure protects the public and defines the specialized type of work.

Licensure for nurses is mandatory; that is, unless a person holds a valid license, he/she cannot practice nursing or use the title of nurse. Each state has a board of nursing that grants licenses and monitors nursing activities. In order to be licensed as a nurse, each candidate must pass the National Council Licensure Examination for registered nurses (NCLEX-RN) or practical nurses (NCLEX-PN).

Registration is a listing of names on an official roster of an agency. Canadian nurses, except in Quebec, are not licensed. They are registered or listed with the provincial board of nursing and the College of Nurses of Ontario. Nurses in the United States are licensed and registered with a state board, hence the term registered nurse. When practical or vocational nurses were required to obtain a license, the term *licensed* became identified with that particular level of nursing.

It is interesting to note that until the early 1900s the practice of nursing was totally unregulated. Although different states enacted laws to license

---

✐ CHARACTERISTICS OF PROFESSIONS

1. Education, usually based on a liberal foundation and extended over a long period.
2. A code of ethics or standards that govern 'right' or proper behaviors.
3. Specialized services are provided.
4. An established theory base that defines abilities and norms.
5. Autonomy in practice is present.

From Etzioni A: *The semiprofessionals and their organizations*, New York, 1961, Free Press.

nurses as early as 1903, it was not until the 1940s that the state boards of nursing united to provide a standard licensing examination for all nurse candidates. Most importantly, these laws regulating nursing licensure were permissive or voluntary until 1980. That means that anyone could practice nursing as long as they did not use the title, Registered Nurse.

State boards of nursing also define the practice of nursing for both RNs and LPNs in their nurse practice acts, approve curricula for schools of nursing, monitor continuing education for nurses, and discipline nurses who do not meet criteria for practice.

Certification. When a nurse becomes certified, he/she meets predetermined standards of nursing competence in a specialized area. To become certified, the nurse must graduate from an approved program, complete a specified amount of work experience, and pass one or more examinations. Nurses who are certified are recognized as specialists within their fields. Certification differs from licensure in two fundamental ways:

1. *Certification is voluntary; licensure is mandatory.* A nurse can choose to be certified, but not to be licensed. Furthermore, a licensed nurse can practice without certification but even a certified nurse cannot practice without being licensed.
2. *Certification is 'private credentialing'; licensure is public credentialing.* This means that the "organization or agency that certifies is nongovernmental, and is usually made up of experts or peers from that particular field" (Kelly, 1991). Public credentialing is the granting of a license and the power to legally prohibit unlicensed people from practicing.

Most certification programs for nurses are conducted by the American Nurses' Association or recognized specialty organizations such as the American Association of Nurse Anesthetists.

Standards of practice. The functions, qualifications and principles of medical–surgical nursing practice were first defined by the American Nurses' Association in 1974. Since then, standards have been developed for many nursing specialties. "Standards of practice provide exact criteria against which clients, nurses, and employers can evaluate care for effectiveness and excellence" (Kozier, Erb, 1987). Standards serve as the yardstick by which the public measures the nursing profession. It is each nurse's legal and ethical responsibility to practice up to standards. (See Chapter 8 for an example standard of practice.)

Policies, procedures, job descriptions. The dimensions of nursing practice and supervision are influenced by each organization's structure and function. **Policies are statements of a course of action or strategy.** For example, "It is this facility's policy to provide oral hygiene at least three times a day." The statement is short, easily understood, and states a course of action. In short, a policy is a statement of what is to be done.

Procedures describe, in detail, the method or technique for performing the stated course of action. Using the above example, the procedure for providing oral care is described. Time frames, such as performing oral care tasks after meals, are included when necessary. Policies and procedures are compiled into a manual that is easily located on every nursing unit in the facility. Refer to them often, especially if unsure. They provide the guidelines for safe, effective nursing practice.

Job descriptions define and specify the functions of a particular job, the qualifications required to do the job, and to whom the employee reports. If the job description is accompanied by performance standards, criteria for monitoring and evaluating are included. Job descriptions are important as they define the scope and limitations of each nursing position. (See Appendix A for a sample job description.) Policies, procedures, and job descriptions all help to standardize care, define and set standards relating to client care, and provide criteria for effective evaluations.

Roles of the nurse

Nurses, as well as other people, have legal rights and obligations. To be an effective nurse, you must also strive to be a good employee and citizen.

Citizen. Nurses have all the rights and responsibilities of all citizens. Good citizens are currently informed, actively participate in community activities, and, perhaps most importantly, exercise the right to vote.

Employee. Nurses, when employed, **enter into a contractual relationship with their employers.** A contract is simply defined as an agreement to do something, but it must contain four specific elements in order to be considered legally binding. The requirements of a contract are

- that the parties have the capacity to contract; that is, they are not incompetent or infants;
- an offer;
- an acceptance of the offer; and
- consideration (Northrop, Kelly, 1987).

Nurses are competent professionals who accept offers to work with various health care organizations in return for consideration in the form of money and benefits.

Contracts may be oral or written, expressed (actually discussed), or implied (no discussion, but a legal contract still exists). For example, nurses have an implied contract with their clients to provide competent care, and clients have an implied contract to provide the nurse with accurate information.

Contractual agreements vary with each institution; therefore, it is wise to consider any expressed or implied contractual obligations before accepting employment. You are legally responsible for meeting the contract's obligations once you communicate acceptance of the offer (Northrop, Kelly, 1987).

Provider of service. Nurses are legally responsible for providing safe, competent care in a manner that prevents harm. As providers of nursing care (and supervisors of that care), nurses are held *liable*, or "legally responsible to account for one's obligations and actions" (Kozier, Erb, 1987).

Nurses are also legally responsible for practicing in accordance with the standards or guidelines established by the state's nurse practice act, nursing associations, and institutional policies, procedures, and job descriptions. Standards of care provide the guidelines within which nurses must practice, and they are used by many lawyers in evaluating nursing actions.

Supervisor/manager. As a manager, supervisor, team leader, lead CNA — regardless of the title, if you supervise the work of one or more people — you are legally responsible for

- providing adequate supervision and evaluation;
- delegated actions;
- determining the competencies of your staff;
- communication;
- advising caregivers; and
- providing safe, professional care.

Guidelines for supervisors will be discussed in detail later in the chapter. For now, remember that the nurse plays many roles. Through roles as citizens, employees, professionals, and supervisors, nurses carry out their personal and professional obligations in a legally responsible manner.

Areas of Potential Liability

Laws are the controls that a society imposes upon itself to maintain order. In this society, the system of laws is based upon four fundamental principles (see box on p. 367). Laws that are derived from the Constitution are

---

✐ FUNDAMENTAL PRINCIPLES OF LAW

1. Law is based on a concern for justice and fairness.
2. Law is characterized by change.
3. Actions are judged on the basis of a universal standard of what a similarly educated, reasonable and prudent person would have done under similar circumstances.
4. Each individual has rights and responsibilities.

---

called *constitutional laws.* When state or federal legislation is enacted, it is known as *statutory law;* and decisions made by the country's courts are referred to as *common law.*

Definitions

Laws help govern relationships. Two types of law pertaining to relationships are public and private law. Public law deals with the relationship between the government and the individual. An important area of public law is called criminal law. Private law focuses on relationships between individuals. Contract law and tort law are two divisions of private law.

Crimes. "The broad aim of criminal law is to prevent harm to society by declaring what conduct is criminal and prescribing the punishment for such conduct" (Northrop, Kelly, 1987). Even if the crime is against only one person, it is considered criminal when an actual or potential threat to the public exists.

Two types of crimes exist in the United States: **felonies** and **misdemeanors.** Felonies are the more serious crimes against society such as homicide, arson, or armed robbery. These offenses are punishable by death, imprisonment of not less than one year, or a fine greater than $1000 (Creighton, 1986). Misdemeanors are less significant crimes that are usually punishable by a fine or less than a year in prison.

Torts. Contract law and tort law are two branches of civil (private) law. Contract law relates to agreements between individuals or organizations. Tort law "defines and enforces duties and rights among private individuals that are not based on contractual agreements" (Kozier, Erb, 1987). A tort is a legal wrong that is committed against the person or the property of another individual. Crimes may be viewed as violations of public rights, whereas torts may be considered as violations of individual rights. Many types of torts exist, but a few are of special importance for health care providers and their supervisors.

Torts relating to nursing

Inherent in the health care profession is the potential for legal violations. Nurses and supervisors must be vigilant if the rights of their clients are to be respected and protected. Torts that are of special interest to health care workers include fraud; invasion of privacy; libel and slander; false imprisonment; assault and battery; and negligence and malpractice.

Fraud. Fraud is defined as the false representation of a fact knowing that the fact will be acted upon. When an individual intentionally gives false information and realizes that someone will act upon the data, he/she is guilty of fraud. To illustrate, if the nurse documents that he/she gave a medication that was not truly administered, a fraudulent act has been committed. The physician, upon seeing the charted medications, acts (based upon the data) to evaluate the client's response, or lack thereof, to the medication. Because the physician acted upon intentionally falsified information, the nurse is guilty of fraud.

Invasion of privacy. Every individual in this society has the right to withhold his life from public scrutiny. The right of privacy includes privacy related to the body, confidential information, and the right to be left alone. Nurses and other health care workers can invade privacy in numerous ways. Releasing confidential information to unauthorized persons, gossiping about clients, opening clients' mail, and intruding in family matters when requested not to are examples. Additionally, invasion of privacy occurs when a caregiver does not knock or request permission before entering a client's unit or private space, exposes body parts unnecessarily, or takes a photograph of the client without his/her permission or knowledge. Health care givers must exercise special caution to protect clients' rights to privacy, and it is the responsibility of the supervisor to ensure that those rights are not violated.

Libel and slander. Defamation of character occurs when information that could damage an individual's reputation is disclosed by another person. When the information is in written form, it is called *libel*. When the information is shared orally, it is referred to as *slander*. For example, a supervisor who tells the nurses in the break room that Mary Jane is drinking too much may be making a slanderous statement. If he/she writes that Mary Jane drinks while on duty on a performance evaluation, he/she may be guilty of libel. Keeping comments about clients or staff on a professional level helps prevent the opportunity for defamation of character.

False imprisonment. Any *unjustifiable* detention that limits an individual's movement against his/her will constitutes false imprisonment. The classic example relates to the use of restraints. Years ago if clients were uncooperative, boisterous, or tended to wander, they were restrained or had their movements restricted. Today, unless the client presents a danger to himself/herself or others, he/she cannot be detained. Forcibly keeping clients in their rooms or intentionally detaining a client for payment of a bill are examples of false imprisonment.

Assault and battery. Although these terms are used interchangeably, each has a distinct meaning. Assault is defined as the "unjustifiable attempt to touch another person or the threat to do so in such circumstances as to cause the other reasonably to believe that it will be carried out" (Creighton, 1986). Simply put, assault is any act that carries a threat with it. If the client *feels* he/she is about to be harmed, assault may have occurred. Actual touching or contact is not required for assault to occur.

Battery is unpermitted contact. It includes carrying out the threat of harm and "violent or negligent touching of another's person or clothes or anything attached to his person or held by him" (Creighton, 1986). Touching the client, his clothing, or his possessions *without his permission* can be grounds for battery. The best prevention for both assault and battery is clear, open, and cooperative communications.

Negligence and malpractice. One of the most important (and publicized) areas of potential liability for nurses and other health care providers is malpractice. Both negligence and malpractice are based upon the 'reasonable and prudent person' theory, which is an important principle for nurses and their supervisors to follow.

Negligence is omitting to do something that a reasonable person in ordinary circumstances would do, or doing something that a reasonable person would not do. The average person or business may be charged with negligence. Professional negligence is called malpractice, and it is defined as "any professional misconduct, unreasonable lack of skill or fidelity in professional . . . duties, evil practice, or illegal or immoral conduct" (Creighton, 1986). It includes any professional misbehavior or unreasonable lack of skills (see box on p. 370).

Malpractice lawsuits can arise from many sources, but nurses are most commonly charged with claims that relate to medication administration, patient falls, perioperative care, equipment (including IVs, catheters, tubes), record keeping, and abandonment (NSO Risk Advisor, 1992). Malpractice lawsuits are also rooted in poor communications, following unclear orders, and omitting routine care (Herrmann, 1980). In essence, grounds for malpractice are present when the nurse does not follow the reasonable and prudent nurse principle and an injury or damages result.

Several areas of potential liability exist today for health care providers and their supervisors. Prudent judgment, based on established standards of care, is our best defense.

MALPRACTICE CRITERIA

1. **Duty** — the nurse owed a duty to the client. Standards of care and expert witnesses help establish the elements of the duty.
2. **Breach** — the nurse did not fulfill the duty.
3. **Proximate cause** — the client was injured as a direct result of the nurse's actions (or inactions), or the nurse's actions were so closely connected that liability exists.
4. **Damages** — the client (plaintiff) must prove that actual loss or damage resulted from the nurse's actions.

From Northrop CE, Kelly ME: *Legal issues in nursing*, St Louis, 1987, Mosby.

Legal Aspects of the Nursing Process

The nursing process has evolved into the foundation for practice. Each step of the process, however, has associated potential liability. As a supervisor/leader, it is your responsibility to minimize any chances for liability. "Errors in *basic* [emphasis added] care are usually at the root of negligence lawsuits" (Calfee, 1991). Legal responsibilities are inherent in each step of the nursing process. A closer examination of these potential liabilities will enhance your ability to prevent problems.

Assessment

The fundamental responsibility of the nurse here is to assess the client's health status and needs and then to appropriately communicate the data derived from the assessment. **Errors of assessment** can arise from three sources: data collection, recognizing significance, and communication.

Data collection. Failure to take accepted steps to gather data can be a basis for suit. When monitoring a client's status, the appropriateness and frequency of nursing actions depend on the client's needs.

Recognizing significance. When a nurse (or his/her supervisor) fails to recognize the significance of the gathered data, as a reasonable and prudent nurse would do, potential liability exists. Examples include "failing to recognize the significance of . . . laboratory values, intake and output measurements, vital signs, and complaints of pain that require immediate attention" (Calfee, 1991). When in doubt about the significance of information, communicate with the physician and document the data.

Communication. The assessed data must be timely communicated, either verbally or in writing, to the appropriate people. Written documentation of initial and ongoing assessments is essential. Both written and verbal communications should be accurate, specific, and complete.

Planning

Although most court proceedings prefer to focus on the implementation phase, errors can and do arise during the care planning process. Four of these errors are based in the plan of care.

Plan of care. Each client, after being assessed, is assigned diagnoses and their appropriate interventions. Mistakes leading to negligence here include a failure to

- include each client's problem on the chart and care plan;
- use understandable language in the care plan;
- follow the plan of care, thus disrupting continuity of care;
- provide understandable, realistic discharge instructions, (Calfee, 1991).

Intervention

The intervention phase of the nursing process brings with it the responsibility of carrying out physician's orders in a timely and prudent manner. Additionally, nurses are legally responsible for their own judgments and interventions. Nursing actions or interventions can be classified as one of three types: dependent, independent, or interdependent (Potter, Perry, 1989).

Dependent nursing actions. These interventions are defined and limited by the physician's orders. They require nursing judgment, and the nurse is responsible for questioning the orders if any doubt exists.

To protect themselves and their clients, nurses should question any order that the client questions, orders that relate to a client's change of condition, verbal orders, and standing orders (Becker, 1983).

Independent nursing actions. Nursing interventions that are implemented without collaboration or consultation are independent nursing actions. They do not require a doctor's order, and they are frequently written as nursing orders. Activities relating to daily living, counseling, health education, and promotion frequently call for independent actions. The best guidelines for independent nursing actions can be found in your state's nurse practice act and your facility's job description's and policy and procedure manual.

Interdependent nursing actions. Those nursing actions that are a result of planning and collaboration with other health care providers are known as interdependent actions. It is important to clearly define each provider's responsibilities when group actions are involved.

Intervention errors. Barbara Calfee (1991), a nurse–lawyer, cites four classic examples of errors associated with the intervention phase. These errors result from a failure to "interpret and carry out a doctor's orders; perform nursing tasks correctly; pursue the doctor if he doesn't respond to telephone calls or to notify your nurse manager if he is unavailable."

Evaluation

The last step of the nursing process, evaluation, is seldom the source for lawsuits because it is based on the results of the assessment, planning, and intervention phases. However, the evaluation phase offers nurses and their supervisors the opportunity to appraise the nursing process from a legal point of view.

Criteria. In order to ward off the possibility of lawsuits ensure that each step of the nursing process meets the following guidelines:

1. Standards of care are used as a basis for providing nursing care.
2. Each step of the nursing process is guided by what a reasonable and prudent nurse would do in a similar situation.
3. Accurate and timely charting (documentation) of the client's condition, nursing actions, and attempts to communicate with the physician prevent many potential problems.

One of the best preventatives is a good client–nurse relationship based on mutual respect and cooperation.

Legal Interests for Nurse Managers

Because supervisors, managers, and team leaders may be responsible for the nursing cares given by others, they must be knowledgeable of the legal concepts of the nurse–client relationship. Six areas that are of special interest to supervisors are informed consent, incident reports, accidents, patients' rights, resuscitation orders, and documentation.

> ### ✒︎ ELEMENTS OF INFORMED CONSENT
>
> 1. The client has the ability to make decisions. As long as the client has not been legally declared incompetent, he/she is presumed to be able to participate in the decision-making process.
> 2. The client was given information relating to the condition, the treatment along with its risks and consequences, any alternatives to treatment, and the probable outcomes if the treatment is not given. Enough information must be given to allow the client to be the ultimate decision maker.
> 3. The consent was given voluntarily. No persuasion or coercion must be used. The client's right to self-determination must be respected.
>
> From Northrop CE, Kelly ME: *Legal issues in nursing,* St Louis, 1987, Mosby.

Informed consents

An informed consent is "an agreement by a client to accept a course of treatment or procedure" (Kozier, Erb, 1987). Its purpose is to provide the client with the information necessary to make decisions regarding his/her care and treatment. Informed consents are usually required upon admission to a health care facility and for any procedures that are invasive or carry a high degree of risk.

Guidelines. Supervisors must ensure that three elements are present in every **informed consent** (see box above). The ultimate responsibility for obtaining informed consent lies with the physician. Delegating this responsibility to the nurse is a questionable practice that increases the potential for liability. However, nurses are frequently called upon to witness an informed consent. When nurses witness a consent form, they are signing a document that states to the best of the nurse's knowledge, based on what the client has told them, the client has been informed. Keep these points in mind because a lack of informed consent can cause treatment, as well as legal, problems.

Incident reports

Records that contain descriptions of any unusual occurrences, including accidents, are called incident reports. They are important data-collection tools that provide statistical and other information useful in preventing future occurrences. Risk-management and quality assurance programs use incident reports to decrease risks and improve nursing care.

Guidelines. Incident reports must contain the following information:

1. Client identification.
2. Date, time, and place of the incident.
3. A description of the *facts* of the incidents. (Value judgments can cause big troubles here.)
4. A description of any involved medications, supplies, or equipment.
5. A description of any associated circumstances.
6. The names and titles of any witnesses.

When completing or reviewing incident reports follow these protective guidelines:

- Complete the report immediately after the incident. Be careful to document the facts accurately and completely.
- Never write in the client's chart that an incident report was filed. Doing this "invokes a legal principle of incorporation by reference — it is referred to and thus becomes an integral part of the medical record, which is discoverable and admissible at trial" (Cushing, 1985).
- Multiple copies of the report should be as few as possible, and access to the data should not be indiscriminately shared. Some hospital policies state that you should not copy the documents at all because this action escalates the chance of violating confidentiality.

Following these guidelines when dealing with incident reports will provide accurate data and help decrease the potential opportunities for legal action.

Accidents

An accident is an unplanned occurrence that may or may not result in injury. To meet the criteria for malpractice, the client must have been injured as a result of the accident *and* because "reasonable standards of care were not followed" (Fiesta, 1991). It is very important for supervisors to be familiar with the facility's policies, procedures, and guidelines for client care and accident prevention. They also become "valuable articles of evidence . . . once a suit is filed" (Fiesta, 1991).

Guidelines. Once an accident has occurred, steps must be taken to prevent further injury and protect the client, the staff, and the organization. The supervisor must make certain that specific nursing actions are taken after an accident (see box on p. 375).

> ### 〰️ POST-ACCIDENT RESPONSIBILITIES
>
> - Assess and protect. Thoroughly assess the client and then take steps to protect him from further injury. Notify:
>   1. appropriate staff members. Follow policies and procedures — usually the physician is notified first.
>   2. the family — follow your agency's policy.
> - Identify witnesses. Also, if possible, ask the client what happened.
> - Assess the circumstances of the accident. Ask yourself what a reasonable and prudent nurse would have done in the same situation.
> - Identify, label, and store any medications, supplies, or equipment. They may be needed later.
> - Document assessments, interventions, and any verbal orders in the client's chart. *Do not chart that an incident report was completed.* Next, fill out an incident report. The primary guideline here is to use objective data. Include all the facts. No impressions, opinions, or conclusions should be involved. Tell the truth and be factual.
>
> From Cournoyer CP: Protecting yourself legally after a patient's injured, *Nursing Life* 5(3):18, 1985.

Patient's rights

Prior to the 1960s, clients assumed the passive role of patient immediately upon entry into the health care system. Treatments were done without prior explanation, and everyone assumed that the doctor knew what was best for the patient. As consumers became more actively involved in assuming responsibility for their own health care, they demanded more control over their bodies through the right of self-determination. The concept of the client–health care provider partnership began to evolve, and in 1972 the American Hospital Association adopted a *Patient's Bill of Rights,* which basically states that the client has a right to respectful care, information, continuity of care, confidentiality, and self-determination. Today, the *Patient's Bill of Rights* serves as a framework for medical and nursing care.

Guidelines. To protect your client's rights, use the following techniques:

Establish a therapeutic relationship. When clients trust their caregivers, they become partners in their care.

Communicate. Inform clients about their caregivers, any procedures, or treatments. Answer questions and allow time for discussions.

Educate. Provide appropriate instruction or education. Make sure the client is equipped (physically, emotionally, and psychologically) to cope with health care changes.

Maintain confidentiality. Be careful to respect the client's right to privacy — personal, written, and verbal. Do not share information unnecessarily.

Respect the client's right to refuse. Do not attempt to coerce or persuade and never take punitive action. Consult the client's physician when needed.

No-code orders

Prior to the use of CPR and other resuscitation techniques, questions about prolonging life were not an issue. Today, with all our modern equipment and practices, physiological life can be maintained indefinitely. Clients and their physicians now need to discuss which measures should be taken to resuscitate or prolong their lives, should the case arise. The physician has the responsibility for writing the code status order (to resuscitate or not). No-code orders are usually written as "Do Not Resuscitate" (DNR) or "No Heroics."

Code, or full-code, orders are presumed unless otherwise written and mean that every attempt to keep the client alive should be made. No-code orders are reserved for clients who are in the terminal stages of an irreversible illness and state that no effort will be made to prolong life. Clients are allowed to die with dignity and respect for their wishes. Recently, orders for "Chemical Code Only" have been written. This means that drugs, but no CPR, will be used to sustain life. Many long-term care facilities now have several levels of resuscitation: no extra measures, chemical measures only, chemical and mechanical measures, and full-code status (CPR plus all other measures).

Guidelines. The supervisor is responsible for making sure that:

The staff knows and follows the policies and procedures for codes.

The physician has a written note on the client's chart.

The staff makes every effort is made to have written documentation of client's status. "A written order will prevent the occurrence of CPR being provided inappropriately" (Vestal, 1987).

The staff communicates the client's status to all caregivers. They have no time to refer to the physician's orders during a cardiac arrest or other emergency situation.

Documentation

One of the most important protections for both caregivers and clients is good documentation. Nurses' notes, along with other sections of the client's record, serve as evidence for the quality of care provided in a court action.

Guidelines. Remember the rule of thumb: If you did not chart it, you did not do it. That rule still holds true in a court of law. (See box below for guidelines.)

Physician's orders. Nurses receive doctors' orders in both written and verbal forms. Obviously, written orders are safer because they provide documentation of the physician's intentions. Whether the order is processed through a computer or unit secretary, the nurse retains the ultimate responsibility for ensuring the accuracy and appropriateness of each order. Additionally, "Nurses may be liable for failing to challenge incorrect orders" (Douglas, 1992).

The use of verbal or telephone orders is discouraged, for the practice has potentially disastrous and legally dangerous consequences. However, there are situations in which they must be used. The following hints will help to eliminate potential problems with **verbal orders:**

Know and follow your facility's policy for receiving verbal orders.
Write the order down as it is being given.
Repeat the order word-for-word, including the client's name, to the physician.

✒ DOCUMENTATION GUIDELINES

1. Document all assessments, problems, nursing actions, and client responses.
2. Be specific. Document objective data. Use quotes when possible to chart client statements.
3. Document all treatments, procedures, observations, and safety measures.
4. Write on every line. Sign all entries. Draw a single line through any spaces left on the written line.
5. Chart late entries or omissions as new entries. Never add to a previous entry.
6. Always do your own charting. Never chart for someone else.

Write the order on the appropriate forms. Sign T.O. for telephone order or V.O. for verbal order. Write the doctor's name and then your own.

Have the physician sign the order as soon as possible, hopefully within 24 hours.

When there is any question about an order, ask the physician who wrote it for clarification.

The legal aspects discussed in this section are important for managers and supervisors of health care delivery. The guidelines will assist you in fulfilling your legal responsibilities and protecting your client's rights.

Implications of Teaching

One of nursing's most fundamental roles is that of teacher. To achieve the highest level of wellness possible, clients must learn and adapt to the changes resulting from the illness or injury. Nurses have a professional duty to teach and counsel, and this applies to long-term as well as acute care clients.

Nurses have a duty to instruct. That duty is expanded to include staff members when the nurse is a supervisor. (Actually, supervisors in most businesses have a teaching role.) Whether the learners are clients or staff members, the **supervisor's (teacher's) legal responsibilities** remain the same.

Duty to know

The obligations of the instructor can be broadly divided into two categories: the duty to know and the duty to instruct. **The duty to know includes two further divisions: the duty to maintain up-to-date knowledge and skills and the duty to know the learning abilities of the client or staff member.**

The first duty is self-explanatory. You cannot teach what you do not know. *You* must be responsible for keeping the professional knowledge relating to your position current.

The duty to know the abilities of the learner relates to assessing the learner's readiness to learn, willingness to learn, level of understanding, and pattern of learning. Some people learn best by doing and some by listening, while others must use their visual sense to learn best. Knowing the abilities of the learner enhances the impact of the teaching.

Competencies. An area of special interest for first-line supervisors is the duty to know the competencies of each staff member. The manager who does not know the skills and capabilities of his/her workers cannot effectively plan, delegate, or supervise. In addition, the legal consequences of such ignorance can be great.

Each new worker should undergo a skills assessment immediately upon employment. The 'return demonstration' method, where an evaluator actually observes the performance of the skill or duty, yields the most accurate data. These data are then used for planning the employee's orientation and continuing education programs. They also assist the supervisor in evaluating the employee's ability to perform skills that will be delegated to him/her. Staff members should be assessed for competencies upon employment, during routine performance evaluations, and whenever a need arises.

Duty to instruct

In order to assist clients in coping with the problems associated with illness or injury, nurses assess and attempt to meet clients' needs for information. Nurses who instruct clients (and supervisors who instruct staff members) are responsible for maintaining accurate, current materials; dated outlines of materials presented with references; learning objectives; evaluation tools; and time tables (Creighton, 1986).

Keep your data simple, but answer these three questions:

- What is to be learned?
- How is it to be learned?
- How will I/we know when it has been learned?

Two other areas of potential liability relating to teaching are giving directions and medication instructions.

Directions. When giving clients or their family members instructions for giving care, assess *and* document the following:

- Who received the instructions?
- What instructions were given?
- How were the instructions given (verbal, written, both)?
- Was the skill practiced and return demonstrated?
- What level of understanding or competency was achieved? (Were objectives met?)

The importance of written instructions for the client cannot be overemphasized. In a lawsuit, written instructions can prove that the client did receive information and that instruction (teaching) was done.

Documentation of the teaching process and the clients response is also of great importance. In many malpractice cases, the nurse actually gave all the right instructions, but the case was lost because the nursing actions were not documented. Charting is great legal protection.

Medications. Providing instructions about medications is fraught with potential liability. Responsibilities frequently overlap between physicians and nurses, but to help clarify the situation, keep these principles in mind:

> Ordinarily, the physician is responsible for instructing the client about the drug and the risks associated with its use.
> The nurse is responsible for instructing the client about the "particulars of care" (Cushing, 1984). The client must be informed about each drug's route, side effects, adverse reactions, special precautions, drug interactions, and instructions for taking the drug. Again, provide written instructions and document the teaching actions.

Providing instructions (teaching) is an essential function of nursing and supervision. By following accepted standards of practice, providing competent instruction, and documenting, quality learning can be fostered within a legally responsible environment.

Implications of Supervision

Managers, supervisors, and leaders have special legal obligations when getting work done through the efforts of others. In fact, a supervisor "may be liable for the negligence of others to whom she or he has assigned certain duties" (Creighton, 1986).

The most important guidelines for supervision lie in the state's nurse practice act, the facility's policies and procedures, and the job descriptions for each staff member supervised. Use them. They are your legal parameters for practice in your institution.

Additional legal implications are rooted in the reasonable and prudent nurse (supervisor) theory and the obligations (duties) of the supervisor.

The reasonable and prudent nurse

The law judges a team leader or any other supervisor by comparing his/her actions with what a reasonable and prudent supervisor would do under similar circumstances. State nurse practice acts and specialty standards of care define what a prudent nurse would do, but supervisors must also rely on their institution's job descriptions, policies, procedures, and authority structure for clarification of their responsibilities.

✐ REDUCING THE RISK OF LAWSUITS

- Know the standards of care, policies for supervision, and job descriptions of your facility. Because the law is broadly written, many courts accept the facility's policies, procedures, and job descriptions as evidence of established standards of care.
- Act with due care toward those you are supervising. The law expects a supervisor to behave in keeping with an average, careful supervisor.
- Maintain the established standard of care. The courts will compare the care received by the plaintiff with accepted standards of care. If the supervisor knowingly allows substandard care to be delivered, the potential for malpractice exists.

Guidelines. To reduce the risk of lawsuits, use the reasonable and prudent nurse theory in daily practice. (See box above for hints on reducing the risk of lawsuits.)

To illustrate, let us say that you are the team leader for a unit that is normally staffed with you (the supervisor), two LPNs, and seven CNAs. Tonight, only one LPN and four CNAs arrived for work. You are obviously understaffed, and the LPN has just threatened to leave. What are the legal implications here?

First, "Refusing to accept patients in a particular unit is not an acceptable solution" (Greenlaw, 1981). This action can endanger patients and may lead to charges of abandonment. Stay with the assignment. Second, the supervisor is obligated to procure sufficient staff to "provide a standard of nursing care equivalent to that which should be available to patients under ordinary circumstances" (Fenner, 1988). Notify your manager and document your actions in personal notes. **Make every effort to secure enough staff to provide care according to standards** but do not abandon your assignment and its responsibilities.

Duties of a supervisor

The legal obligations of supervision can be classified into six general categories or duties. They include the duties to act, advise, communicate, delegate, monitor, and teach.

To act. Supervisors have the duty to act with due care toward clients and employees; that is, they should be adequately prepared to supervise and direct the actions of others. Again, the reasonable and prudent nurse (supervisor) serves as a guideline for action.

To advise. Caregivers must have adequate knowledge to care for their clients. Supervisors are responsible for ensuring that relevant information reaches the appropriate people. Monitoring reports and nursing rounds help the supervisor assess the flow of data. Supervisors also have an obligation to support staff members by being available for advice and instruction when needed.

Recently, new government Occupational Safety and Health Administration (OSHA) regulations have been enacted to make the practice of universal precautions fully enforceable. Supervisors must now also advise employees about the safety practices associated with communicable diseases.

To communicate. Many cases of litigation involve a failure to communicate. Failure to recognize, communicate, or properly respond to significant information are common bases for lawsuits. Review Chapter 2 to brush up on your communication skills. Remember that the best preventative measures for avoiding legal problems are open and effective communications.

To delegate. The ultimate responsibility for any delegated action lies with the supervisor. Chapter 13 discusses the process of delegating in detail. See the box below for legal obligations of the delegating supervisor.

✐ SUPERVISOR'S LEGAL OBLIGATIONS WHEN DELEGATING

1. **Determine the appropriate task to delegate.** Use your nurse practice act and job descriptions as guidelines.
2. **Find the best delegatee.** The most appropriate person is adequately prepared or experienced for the task itself and willing to assume responsibility for the delegated actions.
3. **Match the ability with the assignment.** Supervisors who delegate duties that are beyond the employee's abilities to carry them out may be negligent.
4. **Monitor and evaluate.** You must know the results of the delegated activity. After all, you are the one who is ultimately responsible. Follow up. Make sure the task was done correctly.

To monitor. The duty to determine and monitor the competencies of each staff member lies squarely with the supervisor. Without knowing your staff's skills and abilities, you will be unable to practice effective supervision, provide appropriate client care, or function within legal parameters. You, as the supervisor, are responsible for the efficient functioning of your personnel. You need to be aware of their capabilities.

To teach. The supervisor's duty to teach and develop new skills in staff members remains a primary obligation of the supervisor. Legally speaking, you have the duty to assure that the nursing care being delivered by your staff meets standards. Correcting poorly done tasks and teaching more effective actions can prevent many legal problems.

Providing supervision for health care providers can be challenging and rewarding, but it is not without its responsibilities. Remember your duties as a supervisor and the reasonable and prudent nurse (supervisor) principle. They will serve as very usable guidelines for clarifying many of the legal implications associated with the role of supervisor, manager, or team leader.

Monitors of Quality

Efforts to establish and maintain a high quality of client care are closely associated with the professional and legal responsibility to provide that care according to accepted standards. Monitors of quality are those programs and activities that ensure the delivery of safe and effective health care.

Programs such as quality assurance (QA) and risk management allow employees to move toward providing optimal client care while reducing and controlling risks associated with that care.

Programs

Every health care organization is responsible for meeting established standards. Acute care facilities are accredited by the Joint Commission on Accreditation of Healthcare Organizations (JCAHO), whereas long-term care facilities are federally regulated by Medicare and the Omnibus Budget Reconciliation Act (OBRA). In addition, long-term care facilities must meet state Medicaid regulations. In an attempt to meet these regulations, programs that analyzed the quality of the service were developed.

Quality assurance programs are concerned with providing optimal client care. Activities (e.g., nursing care) are compared to established criteria, problems are defined, and measures are coordinated to improve care. See Chapter 14 for a more detailed discussion of the quality assurance process.

Risk-management programs work closely with QA programs, although each has a different focus. Risk management is "concerned with acceptable care from a legal perspective" (Northrop, Kelly, 1987). The primary focus to identify and implement specific loss prevention activities such as preventing injuries, protecting human and material resources, and identifying potential problems. Together with other programs, opportunities are provided for staff members to identify, monitor, and solve problems relating to the delivery of quality patient care within their facility.

Benefits. Activities that monitor quality have many beneficial effects. First, because QA activities result in data with measurable outcomes, caregivers can see exactly which changes need to be made in order to meet the goal. For example, the QA committee conducted a study that revealed the clients were only drinking about 700 ml of fluid in 24 hours. Standards in your facility state that the client would optimally receive 1500 ml in 24 hours. You now can develop plans and monitoring activities for making sure that each client receives an additional 800 ml of fluid every 24 hours.

Second, monitoring quality ensures that health care providers function within (and up to) their standards of practice. We want to be as effective as possible, but we must function within our legal parameters.

Third, and most important, quality monitoring activities protect the client, for they help ensure the best care possible with the resources available.

Personnel. Monitors of quality are by no means limited to certain programs or specifically labeled activities. **The primary monitors of quality are the facility's employees.** Every employee monitors and evaluates his/her job. If each team leader, supervisor, and manager can open a dialogue with employees, include them in striving for the best care possible, and recognize them for their efforts, quality will be achieved for everyone. To do this, however, involves a commitment.

Commitment. Your commitment to do your best in every situation cannot be legislated, set down in standards, or decreed by regulation. It must come from within you. It is the willingness to try, the confidence to face failures as challenges, and the energy to carry both you and your staff members through change. It is your commitment to quality that builds the fire in others.

We have now come full circle. Chapter 1 of this book began with commitment, and here we end. Between these two discussions lie the principles, skills, tools, and techniques needed to become an effective supervisor and leader, and you already possess all the needed basic personal ingredients within yourself. Now that the elements are here together, one question remains: Are you committed to using them?

ℯↃ **Key Concepts**

- The five characteristics of a profession are an extended education, a code of ethics, specialized services, a theory base, and autonomy in practice.
- Nurses, including supervisors, are legally and ethically accountable for their own actions as well as any delegated actions.
- Licensure is a mandatory legal permit to engage in a particular professional practice.
- Registration is an official listing of names with an agency.
- Each state defines the practice of nursing in its nurse practice act.
- Certification is the voluntary process of meeting predetermined standards of nursing competence.
- Standards of practice describe the qualifications, functions, and principles of a nursing specialty.
- Policies are statements about a course of action or strategy. They state what is to be done.
- Procedures describe how an action is to be performed.
- Job descriptions define the functions, qualifications, and abilities needed for a specific job.
- Standards of practice, state nurse practice acts, policies, procedures, and job descriptions are used to legally define the practice of nursing.
- Nurses and their supervisors have the obligation to be effective citizens, employees, providers of service, and supervisors.
- Laws are controls that a society imposes upon itself to maintain order. Sources of law include the Constitution, state and federal legislation, and the courts.
- Criminal law is a division of public law. Its purpose is to prevent harm to society.
- Contract law and tort law are two divisions of private law.
- Tort law focuses on the rights and duties of relationships between individuals.
- Torts that are of special importance to nurses and their supervisors include fraud, invasion of privacy, libel and slander, false imprisonment, assault and battery, and negligence and malpractice.
- The four elements of a malpractice claim are duty, breach, proximate cause, and damages.
- Each step of the nursing process has associated legal responsibilities.
- Areas of potential liability in the assessment phase of the nursing process are errors in data collection, recognition of the significance of the data, and communication.
- Nurses are legally responsible for their own dependent, independent, and interdependent nursing actions.
- Informed consents are agreements to accept a specific course of action.

- Incident reports are descriptions of unusual occurrences.
- Accidents are unplanned events that may or may not result in injury.
- The *Patient's Bill of Rights* serves as a guideline for medical and nursing caregivers.
- The physician is responsible for writing orders that direct the use of CPR and other resuscitation measures. Orders are classified as code (full-code) or no-code (Do Not Resuscitate [DNR], No Heroics).
- The nurse is responsible for transcribing, questioning, and implementing the physician's orders. Verbal orders need special precautions.
- Legal responsibilities that relate to teaching include the duty to know and the duty to instruct.
- When teaching clients about medications, nurses are obligated to inform them about the particulars of care for each medication.
- The reasonable and prudent nurse (person) principle is an important legal guideline for supervisors as well as nurses.
- The state's nurse practice act, along with the facility's policies, procedures, and job descriptions, act as legal guidelines for supervisors.
- The legal obligations of the supervisor, manager, or team leader include the duties to act, advise, communicate, delegate, monitor, and teach.
- Monitors of quality are those programs and activities that ensure the delivery of safe, effective health and nursing care.
- Quality assurance programs are concerned with providing optimal care.
- Risk-management programs focus on decreasing risk through loss prevention activities.
- The most important monitor of quality is the individual employee.

Learning Activities

1. Obtain a copy of your state's nurse practice act. Analyze it for specific statements relating to supervision.
2. Explain how the reasonable and prudent nurse principle would be used in a legal proceeding.
3. Fill out an incident report for Mrs. J., a 78-year-old female who fell during an assisted transfer from the bed to the chair. Her right leg is twisted, and she is in pain.
4. The doctor has told you not to code Mr. Smith, but no order was written. Mr. Smith's son just told you that family wants everything done in case of an emergency. Describe what you would do in this case.
5. Develop a plan to teach a 60-year-old woman with rheumatoid arthritis about taking aspirin. Include every aspect that may have legal implications.

References

American Nurses' Association: *Code for nurses with interpretive statements,* Kansas City, Mo, 1985, The Association.

Becker M: Five orders you must question to protect yourself legally, *Nursing Life* 3(1):21, 1983.

Calfee BE: Protecting yourself from allegations of nursing negligence, *Nursing 91* 21(12):34, 1991.

Cournoyer CP: Protecting yourself legally after a patient's injured, *Nursing Life* 5(3):18, 1985.

Creighton H: *Law every nurse should know,* ed 5, Philadelphia, 1986, Saunders.

Cushing M: Legal lessons on patient teaching, *American Journal of Nursing* 84(6):721, 1984.

Cushing M: Incident reports: for you eyes only?, *American Journal of Nursing* 85(8):873, 1985.

Douglas LM: *The effective nurse leader and manager,* ed 4, St Louis, 1992, Mosby.

Etzioni A: *The semiprofessionals and their organizations,* New York, 1961, Free Press.

Fenner KM: Nursing shortage: harbinger of increased litigation, *Nursing Management* 19(11):44, 1988.

Fiesta J: Patient falls — no liability, *Nursing Management* 22(11):22, 1991.

Greenlaw J: Understaffing: living with reality, *Law, Medicine and Health Care* 9(9):23, 1981.

Herrmann F: Four kinds of carelessness that can send you to court, *Nursing Life* 1(5):62, 1980.

Kelly LY: *Dimensions of professional nursing,* ed 6, New York, 1991, Pergamon Press.

Kozier B, Erb G: *Fundamentals of nursing: concepts and procedures,* ed 3, Menlo Park, NJ, 1987, Addison-Wesley.

Northrop CE, Kelly ME: *Legal issues in nursing,* St Louis, 1987, Mosby.

NSO Risk Advisor: Legal tips and tidbits, *NSO Risk Advisors* 1(7):1, 1992.

Potter PA, Perry AG: *Fundamentals of nursing: concepts, process and practice,* ed 2, St Louis, 1989, Mosby.

Vestal K: *Management concepts for the new nurse,* Philadelphia, 1987, Lippincott.

Additional Readings

Annas GJ, Glantz LH, Katz BF: *The rights of doctors, nurses, and allied health professionals,* New York, 1981, Avon Books. *This book discusses the rights of clients and health care providers, areas where they overlap, and suggestions for clarifying one's rights in specific situations.*

Bradford EW: Preventing malpractice suits: what you can do, *Nursing 88* 18(9):63, 1988. *Keep legal trouble from falling on you and your hospital, or at least cushion the blow, by taking this attorney's advice.*

Cushing M: First, anticipate the harm, *American Journal of Nursing* 85(2):137, 1985. *This nurse–lawyer points out several legal implications of caring for incapacitated clients.*

Greve P: Documentation: every word counts, *RN* 55(7):55, 1992. *Defensive charting is one of the surest ways to tip the scales of justice in your favor.*

Iyer PW: Thirteen charting rules to keep you legally safe, *Nursing 91* 21(6):40, 1991. *This first of a two-part series gives some helpful tips for protective documentation.*

Iyer PW: Six more charting rules to keep you legally safe, *Nursing 91* 21(7):34, 1991. *The second of a two-part series examines what you should and should not document.*

Kellmer DM: No code orders: guidelines for policy, *Nursing Outlook* 34(4):179, 1986. *As medical technology enables health care professionals to save more lives, they are being forced to make increasingly difficult decisions about the use of life-sustaining treatments.*

Pavalon EL: *Human rights and health care law,* New York, 1980, American Journal of Nursing. *This book provides an overview of pertinent contemporary issues concerning the legal rights of people in various health care situations.*

Rabinow J: Delegating safely within the law, *Nursing Life* 2(9):48, 1982. *To reduce the legal risks of delegation, you need to know what the law expects.*

Regan WA: Verbal orders: invitations to disaster, *RN* 43(7):61, 1980. *Verbal orders leave too much room for error and no time for correction.*

Regan WA: When in doubt, check it out, *RN* 46(5):87, 1982. *If an MD's actions give you "cause to pause," you are legally obligated to take action.*

Performance Standards for
Certified Nursing Assistant

Function: To provide full descriptions of duties as stated in the Job Description for CNA.

DUTIES

A. Assists residents with activities of daily living and allows the residents the opportunity for self-care according to his/her capabilities. Activities of daily living include:

1. Bathing
   a. Tub bath, shower, special tub bath, or bed bath.
   b. Bathing is to include care of the eyes, ears, scalp, nose, face, neck, chest, back, armpits, arms, hands, abdomen, peri area, any body creases, legs, and feet.

2. Hair care
   a. Shampoo as directed or with the first bath of the week unless routinely scheduled with the beauty shop.
   b. Daily grooming—comb hair daily and arrange in pleasing style.
   c. Care of brushes and combs—clean daily, wash weekly, and store in plastic bag in drawer.

3. Shaving
   a. All shaving is to be done with an electric or safety razor.
   b. Male residents, as well as female residents, should be shaved as part of the daily care, if desired.
   c. Bearded residents should have their beards trimmed weekly.

4. Oral care
   To be done after every meal (or at least twice a day with A.M. and h.s. care)
   a. Brush dentures or natural teeth.
   b. Mouth care if without dentures or teeth.
   c. Apply lubricant to lips if dry.
   d. Clean all equipment, dry, and store in bedside drawer.

5. Face care
   a. Clean eyes from inner corner outward, using a new section of face cloth for each eye. Keep eyes free from matter.
   b. Clean inside of nose (nares).
   c. Clean outside of ears (external ear).
   d. Clean glasses or hearing aids daily and as needed.

6. Skin care
   Daily observation for dry areas, rashes, red areas, tears, or scratches; report to supervisor.
   a. Make sure all skin crevices are clean.
   b. Clean skin of contractured hands, arms, or legs daily.
   c. Pad contractures or any areas of skin-to-skin contact.

    d. Apply lotion to any area of dry skin (e.g., elbows, knees, heels, hands, etc.)

    e. Use soap sparingly and rinse well to prevent dry skin.

    f. Apply deodorant sparingly if requested.

    g. Massage gently any reddened areas.

       (1) Report any redness that does not clear with massage.

    h. Position antipressure devices as instructed.

       (1) Turn and position all bedridden patients at least every 2 hours.

7. Peri care

To be done daily with the bath or A.M. care and after every incontinency. To be done every shift for residents with odor problems.

    a. Assure privacy.

    b. For females, cleanse external and internal labia using new area of cleansing cloth for each stroke (front to back).

    c. For males, retract foreskin, cleanse penis, and replace foreskin over head of penis.

    d. Clean and dry anal area last.

    e. Dry areas thoroughly.

8. Nail care

To be done at least twice a month.

    a. Diabetic residents must have nail care done by licensed personnel.

    b. Cut nails straight across and file any sharp edges.

    c. Report any bleeding or nail changes to supervisor.

9. Intake and nutrition

Monitor and encourage fluid and food intake in accordance with the resident's diet and fluid orders.

    a. Unless otherwise ordered, the resident is to receive at least 1500 ml of fluids every 24 hours.

       (1) Offer fluids hourly if resident is awake.

       (2) Note amount each resident drank during your shift on the Intake and Output Monitoring sheet.

       (3) Notify supervisor if resident is not receiving 700 ml on your shift; night shift CNAs are exempt.

    b. Encourage eating by:

       (1) Preparing the meal tray so resident is able to feed self if possible — open milk, cut meat, butter bread, prepare beverage or food.

       (2) Assisting the resident to feed self.

       (3) If needed, feeding the resident in a safe manner.

       (4) Documenting percentage of meal (solid food) eaten.

    c. Maintain accurate Input and Output, using appropriate form, as ordered.

10. Toileting (output) elimination

Monitor and assist residents with bowel and bladder care.

    a. Offer bedpan, urinal, commode, or take to toilet as requested by resident or every two hours (while resident is awake).

    b. Monitor urine for frequency (how often), color, amount, clarity (clear or cloudy), and odor.

    c. Monitor bowel movements for frequency, color, consistency, and amount.

d. Provide bowel and bladder or timed toileting training as ordered.
   (1) Monitor number of incontinencies/shift, chart, and
   (2) Report above data to wing supervisor.
e. Dispose of all briefs, heavily soiled paper towels, or other non-washable items by wrapping and placing in appropriate container.
   (1) Rinse soil from peri rags and place in appropriate container.

11. Dressing
   Assist the residents, as needed, to wear street clothes daily unless bedridden or otherwise indicated.
   a. Remove clothes to appropriate container when soiled, stained, or with odor.
   b. Hang sweaters or clean clothes in closet after the resident undresses.
   c. Monitor all clothing for name labels and label with laundry marker if needed.
   d. If family takes resident's laundry out of facility, place soiled clothes in plastic bag in closet and close bag.

12. P.M. or h.s. care
   Prepare resident for sleep.
   a. Offer and administer back rub.
   b. Assist with oral hygiene and face and hand care.
   c. Perform peri care as indicated.
   d. Straighten bed, prepare quiet environment.

13. A.M. care
   To be done on all residents except those who are bathed before breakfast.
   a. Oral care—clean dentures and place dentures in mouth.
   b. Wash face, peri area, and/or other body areas that may require cleansing.
   c. Dress resident in street clothes unless otherwise noted.
   d. Comb hair.

14. Positioning
   All residents are to be correctly positioned when in bed or wheelchair.
   a. Positions are changed every 2 hours.
   b. Use special devices for positioning as instructed.

15. Linen changes as needed or scheduled

B. Organizes care in order to answer call lights promptly and respond to resident's needs appropriately
   1. If CNA assigned to area is not available, the first available CNA is to answer call light.
   2. Plan care and schedule at the beginning of each shift.

C. Provides a safe environment for resident as well as self. This includes:
   1. Cleanliness of unit, bedside stand, closet, wheelchair, and bathroom of residents. Personal items are to be cleaned and stored in appropriate area.
   2. Knowledge of fire safety, accident prevention, evacuation procedures, and CPR.
   3. Ability to correctly apply and monitor restraints.
   4. Ability to perform the Heimlich maneuver when indicated.
   5. Knowledge of and ability to correctly carry out universal isolation precautions as ordered.

      6. Use of safe body mechanics for self and resident.

      7. Providing appropriate ventilation, warmth, light, quiet, and privacy.

      8. Monitoring of confused or wandering patients.

D. Reports to wing supervisor any pertinent observations, changes, or concerns regarding the resident's condition. Each resident will be monitored for:

    1. Oxygenation–respirations

      a. Note rate, rhythm, any congestion.

        (1) Report presence of congestion to supervisor.

    2. Fluid intake

      a. Note amount and type of liquid consumed.

      b. Note any difficulty in swallowing and report.

    3. Food intake

      a. Note amount and type of food consumed.

      b. Note and report any refusal to eat or difficulty in swallowing.

    4. Output, urine, and BMs

      a. Monitor frequency, color, consistency, clarity, and amount of urine.

      b. Notify supervisor if resident has:

        (1) Not voided for 8 hours.

        (2) Not moved bowels for 3 days.

        (3) Diarrhea or frequent urinations (hourly or more).

    5. Level of consciousness and activity

      a. Note resident's level of consciousness daily and report any changes.

      b. Monitor activity (i.e., wheelchair, ambulation, socialization).

    6. Sleep

      a. Monitor sleep patterns and periods of wakefulness.

      b. Notify supervisor if resident is unable to sleep.

    7. Pain

      a. Note location, type, and severity of pain.

      b. Report any episodes of pain to supervisor.

      c. Use comfort measures to decrease pain (i.e., distraction, change of position).

E. Maintains accurate patient care records on a daily basis

Medical records the CNA is to complete daily include:

    1. Checklist documenting daily nursing care given.

    2. The vital sign sheet.

    3. Intake and output bowel monitoring sheet.

    4. Feeder list noting percentage eaten and ml of fluids taken in.

    5. Check nursing care plan and notify wing supervisor if you feel any changes may be needed.

F. Able to competently perform the following skills:

    1. Vital signs, TPR, and BP, using standard equipment.

    2. Catheter care, both external and indwelling.

    3. Bowel care including administration of enema, return flow enema, and suppository.

    4. Collection of specimens.

    5. Care of urinary equipment (i.e., drainage bags, leg bags, urinals, bedpans, leg bands).

    6. Care of casts and traction equipment.

7. Observation of dressings, duoderm, operation sites, if any. Consult supervisor about sterility of dressing.
8. Monitoring of oxygen as ordered.
9. Use of equipment such as footboards, heel protectors, cradles, walkers, wheelchairs, commodes, Hoyer lift, Century tub.
10. Use of clean technique at all times.
11. Applications of braces, artificial limbs.
12. Admission and discharge procedures.
13. Intake and output monitoring.
14. Post-mortem care.
   NOTE: If CNA feels unprepared to perform the above skills, notify wing supervisor, who will make arrangements for training.
G. Incorporates legal/ethical concepts in relation to self, health team members, patients, and families; respects all confidences; and maintains privacy of resident at all times
   1. Respect all confidences that you may receive from your patients while on duty.
   2. Avoid gossip. Never discuss your supervisor or team workers with other personnel or with patients.
   3. Respect the patient's need for privacy at all times. Screen your patient before all procedures. Provide adequate draping.
   4. The patient's chart is privileged information. The information contained in this chart may be given only to those people directly involved with the patient's care. Refer questions to your nurse supervisor.
   5. Show proper respect for other people at all times. Be loyal to your employer; respect your co-workers and patients.
   6. Practice the nurse aide's code of ethics.
   7. Maintain awareness of the *Patient's Bill of Rights.*
H. Assists residents with transfer, ambulation, range of motion, and other physical activities
   1. Active and passive range of motion at least every shift and when indicated.
   2. Pivot transfers.
   3. Two-, three-, four-person body lifts.
   4. Positioning of resident to prevent contractures.
   5. Application and monitoring of assistive devices (i.e., splints, slings, and braces).
I. Assists social services and activity departments as needed
   1. Prepare resident and transport to scheduled appointment or recreational activity.
   2. Monitor activity calendar for scheduled events and encourage daily attendance.
   3. Prepare and transport resident to beauty shop as scheduled.
J. Assists in meeting psychosocial, love, religious, and belonging needs of the resident
   All people have the need to be loved and belong to a group. The staff at this facility is encouraged to interact in a friendly, therapeutic manner. Appropriate touching and acceptance of the total person builds self-esteem and fosters self-confidence.

1. Never take the place of a religious counselor but be aware of your responsibility in providing spiritual aid for the patient if so required. Advise your supervisor if the patient requests religious attention.
2. Do not discuss your personal or family life and problems with your patients.
3. Loud, noisy behavior is degrading and is annoying to patients and relatives. Walk. Do not run, regardless of the emergency.
4. Discrimination because of race, creed, or color has no place in patient care. Treat each person with equal consideration and respect. Give your best to all.

K. Responds appropriately to instructions and guidance
1. Accept responsibility graciously. Anticipate needs. It is important to never exceed your responsibilities or abilities.
2. Assume the responsibility for your mistakes, errors, or misjudgments. Report them at once to your supervisor. Failure to do so may place you, the patient, and the facility in jeopardy.
3. Offer to assist others when your work is done.

L. Participates in special ongoing projects
Demonstrates professional growth by:
1. Attending monthly staff meetings.
2. Attending workshops and sharing information.
3. Updating nursing skills.
   a. Be available for participation in learning experiences.
4. Promoting healthy interpersonal relations with all staff for enhancement of patient care.

M. Supports philosophy, policies, and procedures of this facility
1. Promotes the philosophy of the facility.
2. Reads and understands information shared during orientation to facility.
3. Refers to policy and procedures manuals as needed.

INDEX